Drug Transit and Distribution, Interception and Control Series

SUBSTANCE WITHDRAWAL SYNDROME

DRUG TRANSIT AND DISTRIBUTION, INTERCEPTION AND CONTROL SERIES

Cooperation with Drug Transit Countries of Illegal Drugs
Benjamin S. Rosen (Editor)
2009. ISBN 978-1-60692-991-9

National Drug Control Strategy
Heather G. Williams (Editor)
2009. ISBN: 978-1-60692-553-9

Substance Withdrawal Syndrome
Janet P. Rees and Olivia B. Woodhouse (Editors)
2009. ISBN: 978-1-60692-951-3

Drug Transit and Distribution, Interception and Control Series

Substance Withdrawal Syndrome

Janet P. Rees

and

Olivia B. Woodhouse

Editors

Nova Biomedical Books

New York

For permission to use material from this book please contact us:
Telephone 631-231-7269; Fax 631-231-8175
Web Site: http://www.novapublishers.com

NOTICE TO THE READER

The Publisher has taken reasonable care in the preparation of this book, but makes no expressed or implied warranty of any kind and assumes no responsibility for any errors or omissions. No liability is assumed for incidental or consequential damages in connection with or arising out of information contained in this book. The Publisher shall not be liable for any special, consequential, or exemplary damages resulting, in whole or in part, from the readers' use of, or reliance upon, this material.

Independent verification should be sought for any data, advice or recommendations contained in this book. In addition, no responsibility is assumed by the publisher for any injury and/or damage to persons or property arising from any methods, products, instructions, ideas or otherwise contained in this publication.

This publication is designed to provide accurate and authoritative information with regard to the subject matter covered herein. It is sold with the clear understanding that the Publisher is not engaged in rendering legal or any other professional services. If legal or any other expert assistance is required, the services of a competent person should be sought. FROM A DECLARATION OF PARTICIPANTS JOINTLY ADOPTED BY A COMMITTEE OF THE AMERICAN BAR ASSOCIATION AND A COMMITTEE OF PUBLISHERS.

Library of Congress Cataloging-in-Publication Data

Substance withdrawal syndrome / [edited by] Janet P. Rees and Olivia B. Woodhouse.
    p. ; cm.
 Includes bibliographical references and index.
 ISBN 978-1-60692-951-3 (hardcover)
 1. Drug withdrawal symptoms. I. Rees, Janet P. II. Woodhouse, Olivia B.
 [DNLM: 1. Substance Withdrawal Syndrome. WM 270 S941995 2009]
 RM302.6.S83 2009
 615'.704--dc22
                    2009017793

Published by Nova Science Publishers, Inc. ✛ *New York*

Contents

Preface   vii

Chapter I   Psychotropic Analgesic Nitrous Oxide [PAN] for Substance Abuse
Withdrawal: Current Status   1
Mark A. Gillman

Chapter II   Selective Serotonin Reuptake Inhibitors Withdrawal Syndromes:
New Insights into Pathophysiology and Treatment   37
Elena Tomba, Emanuela Offidani and Giovanni A. Fava

Chapter III   Benzodiazepine Withdrawal Syndrome and Strategies for
Discontinuing Benzodiazepine Use: Appropriate Treatment
with SSRIs and SNRIs   61
Mutsuhiro Nakao, Kyoko Nomura and Takeaki Takeuchi

Chapter IV   Carisoprodol Withdrawal Syndrome   81
Roy R. Reeves, Randy S. Burke and Mark E. Ladner

Chapter V   Is Aspirin Withdrawal Detrimental for Patients with or at Risk
for Coronary Artery Disease? A Meta-Analysis   93
*Giuseppe G. L. Biondi-Zoccai, Marzia Lotrionte,
Pierfrancesco Agostoni, Antonio Abbate, Massimiliano Fusaro,
Giuseppe M. Sangiorgi and Imad Sheiban*

Chapter VI   Changes Observed in Circulatory and Alimentary Systems
in Alcohol Dependent Patients during the Withdrawal Period   113
*Maria Kłopocka, Jacek Budzyński, Grzegorz Pulkowski
and Marcin Ziółkowski*

Chapter VII   The Effects of Acute, Chronic and Withdrawal from Chronic
Ethanol on Emotional Learning   169
Danielle Gulick and Thomas J. Gould

Chapter VIII   Topographic Brain Mapping of Caffeine Use and Caffeine Withdrawal   197
Roy R. Reeves and Frederick A. Struve

Short Communication

Craving, Leptin and Metabolic Assessment in Subjects with Cocaine Abuse
Dependence: Results from an Original Study   **211**
*S. Andreoli, G. Martinotti, M. Mazza, M. Di Nicola, F. Tonioni
and L. Janiri*

Index   **221**

Preface

Substance Withdrawal Syndrome refers to the physiological and psychological symptoms associated with withdrawal from the use of a drug after prolonged administration or habituation. The concept includes withdrawal from smoking or drinking, as well as withdrawal from an administered drug. This new book presents the latest research in the field.

Chapter I - PAN is high concentrations of oxygen (O_2) plus low concentrations of nitrous oxide (N_2O) individually titrated to an endpoint where the subject is relaxed and at which they are fully conscious and co-operative throughout inhalation of the gases. PAN is not merely administering nitrous oxide/oxygen. It also specifically excludes using nitrous oxide at a fixed preconceived dose. Instead, PAN uses titration to provide the nitrous oxide using the individual clinical response of each patient as the guide to the optimal concentration required. Thus, optimal concentrations of nitrous oxide vary widely from individual to individual. Titrating to the correct endpoint usually requires hands-on training or very careful attention to the instructions given in previous papers or in a textbook dealing with dental conscious sedation with nitrous oxide, because the inhaled concentrations of N_2O required to achieve the correct endpoint varies between 10-70%. Although this technique has been used safely and effectively in South Africa (S.A.) for more than 25 years and in Finland for over a decade, there has been strong published criticisms of the technique, from armchair academic critics in S. A., Finland and Sweden. Despite their widely published opposition on theoretical grounds alone, it took almost 10 years before the Finnish group attempted to replicate the use of PAN for treating alcoholic withdrawal states. However, although they used nitrous oxide, they failed to use the PAN technique correctly. This review will cover the published criticisms and work on PAN for alcohol withdrawal, as well as detailing with the latest research supporting its efficacy. Evidence will be presented that the PAN therapy is safe and rapidly effective and can be applied by a trained registered nurse, without direct physician supervision, making PAN an ideal cost-effective method for First and Third World countries, saving unnecessary in-patient admissions. Although more controlled trials using the correct method are needed, evidence will be presented that PAN is an effective treatment of the acute withdrawal state from most substances of abuse including alcohol, opioids, cannabis, cocaine, methaqualone/cannabis combinations, nicotine and polydrug abuse. PAN is recognised by the Health Professions Council of South Africa (official tariff code: 0203/0204) and is therefore accepted by medical insurance organisations in S.A.. Because it has been used safely (with no more than trivial adverse effects) and effectively on thousands of outpatients in S.A. and Finland the review will highlight how potentially large cost-savings can be made because many more patients can be treated safely as outpatients than with the currently favoured sedative therapies because the:

1. Patient improves within minutes of administration and is often well enough to have the next meal;
2. Use of addictive sedative medications such as the benzodiazepines (e.g. diazepam) are reduced by 90% plus. This obviates the danger of secondary addiction in this highly susceptible group;
3. Extreme rapidity of recovery enables nurses/physicians to distinguish those patients requiring intensive inpatient therapy from those that do not; since 90% plus patients respond positively to one administration of the gases, usually on admission;
4. Rapidity of response enables the patient to abandon the sick role speedily (often within an hour of gas treatment) and enter the essential next phase of rehabilitation; usually requiring social, psychological and/or psychiatric therapy;
5. Placebo (oxygen) alone ameliorates withdrawal in approximately 30-50% of patients who require no further pharmacological therapy.

PAN is usually given on one occasion only for inpatients. Depending on the drug of abuse, out-patients may require more than one application of the gases, but usually no more than 2 applications during the first week of withdrawal. PAN has been used successfully on more than 50,000 patients in South Africa, Finland and the USA. The rationale for using PAN, as a gaseous partial opioid agonist will be discussed. The review concludes by placing the PAN method in the wider perspective of substance withdrawal states and craving, dealing with its current status and ending with an appeal for more studies to be done on this promising therapy.

Chapter II - There has been increasing awareness of the withdrawal syndromes which may occur with discontinuation of the selective serotonin reuptake inhibitors (SSRI). The literature that is surveyed indicates that they are frequent, may vary from one SSRI to another, occur with either abrupt or gradual disconfirmation, and are not necessarily reversible. These phenomena may be explained on the basis of the oppositional model of tolerance.

Continued drugs treatment may recruit processes that oppose the initial acute effect of a drug. When drug treatment ends, these processes may operate unopposed, at least for some time, induce withdrawal symptoms and increased vulnerability to relapse.

The model may provide an explanation also for other clinical findings in depression treatment: tolerance to the effects of antidepressants during long-term therapy, onset of resistance upon rechallenge with the same antidepressant drug, paradoxical effects of antidepressants in some patients, switching and cycle acceleration in bipolar disorder, very unfavourable long-term outcome of major depression treated by pharmacological means. The implications for treatment of depression are considerable.

Chapter III - Although benzodiazepines are among the most commonly prescribed medications, owing to their roles in multiple areas of therapeutic action as anxiolytics, sedative hypnotics, anticonvulsants and muscle relaxants, they are also highly addictive.

Long-term use can lead to dependency, rebound anxiety, memory impairment, and withdrawal. Excessive prescription of benzodiazepines has emerged as a major clinical issue in Japan. The number of people taking these medications has been increasing, and the costs associated with benzodiazepine use are substantial. In our recent study, we showed that a minimal dose of a selective serotonin reuptake inhibitor (SSRI) increased the success rate of a benzodiazepine discontinuation program among chronic benzodiazepine users, without association with major depression. Ten subjects (45.5%) in the SSRI-assisted benzodiazepine-reduction group (n = 22) succeeded in becoming benzodiazepine-free after completing the program, whereas only four (17.4%) in the simple benzodiazepine-reduction group (n = 23) succeeded. SSRI use significantly predicted the success of becoming benzodiazepine-free (P = 0.023), controlling for the effects of age, sex, duration of benzodiazepine use, and baseline scores on the Hamilton Rating Scales for Depression and Anxiety. However, the SSRI itself might cause a withdrawal syndrome; indeed, one participant who received a minimal dose of SSRI suffered from SSRI withdrawal syndrome after changing to a tricyclic antidepressant. Benzodiazepines are much more frequently prescribed in Japanese hospitals and clinics than SSRIs and serotonin and noradrenaline reuptake inhibitors (SNRIs), especially among physicians practicing internal medicine. For example, among the 644,444 prescriptions emanating from our university hospital in 1 year, 76,563 (11.9%) ordered benzodiazepines and 10,627 (1.6%) ordered SSRIs and SNRIs. Although future studies should collect multi-institutional data, the dissemination of relevant medical knowledge to internists and primary care physicians about the clinical issues accompanying benzodiazepine use and the suggested alternative medications, such as SSRIs, represents one public health approach to this imbalance between benzodiazepine and SSRI/SNRI prescriptions. In this paper, we discuss the difficulties attending benzodiazepine withdrawal and the appropriate use of benzodiazepines, SSRIs, or SNRIs, as demonstrated in our clinical studies.

Chapter IV - Carisoprodol (N-isopropyl-2 methyl-2-propyl-1,3-propanediol dicarbamate; N-isopropylmeprobamate) is a commonly prescribed centrally acting skeletal muscle relaxant. The drug is structurally similar to meprobamate, a Schedule IV controlled substance at the Federal level with known risk for causing addiction. In fact, carisoprodol is metabolized to hydroxycarisoprodol, hydroxymeprobamate, and meprobamate, with meprobamate being the primary active metabolite. The abuse potential of meprobamate is equal to, if not greater than, that of benzodiazepines. With meprobamate having this degree of abuse potential, one might expect a risk of misuse of carisoprodol. A number of reports suggest this to be a valid concern. Carisoprodol has been abused (usually in amounts much larger than the recommended daily dose of 350 mg three or four times daily) for its sedative and relaxant effects, has been used to augment or alter the effects of other drugs (e.g., to increase the sedating effects of benzodiazepines or help calm persons after cocaine use), and has been combined with other prescribed medications (e.g., tramadol) to produce euphoric effects. It appears to be somewhat less difficult to obtain prescriptions for carisoprodol than for controlled substances. Carisoprodol abuse has increased significantly during the past decade, particularly in the southern US.

Because of the abuse potential of the drug, withdrawal symptoms might be expected to occur with cessation of intake of large doses of carisoprodol. As the misuse of carisoprodol has increased, descriptions of a carisoprodol withdrawal syndrome have begun to emerge. Symptoms typically encountered during this withdrawal syndrome include anxiety, tremulousness, jitteriness, and muscle twitching. Psychotic symptoms such as hallucinations occur in some patients. These symptoms are similar to those previously described during meprobamate withdrawal. Because of these similarities, symptoms occurring during carisoprodol withdrawal may be postulated to be due to withdrawal from accumulations of meprobamate present as a result of taking excessive amounts of carisoprodol.

Carisoprodol is metabolized to a controlled substance, has clear evidence of abuse potential and increasing incidence of abuse, and has shown evidence of a withdrawal syndrome with abrupt cessation from intake of large amounts of the drug. Carisoprodol has been assigned a Schedule IV controlled substance status in several states. These facts have caused some to conclude that it is time for carisoprodol to become a controlled substance at the Federal level. This article will discuss the abuse potential of carisoprodol and recent descriptions of a carisoprodol withdrawal syndrome, and will explore the clinical implications of these occurrences.

Chapter V - The protective role of aspirin in the management of patients with or at risk of coronary artery disease has been established for several years. The clinical appropriateness of aspirin therapy depends however on the risk-benefit balance between its potential adverse effects, namely bleeding, and its benefits. Indeed, it is not uncommon for patients to discontinue aspirin according to physician advice or unsupervised, eg before an invasive procedure.

The hazards inherent to aspirin discontinuation in such patients are however incompletely defined. We thus undertook a systematic review and meta-analysis of clinical studies reporting on the impact of aspirin withdrawal in subjects with established coronary artery disease or at moderate-to-high risk for coronary events.

We searched PubMed for pertinent studies, without language restrictions. Study designs, patient characteristics, and outcomes were formally abstracted. Pooled estimates were computed according to random effects methods, when appropriate.

From the 612 studies screened for selection, we finally included in the analysis 6 studies, enrolling a total of 50279 patients. One study involved 31750 patients on secondary prevention for coronary artery disease, 2 studies enrolled 2594 subjects admitted for acute coronary syndromes, 2 studies were focused on 13706 patients undergoing coronary artery bypass grafting, and an additional study involved 2229 patients who had underwent percutaneous coronary revascularization with intracoronary drug-eluting stent implantation. Overall, aspirin withdrawal was associated with a 3-fold higher risk of major adverse cardiac events (3.14 [95% confidence interval 1.75-5.61], P=0.0001). This risk was magnified in patients with intracoronary stents, as such discontinuation of antiplatelet treatment was associated with an even higher risk of adverse events (89.78 [29.90-269.60]).

This systematic overview suggests that aspirin withdrawal has ominous prognostic implication in subjects with or at moderate-to-high risk for coronary artery disease. Such information should be borne in mind when advising patients under such treatment, and aspirin discontinuation should be advocated only when the risk of bleeding or other adverse effects clearly overwhelms that of cardiovascular atherothrombotic events.

Chapter VI - This chapter includes up-to-date information concerning the most important changes in morphological and functional status of cardiovascular system and gastrointestinal tract, observed in alcohol dependent patients after alcohol withdrawal. The results of our own studies on this subject are also presented and discussed.

Alcohol abuse is associated with well-known psychosomatic health and social problems. It leads to multi-organ, especially cardiovascular system, alimentary tract, liver, pancreas and immunologic system dysfunction. Therefore withdrawal and anti-relapse therapy should be undoubtedly undertaken in every case. Nevertheless our knowledge on alcohol withdrawal consequences is still insufficient. Within abstinence period, especially during the first month, not only psychiatric, but also systemic and metabolic (mainly endocrine, haemostatic and immunologic) changes occur. As a result of such changes, some differences in circulatory system function, exercise capacity and autonomic nervous system activity can be observed. Some of them may be even life-threatening, leading to sudden cardiac death or acute cardiovascular events.

The most expressed alterations in cardiovascular diseases risk factors values occur within first four weeks after alcohol misuse period, although, as it was proved in our studies, they can be also noted after six months of observation. In such long abstinence period pro-atherogenic metabolic changes expressed by the decrease of HDL and increase of LDL-cholesterol plasma concentration occurred. These unfavorable changes were less expressed in patients treated with naltrexone, what probably should be taken into consideration, when anti-relapse pharmacotherapy is planned. Other factors important in atherosclerosis progression and acute coronary syndromes pathogenesis are platelets activation and plasma blood coagulation and fibrinolysis system function. In our studies some indirect markers of platelets activation were determined in the early abstinence period. The highest level of fibrinogen, thrombomodulin, antithrombin, markers of trombinogenesis activation in vivo (thrombin- antithrombin, TAT complexes), tissue type plasminogen activator antigen (t-PA:Ag), antigen of plasminogen activator inhibitor type 1 (PAI-1:Ag), markers of fibrinolysis activation in vivo, such as D-dimers, plasmin- alpha2- antiplasmin (PAP) complexes were recorded shortly after alcohol drinking cessation. Mentioned changes were strongly expressed in patients with determinable TNF-alpha plasma level. Abstinence keeping improved effort capacity and positively modulated autonomic nervous system activity via vagal nerve influence on heart rate variability.

Similarly, in alcohol withdrawal period can be observed some morphological and functional changes in alimentary tract, although they are less expressed and mostly beneficial as a result of cytotoxic action cessation. The most important clinical manifestations of alcohol abuse are mucosal leasions in the upper part of the gastrointestinal tract, motility disorders, pancreatitis and liver function impairment. In our studies some changes in examined parameters values, which occurred within the withdrawal period were estimated by endoscopic examinations, esophageal and gastric pH-metry, esophageal manometry, abdominal ultrasonography and blood samples biochemical analysis. Favorable effect of alcohol withdrawal on liver function tests values was affected by pituitary-thyroid and pituitary- gonadal axes hormones level, cytokine TNF-alpha serum level, nutrition status, Helicobacter pylori infection presence and gastric acidity value.

The results of our analysis also indicated, that some of studied haematological and biochemical parameters, such as mean platelets volume and nitric oxide metabolites plasma level may be taken into consideration as new, potentially valuable markers of alcohol abuse as well as drinking relapse predictors.

Conclusion: Alcohol withdrawal and early abstinence is a dynamic period with potentially harmful health consequences, especially in cardiovascular system. In some cases appropriate treatment, also pharmacologic, should probably be recommended. The results of latest papers on the alcohol withdrawal benefit and harmful effects suggest the necessity of scrupulous multicentre studies to estimate the real clinical importance of occurring changes and cost- benefits analysis of selected interventions.

Chapter VII - Alcohol is the most commonly used and abused recreational drug, and one effect of ethanol administration, regardless of whether it is acute or chronic, is the disruption of learning and memory. Although recent studies have demonstrated that ethanol does not produce global deficits but, rather, acts on specific substrates to alter neural function, our understanding of the effects of ethanol on cognitive processes remains incomplete. The studies discussed herein offer support for the specificity of the effects of ethanol on learning-related processes and examine how these effects vary with both the task and the phase of ethanol administration examined. Acute ethanol impairs emotional learning as measured by standard contextual and cued fear conditioning, as well as trace fear conditioning and passive avoidance. However, the effects of acute ethanol on these tasks are influenced by multiple factors, such as genetics and age. Furthermore, as ethanol administration transitions into chronic and withdrawal from chronic ethanol, the pattern of impairments in emotional learning changes. This suggests that acute, chronic, and withdrawal from chronic ethanol differentially alter behavior and therefore may also differentially alter neuronal function. Thus, the current review compares and contrasts the effects of acute, chronic, and withdrawal from chronic ethanol within fear conditioning and passive avoidance tasks, and across these two models of aversive/emotional learning.

Chapter VIII - Caffeine is a widely used psychoactive substance consumed daily by the majority of Americans. Saletu showed that 250 mg of caffeine can produce a transient reduction of EEG total absolute power in normal persons. Additional studies have confirmed this phenomenon. Overall, however, studies of EEG changes following caffeine exposure have reported variable results. Studies have been done in individuals who are not caffeine naïve and the effect of previous caffeine usage (often for years) on EEG is unknown. It is postulated that this confound may contribute to the variations in results between studies of caffeine exposure.

Several studies have shown that persons consuming even low or moderate amounts of caffeine (in some cases, as low as 100 mg per day) may develop a withdrawal syndrome with caffeine cessation with symptoms such as headaches, lethargy, muscle pain, impaired concentration, and physiological complaints such as nausea or yawning. Preliminary studies of individuals abstaining from caffeine have demonstrated significant changes relative to when they were consuming the drug in a number of EEG variables, including: 1.) increases in theta absolute power over all cortical areas, 2.) increases in delta absolute power over the frontal cortex, 3.) decreases in the mean frequency of both the alpha and beta rhythm, 4.) increase in theta relative power and decrease in beta relative power, and 5.) significant changes in interhemispheric coherence. Additionally, caffeine cessation appears to increase firing rates of diffuse paroxysmal dysrhythmias in some individuals. Preliminary data also suggests that caffeine withdrawal has some effect on cognitive P300 auditory and visual evoked potentials.

Short Communication - *Introduction*: Leptin is a 16-kDa protein secreted from white adipocytes; it acts by binding to specific hypothalamic receptors to alter the expression of several neuropeptides regulating neuroendocrine function, food intake and the body's entire energy balance. Leptin receptors have been found in several brain areas, including the cerebellum, cortex, hippocampus, thalamus and in peripheral tissues including the liver, pancreas, adrenals, ovaries, and hematopoietic stem cells. Leptin regulates and is regulated by several neuropeptides and hormones, such as Neuropeptide Y, melanocyte-stimulating-hormone, Agouti-related-hormone, pro-opiomelanocortin, orexin, cocaine- and amphetamine-regulated transcript, melanin-concentrating-hormone, insulin, IGF-system, sympathetic/parasympathetic tone, immune function and hemopoiesis (cytokines), the hypothalamic-pituitary-gonadal axis and the thyroid and adrenal axes (CRH, TSH). Actually, leptin is considered a modulator of withdrawal-induced craving in alcoholic subjects. During detoxification, craving can shift towards other kinds of craving (e.g., food or smoking), but if plasma leptin increases during withdrawal this shift can be attenuated, and consequentially appetite decreases and alcohol craving can be enhanced, determining possible relapses in alcohol consumption. Leptin is involved in the brain reward circuitry together with the CART-system, regulated by leptin itself; CART may be an important connection between food- and drug-related rewards. We studied the hypothesis that leptin might modulate cocaine craving in cocaine-detoxified addicts, evaluating any possible correlation with metabolic, hormonal and psychometric parameters.

Methods: A sample of 12 cocaine-dependent subjects, according to DSM-IV-TR, was evaluated as follows: height, weight (BMI), blood pressure, heart rate, substance and drug consumption, triglicerides, cholesterol, plasma leptin value, cortisol, insulin, ACTH, FT3, FT4, and TSH; and SHAPS, VASc/f/s (Visual-Analogue-Scale for cocaine/food/sex), CCQ (Cocaine-Craving-Questionnaire), Barratt Impulsiveness Scale, HAM-D, and HAM-A at baseline and after 15 days of abstinence.

Results: Leptin results positively correlated with VASc, CCQ and HAM-A; VASc was positively correlated with CCQ and HAM-D. VASf was negatively correlated with cholesterol (as attended) and positively with VASs and TSH. CCQ was positively related with HAM-D and the plasma leptin mean levels in the male subsample were higher with respect to controls. Data is expressed as mean, standard deviation and Pearson correlation coefficiency.

Conclusions: In our sample, leptin correlates with cocaine craving measured by VASc and CCQ independently from BMI or the hypothalamic-pituitary-adrenal axis. At baseline, VASc (mean) was less than VAS f and s mean score, confirming the shifting craving phenomenon. Cocaine craving is correlated with depressive symptoms and leptin correlates with anxious symptoms. Although our data confirm the correlation between leptin and cocaine craving, further studies are requested.

In: Substance Withdrawal Syndrome
Editors: J. P. Rees and O. B. Woodhouse

ISBN 978-1-60692-951-3
© 2009 Nova Science Publishers, Inc.

Chapter I

Psychotropic Analgesic Nitrous Oxide [PAN] for Substance Abuse Withdrawal: Current Status

Mark A. Gillman
South African Brain Research Institute,
Johannesburg, South Africa

Abstract

PAN is high concentrations of oxygen (O_2) plus low concentrations of nitrous oxide (N_2O) individually titrated to an endpoint where the subject is relaxed and at which they are fully conscious and co-operative throughout inhalation of the gases. PAN is not merely administering nitrous oxide/oxygen. It also specifically excludes using nitrous oxide at a fixed preconceived dose. Instead, PAN uses titration to provide the nitrous oxide using the individual clinical response of each patient as the guide to the optimal concentration required. Thus, optimal concentrations of nitrous oxide vary widely from individual to individual. Titrating to the correct endpoint usually requires hands-on training or very careful attention to the instructions given in previous papers or in a textbook dealing with dental conscious sedation with nitrous oxide, because the inhaled concentrations of N_2O required to achieve the correct endpoint varies between 10-70%. Although this technique has been used safely and effectively in South Africa (S.A.) for more than 25 years and in Finland for over a decade, there has been strong published criticisms of the technique, from armchair academic critics in S. A., Finland and Sweden. Despite their widely published opposition on theoretical grounds alone, it took almost 10 years before the Finnish group attempted to replicate the use of PAN for treating alcoholic withdrawal states. However, although they used nitrous oxide, they failed to use the PAN technique correctly. This review will cover the published criticisms and work on PAN for alcohol withdrawal, as well as detailing with the latest research supporting its efficacy. Evidence will be presented that the PAN therapy is safe and rapidly effective and can be applied by a trained registered nurse, without direct physician supervision, making PAN an ideal cost-effective method for First and Third World countries, saving unnecessary in-patient admissions. Although more controlled trials using the correct method are needed, evidence will be presented that PAN is an effective treatment of the acute withdrawal state from most substances of abuse including alcohol, opioids, cannabis, cocaine, methaqualone/cannabis combinations, nicotine and polydrug abuse. PAN is recognised by the Health Professions Council of South Africa (official tariff code: 0203/0204) and is therefore accepted by medical insurance organisations in S.A.. Because it has been used safely (with no more than trivial adverse effects) and effectively on thousands of outpatients in S.A. and Finland the review will highlight how potentially large cost-savings can be made because many more patients can be treated safely as outpatients than with the currently favoured sedative therapies because the:

1. Patient improves within minutes of administration and is often well enough to have the next meal;
2. Use of addictive sedative medications such as the benzodiazepines (e.g. diazepam) are reduced by 90% plus. This obviates the danger of secondary addiction in this highly susceptible group;
3. Extreme rapidity of recovery enables nurses/physicians to distinguish those patients requiring intensive inpatient therapy from those that do not; since 90% plus patients respond positively to one administration of the gases, usually on admission;
4. Rapidity of response enables the patient to abandon the sick role speedily (often within an hour of gas treatment) and enter the essential next phase of rehabilitation; usually requiring social, psychological and/or psychiatric therapy;
5. Placebo (oxygen) alone ameliorates withdrawal in approximately 30-50% of patients who require no further pharmacological therapy.

PAN is usually given on one occasion only for inpatients. Depending on the drug of abuse, out-patients may require more than one application of the gases, but usually no more than 2 applications during the first week of withdrawal. PAN has been used successfully on more than 50,000 patients in South Africa, Finland and the USA. The rationale for using PAN, as a gaseous partial opioid agonist will be discussed. The review concludes by placing the PAN method in the wider perspective of substance withdrawal states and craving, dealing with its current status and ending with an appeal for more studies to be done on this promising therapy.

Introduction – Distinguishing between Psychotropic Analgesic Nitrous Oxide and Anaesthetic Nitrous Oxide

Since its first use in the late 18th century, nitrous oxide has had a rather chequered history punctuated by periods of acceptance and rejection [Frost, 1985]. The times when it has fallen into disrepute have usually been caused by ignorance of the biological properties of the gas and false perceptions of how it should be administered [Frost, 1985].

As will be seen below, history has a habit of repeating itself. Thus, to get a balanced picture, any discussion on the current status of nitrous oxide needs to be placed in the context of the existing perceptions, which in certain cases have been divorced from the scientific facts. Unfortunately, it is often perceptions not facts that guide peoples' attitudes on a subject. Surprisingly perhaps, this applies equally to scientists (Gillman, 1996).

The modern history of nitrous oxide is a case in point. A number of prominent and influential people, working in the substance abuse field, have based their perceptions on the use of psychotropic analgesic nitrous oxide (PAN) for treating substance abuse withdrawal states, on misconceptions and not on the scientific facts. Unfortunately, these misconceptions have driven negative attitudes to PAN. I shall present evidence that these individuals are currently attempting to block the clinical use of PAN for ameliorating acute withdrawal states. They are also, by virtue of their prominence, de facto, blocking further research into this potentially useful therapy. These workers have played a significant role in retarding the progress of the use of the PAN therapy and are continuing to do so. No discussion on the current status of PAN is complete, without dealing with this aspect. Many researchers would eschew such a discussion because they are under the illusion that science is free of personal animus and prejudice. Those scientists labour under this misconception, at a cost, not only to themselves but also science [Gillman, 1996]. Furthermore, one of the most important goals of this review is to disabuse those who believe that science is the disinterested and passionless pursuit of knowledge.

The other more obvious key aim of this paper is to highlight the existing scientific knowledge on nitrous oxide in the context of PAN and the treatment of acute substance withdrawal states.

We introduced the term PAN in order to clearly distinguish the psychotropic effects of nitrous oxide from the anaesthetic effects of nitrous oxide [Gillman and Lichtigfeld, 1994a]. We were constrained to do so because when nitrous oxide is mentioned most medical professionals, with the possible exception of dentists, immediately assume that the anaesthetic properties of the gas are under consideration [Gillman and Lichtigfeld, 1994a; Gillman and Lichtigfeld, 2006]. Many health professionals do not realise that the low concentration of nitrous oxide diluted with high concentrations of oxygen, consistent with conscious sedation with nitrous oxide/oxygen (synonymous with PAN), produce very different pharmacological effects as compared to the much higher concentrations that produce surgical anaesthesia [Gillman and Lichtigfeld, 1994a]. Apart from its well-known analgesic and anaesthetic actions PAN also produces emotional changes. These emotional effects, which occur at low concentration of nitrous oxide, where the subject is always conscious, include mood elevation, anti-stress and anti-craving effects, most of which are inextricably involved in PAN's usefulness for ameliorating acute substance abuse withdrawal states [Gillman and Lichtigfeld, 1994a].

In contrast, as higher concentrations of nitrous oxide are given these produce preanaesthetic excitation and as the concentration increases further, unconsciousness and surgical anaesthesia supervene [Malamed, 1989; Gillman and Lichtigfeld, 1994a]. Although the anaesthetic actions of nitrous oxide have been extensively studied, its emotional effects have not. A phenomenon that might well be related to the fact that the use of nitrous oxide has been mainly confined to anaesthesia, where the anaesthesiologist is anxious to anaesthetise the patient as rapidly as possible and therefore keeps the period of consciousness to a minimum [Marshall and Wollman, 1985].

To avoid preanaesthetic excitation [and anaesthesia] and to obtain the goal of relaxation, PAN is always titrated to the requirements of each individual patient and a predetermined dose should *never* be used [Langa, 1976; Bennet, 1978; Skelly, 1998; Malamed, 1989a; Clark and Brunick 2008; Gillman and Lichtigfeld 2004a;b;c; Gillman and Lichtigfeld, 2006]. The array of doses that are effective range from 10% to 70% inhaled, with 70% of patients responding at inhaled concentrations of between 30%-40% [Malamed, 1989]. Skelly [1998] have suggested a range 'between 20% and 40%...although the effective sedation concentrations varies considerably between individuals and may occasionally be as low as 5-10% or as high as 60-70% N_2O in oxygen.' My colleague and I [Gillman and Lichtigfeld, 1990], have suggested a similar range to that of Skelly [1998]. The concentration can be as low as 5% or as high as 70% in very rare hyper or hypo responders [Gillman and Lichtigfeld, 1990]. Indeed, as can be seen above, the amount of nitrous oxide consistent with PAN is so variable across a cohort, there is no universal agreement, even among experts[Langa, 1976; Bennet, 1978; Malamed, 1989; Skelly, 1998; Gillman and Lichtigfeld, 1990; Clark et al, 2006; Clark and Brunick, 1999; 2003; 2008], as to what the average dose is.

Crucially, all workers who have a good understanding of the technique of dental conscious sedation with nitrous oxide/oxygen (which is synonymous with PAN) emphasise the importance of titration to the patient's own individual dose.

If a predetermined dose is chosen, some patients will be oversedated and approach or enter stage II of anaesthesia (or the excitation stage of anaesthesia) [Beirne and Smith, 1985; Malamed, 1989]. This is not only potentially dangerous, but unethical. Malamed [1989] states: 'Only procedures of short duration should be contemplated in stage II and then only by persons who have been thoroughly trained in general anesthesia… Because reflexes are hyperactive in this stage… …laryngospasm may be produced.' Malamed [1989] also indicates that *another* well-trained person should be present to ensure maintenance of the patient's airway. It is therefore not surprising that, 'Anesthesiologists try to reduce the duration and intensity of this stage to the minimum.' [Marshall and Wollman, 1985]. Cohen [1975] goes further '..the duration and the intensity of this stage should be reduced to a minimum for patients in substandard health.' Presumably this includes chronic alcoholics, who are often malnourished and debilitated [Edwards, 1991].

Indeed, the correctly trained practitioner will always titrate PAN slowly to the patient's clinical response and to obtain relaxation. As the point of relaxation is approaching smaller doses of nitrous oxide are added until the clinical endpoint of relaxation is obtained. This clinical endpoint is well before stage II anaesthesia (excitation) and indeed the entire point of hands-on training is to enable the practitioner to obtain the definite but subtle clinical endpoint without straying into the excitation stage of anaesthesia (stage II). This is the case, since the training inculcates the importance of titration to the individual's unique concentration. Furthermore, it would seem that even among individuals, the concentration required may vary from day to day i.e. it is a state rather than a trait phenomenon [Gillman and Lichtigfeld, 1987].

A classical example of the dangers of choosing a predetermined concentration of nitrous oxide, and not titrating to the individual clinical response, is shown in some recent work [Alho et al, 2002; 2003]. These workers refused offers of hands-on training and instead were guided by an anaesthetist on their team who did not understand the PAN technique [Gillman and Lichtigfeld, 1997; Gillman and Lichtigfeld, 2004a]. They assumed wrongly, despite verbal warnings from Reijo Ojutkangas [personal communication, Ojutkangas 1999] and myself that an anaesthetist would not be well schooled in all applications of nitrous oxide.

Unfortunately, under the guidance of this anaesthetist, they not only chose a predetermined concentration of nitrous oxide i.e. 30% end tidal volume [or 60% inhaled] but instead of titrating to the clinical response, they titrated to their predetermined target concentration of nitrous oxide, which they only decreased when the patient was about to fall unconscious [Alho et al, 2002; 2003]. Clearly, almost all the study group within their cohort of 105 patients were held in a state either in, or very close to the excitation stage of anaesthesia. That their patients were not relaxed (which is the hall mark of correctly used PAN) and indeed in the excitation stage (stage II anaesthesia) is recorded in their paper, in that the majority of patients receiving nitrous oxide exhibited increased facial muscle tone as measured by electromyography as compared to controls [Alho et al, 2002]. These patients also showed evidence of increased sympathetic tone [Alho et al, 2002]. Increased muscle tone and sympathetic activity are classical signs of the excitation seen in the vicinity of the excitement stage of anaesthesia (i.e. stage II) [Cohen, 1975]. This must have been extremely uncomfortable and stressful for their patients [Alho et al, 2002; 2003], already suffering from a condition (alcohol withdrawal) characterised by a tense trembling hyperadrenergic state [Lichtigfeld and Gillman, 1982; Gillman and Lichtigfeld, 1983; Edwards, 1991] but is clearly not appropriate in terms of PAN. Thus, it would not surprise the reader that Morris Clark the senior author of the current gold-standard textbook on conscious sedation [Clark and Brunick, 2008] with nitrous oxide wrote, regarding the work of Alho et al [2002; 2003] as follows [Clark et al, 2006]:

'It has been the authors' experience that nitrous oxide/oxygen has been commonly misused [Alho et al.,2002; 2003] to achieve desired outcomes for a specific procedure or patient.'

Clark et al [2006] are at pains to emphasise the importance of titrating to the patients' clinical state, using different concentrations of nitrous oxide for each patient [Clark et al, 2006]; a fact stressed in the textbook as well [Clark and Brunick, 1999; 2003; 2008]. Clark and Brunick [1999; 2003; 2008] also highlight the importance of correct training in the technique of conscious sedation with nitrous oxide, which as mentioned earlier is a synonym for the PAN method.

From this, it will be clear to the reader why it is important to have brief hands-on training [Gillman and Lichtigfeld, 1990; Gillman and Lichtigfeld, 1997]. I have deliberately spent considerable time making the distinction between PAN and anaesthetic nitrous oxide in order to forewarn other workers who might be interested in repeating our work [Gillman and Lichtigfeld, 1990; Gillman and Lichtigfeld; 2006], because a wrong technique and dose (like any other medication), guarantees failure [Gillman and Lichtigfeld, 2004a;c].

Needless to say Alho et al [2002, 2003] were unable to repeat our work because their technique was incorrect [Langa, 1976; Bennet, 1978; Malamed, 1989; Clark et al, 2006; Clark and Brunick, 1999; 2003; 2008; Gillman and Lichtigfeld, 2004a,b,c; Gillman and Lichtigfeld, 2006; Gillman et al, 2007] and because they used a predetermined, excessively high concentration of nitrous oxide, which was well above the doses that the majority of subjects would need to achieve concentrations of nitrous oxide consistent with PAN [Skelly, 1998; Gillman et al, 2007].

Clearly, PAN is not just the use of any predetermined concentration of nitrous oxide, but rather a specialised technique [Gillman and Lichtigfeld, 2006]. A technique of using various concentrations of nitrous oxide at concentrations determined by the individual requirements of each patient, slowly and carefully titrated to a clinical endpoint characterised by relaxation and nowhere near stage II anaesthesia.

When the technique is correctly applied in the hands of trained medical professionals, it is possible to rapidly treat acute substance withdrawal states from alcohol [Lichtigfeld and Gillman, 1982; Gillman et al, 2007]; cocaine [Carey et al, 1991; Gillman et al, 2006b] cannabis [Carey et al, 1991; Daynes and Gillman, 1994]; nicotine [Gillman and Shevel, 1988; Daynes and Gillman, 1994; Bayrakdarian, 2000], opioids [Kripke and Hechtman, 1972; Gillman and Lichtigfeld, 1985; Carey et al, 1991] and combinations of cannabis plus methaqualone [Gillman et al, 2006a].

The PAN therapy was first used in South Africa (S.A.) in 1979. Despite considerable opposition from academics [Gagiano, 1994; Emsley, 1994] and others [Openshaw, 1986] it was accepted as a standard therapy for substance abuse withdrawal states by the South African Medical Association and the Health Professionals Council of South Africa. It has an official fee and tariff code and for this reason is accepted for medical aid (insurance) claims in S. A. [Gillman, 2006]. The PAN therapy is therefore not regarded as an experimental technique in S.A. Furthermore, registered nurses who have been trained to use the gas, are able to treat substance withdrawal, without direct medical supervision, once it has been prescribed by a physician [Gillman and Lichtigfeld, 2006] or in the case of nicotine dependence, by a dentist[Gillman, 2008].

How PAN Ameliorates Substance Abuse Withdrawal States

Right from the very first paper we hypothesised that PAN acted on the endogenous opioid system to produce its therapeutic effect in withdrawal states [Lichtigfeld and Gillman, 1982]. Since then, additional experimental evidence has appeared showing that PAN has opioid properties [Gillman and Lichtigfeld, 1994a; Gillman and Lichtigfeld, 2006].

Not long after we published our initial paper [Lichtigfeld and Gillman, 1982], we suggested that mutually antagonistic κ-opioid and μ-opioid systems were involved in the pathogenesis of substance abuse [Gillman and Lichtigfeld, 1984; 1994a; Lichtigfeld and Gillman, 1996]. Experimental evidence from rodents and primates showed that μ-opioid agonists applied to the mesolimbic dopamine system stimulate dopamine release in the nucleus accumbens [Lichtigfeld, and Gillman, 1996]. In contrast, administration of κ-opioid agonists to the mesolimbic dopamine system have the opposite effect, in that dopamine release is inhibited in the nucleus accumbens [Lichtigfeld, and Gillman, 1996].

There is also evidence that PAN activates both κ-opioid and μ-opioid receptor systems [Gillman and Lichtigfeld, 1994a; Lichtigfeld and Gillman, 1996]. Thus, it is possible that

PAN, by differentially acting on the μ-opioid and κ-opioid receptor systems interacts to rapidly restore the homeostatic balance that has been disturbed as a result of alcohol abstinence, during the alcoholic withdrawal state [Gillman and Lichtigfeld, 1994a; Lichtigfeld and Gillman, 1996]. This hypothesis could also be invoked to explain the 'minute'[Gillman, 1995] abuse potential of PAN and its lack of secondary abuse potential observed in over 25,000 (now over 50,000) cases of substance abuse treated by us and others, since 1979 [Gillman, 1992; Gillman and Lichtigfeld, 1994a; Lichtigfeld and Gillman, 1996, Gillman, 2006].

It is possible that the modulation of the μ-opioid and κ-opioid receptor systems by PAN underlies its efficacy in ameliorating all forms of acute substance abuse withdrawal including that from alcohol [Lichtigfeld and Gillman, 1982; Gillman et al, 2007]; cocaine [Carey et al, 1991; Gillman et al, 2006b] cannabis [Carey et al, 1991; Daynes and Gillman, 1994]; nicotine [Gillman and Shevel, 1988; Daynes and Gillman, 1994; Bayrakdarian, 2000], opioids [Kripke and Hechtman, 1972; Gillman and Lichtigfeld, 1985; Carey et al, 1991] and combinations of cannabis plus methaqualone [Gillman et al, 2006a].

Above, I have dealt in some detail with the differences of using nitrous oxide for obtaining anaesthesia as opposed to PAN. I have also highlighted the crucial pitfalls that occur, if these differences are not fully understood and the operator does not have the basic theoretical knowledge to appreciate these differences, before embarking on a study of PAN [Alho et al, 2002; 2003; Clark et al; 2006].

Nonetheless, I have not outlined in detail the method of administering it. Details of the technique can be found in various papers [Gillman and Lichtigfeld, 1990; 2006; Clark et al, 2006] and for those interested in repeating the work, in any textbook devoted to the subject [Langa, 1976; Bennet, 1978; Malamed, 1989; Clark and Brunick, 2008].

PAN for Treating Alcohol Withdrawal States

Alcohol Withdrawal States

At the outset I would like to emphasise that all our studies on the alcoholic withdrawal states excluded any patients suffering pre-delirium or worse. We did so because severe alcoholic withdrawal states can have severe sequelae including death, and there are tried and trusted sedative therapies such as the benzodiazepines [Saitz et al, 1994] that should immediately be used in such cases, rather than exposing patients' that are seriously ill to a clinical trial.

Our first study started in 1979, tested the effects of nitrous oxide against oxygen single-blind. Here, the nurse administering the gases was aware of which gas she was giving but not the patient.

Oxygen was first administered to each subject for 20 minutes. Immediately thereafter, nitrous oxide was slowly added to oxygen until the concentration of nitrous had been titrated to achieve levels consistent with PAN. The average time for titration, ranges between 2-12 minutes, depending on the dose required for each patient. I would like to emphasise, once again, that the use of a predetermined dose, as used by Alho et al. [2002; 2003] is totally unsuitable when using PAN [Gillman and Lichtigfeld, 2004a;b;c] because the concentration of nitrous oxide required to achieve relaxation (the goal of using PAN), differs so markedly between subjects [Langa, 1976; Malamed, 1989; Bennet, 1978; Gillman and Lichtigfeld, 1994a; Clark and Brunick, 1999; 2003; 2008].

The reader should note that regardless of the time taken to obtain the correct dose for each patient, all cases received nitrous oxide for a total of 20 minutes, which includes the titration time [Gillman and Lichtigfeld, 1990]. The goal of the PAN and the hallmark of its effects are relaxation of the patient, without signs of sedation [Gillman and Lichtigfeld, 1990]. After the 20 minute period of PAN administration a washout with 100% oxygen was given [Lichtigfeld and Gillman, 1982].

There were ninety eight patients in this first study [Lichtigfeld, and Gillman, 1982]. After the first exposure to oxygen for 20 minutes the initial aggregate symptom score of 518 was reduced to 188. Nonetheless, PAN reduced the after oxygen score of 188 to 57 [Lichtigfeld and Gillman, 1982]. We concluded from this open study that both PAN and placebo gas [oxygen] were therapeutic.

Two later trials examined the effects of placebo gas [medical air] against oxygen [Lichtigfeld Gillman, 1989a] and oxygen and carbogen [95% oxygen plus 5% carbon dioxide] [Gillman and Lichtigfeld, 1991a]. In the latter studies, the placebo response ranged from 30-50% [Lichtigfeld and Gillman, 1989a; Gillman and Lichtigfeld, 1991a]. We observed a difference in the percentage of placebo responders in each study. However, the placebo gases when compared against each other within each trial did not show a statistically different therapeutic effect. Both these trials were undertaken randomised and double-blind. All placebo *non*-responders from each trial were then exposed to PAN, with most of these subjects responding positively to PAN [Lichtigfeld and Gillman, 1989a; Gillman and Lichtigfeld, 1991a].

Our next step, because of the large placebo response [Lichtigfeld and Gillman, 1982; 1989a; Gillman and Lichtigfeld, 1991a] was to try and demonstrate that PAN was statistically better than placebo. We examined 100 patients who had been randomly given either medical air or oxygen double-blind. 48 patients from these 2 groups did not respond to either air or oxygen. These non-responders were then immediately given PAN single-blind. Of these 48 patients, 42 responded positively to PAN, with 6 not responding.

In order to make the statistical analysis as fair as possible, we assumed that at least 50% of the placebo non-responders (that is 24 of the 48 patients) would have improved by 50% (or more) if given an additional 20 minutes of placebo [oxygen or air]. We then conducted the chi-square test on these results. We did this despite knowing, from previous clinical experience, that exposure of placebo non-responders to a further 20 minutes of placebo gas did not ameliorate alcoholic withdrawal states above that achieved by the initial 20 minute exposure [Gillman and Lichtigfeld, 2006]. Even using this statistical assumption, the results of the chi-square test showed PAN to be significantly better than placebo at the 0.01% level [Lichtigfeld and Gillman; 1989b]. Work published latter supported the latter findings [Gillman and Lichtigfeld; 1991a]. We believed that these studies demonstrated that PAN could rapidly, safely and effectively improve mild to moderate alcohol withdrawal states [Lichtigfeld and Gillman, 1982; 1989b; Gillman and Lichtigfeld, 1986; 1991a].

One of the things that struck us from the very first study was that the maximum therapeutic effect occurred extremely rapidly. Indeed, in most cases, the maximum therapeutic response was observed within 60 minutes of initial gas administration and often well before an hour had elapsed [Lichtigfeld and Gillman, 1982; 1989a;b; Daynes, 1989; Ojutkangas, 1991]. We have also found that a single 20 minute exposure to PAN for inpatients, usually on admission, is adequate in more than 90% of cases for the total 7 day in-patient stay [Lichtigfeld and Gillman, 1982; Gillman and Lichtigfeld, 1990]. Later work in an out-patient setting showed that a single gas exposure is usually all that is required for outpatients in more than 85% of patients [Ojutkangas and Gillman, 1994]. These observations have been confirmed by other investigators [Daynes, 1989; Ojutkangas, 1991; Carey et al, 1991].

We soon realised, with our work with nitrous oxide and withdrawal states, that it would be very difficult to compare an agent that exerts its maximal effect within 60 minutes to sedative agents such as the benzodiazepines, which when used in a standard manner usually take a day or two to exert an equal effect [Goldstein, 1983; Gillman and Lichtigfeld, 1991a; Saitz, et al, 1994; Gillman and Lichtigfeld, 2006].

There are also difficulties when trying to compare different physical formats i.e. a tablet format [such as a benzodiazepine] with a mixture of gases such as PAN. Initially we did not believe this to be a problem, because the effect of PAN was so rapid and obviously superior to sedative detoxifications, that at first we thought it unnecessary to conduct a double-blind trial. Indeed, the therapeutic effect was so dramatic that when we had finished our initial trial, we arrived at the detoxification centre to pack up the equipment, believing that the nursing staff would be happy to return to their previous use of the benzodiazepines and other sedatives. We were quite mistaken. While we were packing, the senior nurse and matron, came into the ward and remonstrated with us. They said that the PAN treatment was so superior to anything they had ever used, that they wanted to adopt it as the treatment of choice for their facility (Rand Aid Association, Wedge Gardens, Edenvale Johannesburg, S. A.).

This was a great compliment for the PAN method because some of these nurses at the Wedge Gardens had been in the field of alcoholic detoxification for over 20 years. These very experienced nurses had therefore seen many different therapies come and go. The gamut of treatments for alcoholic withdrawal states that they had observed over the preceding 20 years included intravenous ethanol drips (in the very early days), and later barbiturates, chlormethiazole and then the advent of the benzodiazepines. Despite the vast superiority of the benzodiazepines when compared to the barbiturates and ethanol drips, they now believed that PAN was superior to the benzodiazepines. Their reasoning was as follows [Gillman, 2006] the:

1. most patients improved within minutes of gas treatment and were often well enough to enjoy the next ward meal;
2. use of addictive sedative medications such as the benzodiazepines (e.g. diazepam) are reduced by 90% plus. This obviates the danger of secondary addiction in this highly susceptible group;

3. extreme rapidity of recovery enables nurses/physicians to distinguish those patients requiring intensive inpatient therapy from those that do not; since 90% plus patients respond positively to one administration of the gases, usually on admission. It has been our experience that those who do not respond by an improvement of 50% or more on a withdrawal instrument after the initial administration of PAN, almost always require aggressive inpatient therapy. It therefore would seem to be a unique method of screening those who can safely be treated as outpatients from those who require inpatient therapy;

4. rapidity of the therapeutic response enables the patient to abandon the sick role speedily and enter the essential next phase of rehabilitation; usually requiring social, psychological and/or psychiatric therapy;

5. placebo (O_2) alone ameliorates the withdrawal state in approximately 30-50% of patients who require no further pharmacological therapy. It is therefore the only detoxification treatment as far as I am aware, that maximises the placebo response.

As the benefits of the PAN therapy became more widely known through various scientific publications and university dissertations [Lichtigfeld and Gillman, 1982; Lichtigfeld and Gillman, 1983a;b; Kahn, 1983; de Rooster, 1983; Edwards, 1985; Myles, 1984; 1994; Gillman, 1985; Gillman and Lichtigfeld, 1983; 1986] other clinicians came to Wedge Gardens and availed themselves of the opportunity to view patients being treated with PAN. After observing one or two patients themselves they became convinced that the PAN therapy had a place in the treatment of withdrawal states and deserved to be researched further [Carey et al, 1991; Daynes, 1994; Fourie, 1994; Ojukangas, 1991]. All these practitioners, including one from Finland (Ojutkangas) soon came to Wedge Gardens for the brief hands-on training and then went on to continue using it successfully at their treatment centres. In short, after seeing for themselves the rapidity of the therapeutic response following an hour of PAN and viewing the scientific work on which it was based [Lichtigfeld and Gillman, 1982; Lichtigfeld and Gillman, 1983a;b; de Rooster, 1983; Christian, 1991; Myles, 1984; 1992; Gillman, 1985; Gillman and Lichtigfeld, 1983; 1986] they were convinced. They did not need a double-blind trial to show them that the PAN treatment had merit – the face validity was good enough for them.

Unlike these open-minded clinicians, the academic community in S. A. and Finland refused to come and see for themselves, although by then, PAN was being used at widely dispersed geographical site in South African and in Finland. The academic resistance was led by the President of the Society of Psychiatrists of S.A. [Gagiano, 1994] and his Vice-President [Emsley, 1994] and by the Dean of Medical Education of Helsinki University Mikko Salaspuro [Salaspuro and Alho, 1997; Metheun et al, 1997]. Moreover, it became apparent that none of these academics were prepared to believe the published work of other investigators [Myles, 1984; 1992; de Rooster, 1983; Daynes, 1989 Christian, 1991] and ourselves [Lichtigfeld and Gillman, 1982; Lichtigfeld and Gillman, 1983a;b; Gillman, 1985; Gillman and Lichtigfeld, 1980; 1983; 1986; 1990; 1991a; 1994a].

Naively (as will be discussed later), we assumed that these scientific purists still required a double-blind randomised study, before being convinced that the PAN treatment might have some merit, or to actually visit one of the sites in S. A. where the treatment was being used successfully. We were therefore obliged, to embark on a double-blind study [Gillman and Lichtigfeld, 2002; 2004d] after more than twenty years of safe and successful use of PAN, in many thousands of patients, without significant side-effects, or evidence of secondary addiction to PAN [Gillman and Lichtigfeld, 1990; 1997; 2002; 2006] or sequelae [Gillman and Lichtigfeld, 1990; 1997; 2002; 2006].

Double-Blind, Randomised Trials with PAN versus A Benzodiazepine

As discussed above, in order to design randomised double-blind studies we had to overcome the following practical problems arising from the:

1. rapidity of the effects of the gases, which occurred within minutes and certainly within a maximum of 60 minutes, in cases where the gas or gases were effective. The benzodiazepines take much longer to act than an hour [Gillman, 2006; Gillman and Lichtigfeld, 2006];
2. fact that we were testing physically different agents, in this case tablets versus gases [Gillman, 2006; Gillman and Lichtigfeld, 2006].
3. positive effects of the placebo gas, which on its own, produced such a good therapeutic response that exposure to PAN was not required, for between 30-50% of patients [Gillman, 2006; Gillman and Lichtigfeld, 2006];

I will now describe how we overcome these difficulties by randomly assigning the cohort into 2 different groups and administering the gases double blind and randomly.

All patients that signed informed consent for the trial were given placebo gas for 20 minutes, in order to exclude placebo responders. Thus, those who responded by a 50% or more on a modified Gross scale were then excluded from further study. In this way we were able to minimise the effects of the placebo response [Gillman and Lichtigfeld, 2002; 2004d]. Despite this, we cannot exclude the possibility that a placebo response may have played some part in the therapeutic response measured because each group did eventually receive a placebo [Gillman and Lichtigfeld, 2006].

To eliminate the problems of double-blinding a gas and a tablet that acted at such different speeds we measured the therapeutic response at 2 hours after the start of treatment and we randomly assigned each group (using a random number table) as follows:

1. the one group received carefully titrated placebo gas [oxygen] and active benzodiazepine tablets (diazepam) and;
2. the other group received active gas (carefully titrated PAN) and placebo tablets (dummy tablets, identical in all other respects to the active tablets).

As mentioned above, only non-placebo responders were entered into the double-blind randomised stage of the trial. These patients were given the gases, through identical gas flowmeters (MDM Qauntiflex Matrx, Medical) marked 'A' and 'B'. The gas supply to each flowmeter was hidden, so that neither the administering nurse nor the patient were able to identify which treatment was given. The diazepam and placebo tablets were identical in appearance. One of these flowmeter heads was modified so that the nitrous oxide port at the rear of the machine was connected to the oxygen supply, so that both ports received oxygen.

All subjects entering the trial met the DSM-IV (1994) criteria for alcohol dependence and were actively withdrawing. Patients were excluded if they were suffering from delirium tremens or any of the following; chronic obstructive pulmonary pathology; or any other severe chronic organic or psychiatric pathology [Gillman and Lichtigfeld, 2002; 2004d].

The South African Medical Research Council (MRC) granted ethical approval for the studies and all subjects provided written informed consent.

In the first study [Gillman and Lichtigfeld, 2002] we observed 23 patients who were admitted fairly early on the day of the trial and were given no medication until the double-blind phase of the trial.

The code was broken only after all the data had been collated and analysed.

Of the total of 23 subjects, 11 had been given gas A (PAN plus placebo tablets) and 12 gas B (placebo gas and active tablet). In the group that received PAN plus placebo tablet, 10 subjects responded positively, while the group that received placebo gas plus active diazepam, 8 responded positively.

Despite the small sample used (n=23) PAN was significantly more effective than the benzodiazepine at p=0.05 level when compared at 120 minutes.

After the initial 120 minutes all patients were followed up for the full remainder of the 7-day inpatient detoxification program. Patients who had responded positively to PAN required small doses of oxazepam (30 mgs) nocte on the first and second day only. The remaining patients (i.e. those who had received placebo gas and active tablet), including the single patient who had not responded to PAN, were given a standard benzodiazepine detoxification i.e. diazepam 5 mgs tds for day 1-3; 5mg bd for day 2-5 and 5 mg once only for day 6. Oxazepam nocte was required for all the latter patients [Gillman and Lichtigfeld, 2002].

In the second study [Gillman and Lichtigfeld, 2004d] we pooled the above results with 28 subjects who had received diazepam the previous night, because they had arrived at the alcohol facility too late to be entered into the trial that day. We did so in order to see whether an extra dose of diazepam would make a significant difference to the result of the first study [Gillman and Lichtigfeld, 2002].

After the code had been broken, 23 subjects of the 51 had received PAN plus placebo tablet and 28 placebo gas plus active diazepam.

21 subjects responded positively to active gas plus placebo tablet, while 19 responded positively to placebo gas and active tablet.

There were 10 positive responses in the group who had been given PAN and who had not received diazepam the prior night and 1 negative response. Those in the PAN group who did receive a benzodiazepine the previous night, showed 11 positive and 1 negative responses. Thus in the PAN plus placebo tablet cohort, a total of 21subjects manifested a positive response while 2 had a negative response.

In the other cohort (i.e placebo gas plus diazepam) those not receiving a benzodiazepine the prior night had 8 positive and 4 negative responses. Those in this group that had received a benzodiazepine the night before showed 11 positive and 5 negative responses. Thus in this cohort there were 19 positive and 9 negative responses.

We found that even with an additional dose of diazepam the previous night, superimposed on the same protocol as in the first study [Gillman and Lichtigfeld, 2002], PAN plus placebo tablet is superior to placebo gas plus active diazepam at p=0.05 level [Gillman and Lichtigfeld, 2004d].

As was the case with the patients in the earlier study [Gillman and Lichtigfeld, 2002] all patients were followed up for 7 days. Those patients, who had responded positively to PAN, needed no further treatment except oxazepam [30 mgs] for night sedation usually for day 1 and 2 only. All the remaining patients i.e. those consigned to the group who had received placebo and diazepam plus the 2 non-responder to PAN were given a standard benzodiazepine regimen as described above [Gillman and Lichtigfeld, 2002]. All those detoxified with benzodiazepines required night sedation with oxazepam for 7 days [Gillman and Lichtigfeld, 2004d].

Our double-blind trials [Gillman and Lichtigfeld, 2002; 2004d] have been criticised as poorly designed and therefore useless, on the basis that 'two hours may not have been a sufficient amount of time for diazepam to exert its full therapeutic effect before symptom assessment.'[Prince and Turpin, 2008]. A criticism that is invalid, since diazepam is 'absorbed rapidly, reaching peak concentrations in about an hour' [Baldessareni, 1996]. Greenblatt and Shader [1985] note that diazepam is one of the most rapidly absorbed oral benzodiazepines 'reaching peak concentrations in the blood within one hour after dosage.' Thus, there was at least an extra hour to cover pharmacokinetic differences that may have manifested over the cohort, and ensuring that all subjects were exposed to peak active levels of diazepam by the time the ratings were taken [Gillman and Lichtigfeld, 2002; 2004d]. Furthermore, the additional dose of diazepam, given the previous night [Gillman and Lichtigfeld, 2004d], was ignored and therefore was discounted [Prince and Turpin, 2008]. The extra dose is relevant because it is likely to have potentiated the diazepam given two hours before ratings were taken [Gillman and Lichtigfeld, 2004d] since diazepam has a long half-life, which is applicable with a multidosing schedule [Greenblatt and Shader, 1985; Baldessareni, 1996].

Furthermore they [Prince and Turpin, 2008] indicate, wrongly, that no outcome was reported after two hours. As can be seen from the description of these trials above, the benzodiazepine requirements for the PAN group was much reduced as compared to those who had been given placebo gas plus active diazepam [Gillman and Lichtigfeld, 2002; 2004d]. They also wrongly state that 'Oxazepam 30 mg was administered to subjects in both groups at bedtime.' While oxazepam was needed for a night or two for the PAN group, it was required every night for the benzodiazepine group [Gillman and Lichtigfeld, 2002; 2004d]. Prince and Turpin [2008] note that our studies did not address adverse outcomes. A recent Cochrane Review, mentions that the review did not 'indicate any causes for concern that PAN is more harmful than the benzodiazepines' [Gillman et al, 2007], showing that adverse effects of PAN are no worse than those found with benzodiazepines. In agreement with the Cochrane Review [Gillman et al, 2007] our experience with thousands of cases is that adverse effects are trivial. Alho et al (2002) used double the inhaled concentration of nitrous oxide than that would (on average) be required for PAN and yet they also reported only minor side-effects.

Of course, when PAN is used at the correct dose, there is no evidence of excitation, as reported by Alho et al [2002]. Obviously, excitation should be avoided in any tremulous, hyperadrenergic state such as alcohol withdrawal [Gillman and Lichtigfeld, 1983; Edwards, 1985]. The excitation found by Alho et al [2002], which is avoided when PAN is used at the correct dose titrated for each individual patient, was clearly due to the excessively high doses of nitrous oxide used [Alho et al, 2002].

Although Prince and Turpin [2008] note in their review that nitrous oxide is 'commonly used... ...in outpatient dentistry'. Nonetheless, rather illogically, they assume that PAN 'is not a practical option in the outpatient treatment of alcohol withdrawal.' The latter assumption flies in the face of the existing evidence where it has been used on outpatients for thousands of cases in S.A. [Carey et al, 1991; Gillman and Lichtigfeld, 2006] and Finland [Gillman and Ojutkangas, 1994].

Prince and Turpin [2008] have also ignored all the other work indicating that PAN is useful for alcohol withdrawal states [Lichtigfeld and Gillman, 1982; Lichtigfeld and Gillman, 1983a;b; de Rooster, 1983; Christian, 1991; Myles, 1984; 1992; Carey et al, 1991; Gillman, 1985; Gillman and Lichtigfeld, 1986; 1990; 2002; 2004d] on the basis that none of these are randomised and double-blind. Face validity does not seem to have a place in their reckoning. Obviously it is better to have double-blind randomised trials, but that does not discount clinical observations. Observations, without such controls are still valid [Gillman and Lichtigfeld, 1997]. For instance '.....it takes only two minutes to establish the mind-blowing effect of cocaine!' [Pfeiffer, 1987]. Furthermore, a Harvard psychiatry professor states 'If something works it certainly is important to study it, but doesn't mean that people should stop using it just because it has not been proven efficacious in a double-blind study., ...' [Liu, 1996] A truth that is even more cogent when examining a treatment that on observation has obvious advantages over the 'gold-standard'. Indeed, it was this very fact, which complicated the search for a suitable double-blind technique [Gillman and Lichtigfeld, 1997; 2002; 2004d]. It is clearly dangerous to be bound slavishly to any phenomenon in medicine including double-blind studies.

Although there is no doubt that further good quality studies on the efficacy of PAN are necessary [Gillman et al, 2007; Prince and Turpin, 2008] it is clearly premature to assert that 'Nitrous oxide should not be used in the treatment of alcohol withdrawal because reputable clinical trials are lacking and its administration requires training and specialized devices.' [Prince and Turpin, 2008]. Furthermore, to assert that any health care intervention 'should not be used' because 'its administration requires training and specialized devices.' would banish much of medicine, including all surgery. This is clearly an overkill as is their concluding statement 'nitrous oxide should be avoided for this indication.' The most that these workers can say is that further work is needed before a decision can be taken on the use of PAN.

The work of Alho et al [2002; 2003] can be discounted because although they used nitrous oxide, their technique does not fulfil the criteria for PAN [Clark et al, 2006; Gillman and Lichtigfeld, 1990; Gillman and Lichtigfeld, 2004a;b;c; Gillman et al, 2007]. Their concomitant use of benzodiazepines in all groups studied [Alho et al., 2002; 2003] also disqualifies this work. By adding daytime diazepam, their study [Alho et al., 2002; 2003] 'became not analgesic nitrous oxide against a placebo, but rather nitrous oxide combined with diazepam versus placebo plus diazepam.'[Gillman and Lichtigfeld, 2004a]. Other workers have also criticised Alho et al [2002; 2003] for this poor design feature, rendering their results meaningless [Prince and Turpin, 2008]. Thus, our double-blind randomised studies [Gillman and Lichtigfeld, 2002; 2004d] supports our earlier work [Lichtigfeld and Gillman, 1982; Gillman and Lichtigfeld, 1986;1990] that PAN 'is a safe, rapid and effective therapy for acute mild to moderately severe withdrawal states' and that there is a reduction in the amount of sedative medication required when PAN is used [Lichtigfeld and Gillman, 2004d].

PAN for Treating Other Substances of Abuse Apart from Alcohol

Opioids

Kripke and Hechtman [1972] were the first workers to report after successfully treating a case of substance abuse withdrawal with concentrations of nitrous oxide consistent with PAN. Although the inhaled concentration of nitrous oxide was consistent with PAN, their technique was different because they did not titrate but rather used a proprietary 50:50 mixture of oxygen and nitrous oxide. They described using nitrous oxide/oxygen to wean a patient heavily addicted to pentazocine. The patient had used daily doses of pentazocine ranging from 700-1000mg over 2 years. The rationale for trying nitrous oxide was to treat severe gastro-intestinal problems using the well-known analgesic properties of the gas. PAN was used daily for at least 6 hours per day for 200 days. And for the first 30 days she was given PAN for 24 hours each day, to control the intense dysphoria associated with opioid withdrawal. Apart from good pain control was the incidental finding that the PAN enabled the patient to be withdrawn from her addiction.

Another important observation by Kripke and Hechtman [1972] was that despite the chronic exposure of the patient to nitrous oxide for 200 days, there was no sign of agranulocytosis. In fact she had developed pneumonia during the 200 days of exposure but responded with lymphocytosis in response to the infection. This is suprising because some patients develop signs of dyshaemopiesis following chronic long-term exposures to nitrous oxide [Gillman, 1987], which clearly was not the case with this patient. This work was the first to demonstrate that PAN could reduce the signs and symptoms of an abstinence syndrome from an opioid. More recently, these findings have been confirmed by other workers, indicating the usefulness of PAN for treating opioid withdrawal [Gillman and Lichtigfeld, 1985b; Carey et al., 1991; Ojutkangas, 1991].

This work has been repeated at a number of treatment centres under the auspices of the South African. National Council for Alcoholism and Drug Dependence (S.A.N.C.A.). The latter is the largest NGO dealing with the treatment and prevention of substance abuse in S.A. One of their associated centres (Family Outreach) specialises in opioid dependency withdrawal. This centre is located in the centre of South Africa 50 miles north of Graaf Reneit in the Western Cape Province. This centre has been using PAN as the treatment of choice for opioid withdrawal for nearly 3 years and reports high levels of success on numerous patients treated there, since the introduction of PAN in 2005.

Some recent animal work, using a place preference paradigm, has provided further evidence supporting the use of PAN for treating opioid abuse. Although nitrous oxide did not itself induce conditioned place preference it reduced the expression of morphine-induced place preference [Benturquia et al, 2007]. Furthermore, in another study the increase in extracellular levels of dopamine produced by placing rats and mice in a morphine-paired compartment was blocked by nitrous oxide [Benturquia et al, 2008].

Cocaine

Cocaine abuse has only become a problem in South Africa over the last 10 or so years. Until then, it was relatively rare and limited to the rich upper classes. Indeed, by 1988 crack abuse was insignificant in S.A. [Searll, 1989]. However, since then, the proportion of those seeking treatment for cocaine, including crack cocaine, has increased as a proportion of the total demand for treatment for substance abuse in S.A. [Parry et al., 2002]. As a result, those SANCA Societies using PAN have been increasingly using PAN to treat the acute withdrawal state arising from cocaine abstinence. These SANCA Societies have reported good results when using PAN to treat cocaine abstinence syndromes.

A recent single-blind study [Gillman et al, 2006b] examined 33 subjects [25 males; 8 females] with cocaine withdrawal symptoms that were treated at the SANCA Port Elizabeth outpatient clinic with an average age of 28.1 years [range 21-42 years].

Baseline recordings using a withdrawal scale were taken and then 100% oxygen was given to eliminate placebo responders. Carefully titrated PAN was then given for 20 minutes and the withdrawal instrument applied again. A reduction in symptom score of 50% or more was taken to be a positive response, since clinical experience has shown a 50% improvement is synonymous with observed recovery. 31 of the 33 cases responded by a decrease of symptom scores of 50% or more,

5 subjects responded positively to oxygen alone and did not improve further with PAN. 11 subjects did not improve with placebo but did respond positively to PAN. 15 subjects responded positively to Oxygen but then improved by a further 50% or more after breathing PAN. 2 patients failed to respond to either oxygen or PAN. Interestingly, neither of these non-responders was suffering from the most severe withdrawal state amongst those treated. All subjects had abused crack cocaine or cocaine.

Placebo reduced craving, depression, remorse, guilt which was further decreased following PAN. Oxygen plus PAN decreased baseline scores 'by 81%, 89%, 91%, 90% and 87% respectively.' [Gillman et al, 2006b].

Thus 93.9% of the subjects were improved by the use of PAN and /or O_2 alone.

These findings confirm the empirical findings reported by the various centres using PAN to treat acute cocaine withdrawal, which appears to be worth investigating further; in particular with a double-blind randomised trial.

As discussed above, we postulated that during the pathogenesis of substance abuse withdrawal states an inbalance develops between the κ and μ opioid systems [Gillman and

Lichtigfeld, 1984; Lichtigfeld and Gillman, 1996]. It is therefore significant that Mash and Staley [1999] have provided evidence that the κ_2 opioid system is upregulated during withdrawal from cocaine. It is therefore possible that PAN restores homeostasis by differentially activating the mu and kappa systems which could account for its beneficial effects during withdrawal states [Lichtigfeld and Gillman, 1996].

There is now further evidence from animal studies indicating that PAN is useful for treating substance abuse. For instance, when rats receive nitrous oxide (in subanaesthetic concentrations) in combination with amphetamine, locomotor sensitization is attenuated [Abraini et al, 2005]. Furthermore, as mentioned above for opioids, a place preference paradigm, has provided further evidence supporting the use of PAN for treating substance abuse, in this case cocaine abuse [Benturquia et al, 2007]. Although nitrous oxide did not itself induce conditioned place preference it reduced the expression of cocaine-induced place preference [Benturquia et al, 2007].

Nicotine

There have been reports that PAN can be used to ameliorate the acute nicotine withdrawal state [Shevel and Gillman 1988; Daynes and Gillman, 1994; Bayrakdarian, 2000]. In the first study, which was conducted single-blind, 35 heavy smokers (20 cigarettes/day for a minimum of 10 years), both male and female ceased smoking 24 hours before the trial started. Baseline scores were taken using a nicotine withdrawal instrument [Glassman et al, 1984] prior to titration of PAN. PAN was then titrated and the patients re-rated. All symptoms were greatly reduced (see Table 1).

Table 1. PAN for Acute Withdrawal from Cigarettes

	Before Treatment		After Treatment	
Symptoms	Group Score	Average	Group Score	Average
Craving	316	9.02	18	0.51
Headache/ Headpressure	181	16	0	0
Anxiety	155	4.43	0	0
Irritable	202	5.77	0	0
Tension	193	5.51	0	0
Sad/Tearful	35	1.00	5	0.14
Drowsy	159	4.54	34	0.97
Unable to				
Concentrate	154	4.4	0	0
Restlessness	157	4.48	0	0
Dizziness	36	1.03	8	0.23
Sweating	46	1.31	0	0
Butterflies in Stomach	57	1.63	0	0

Daynes and Gillman [1994] have also examined the effects of PAN on craving for tobacco (see below under section dealing with craving).

Bayrakdarian (2000) undertook an open trial to establish whether PAN could reduce cigarette smoking in a small sample (n=7). Urine cotinine samples were taken daily as an objective test of abstinence. Following PAN, cigarette use decreased from 17.1(sd=7.6) before N20 to 2.6(sd=3.42) (t=9.04, df=6, P<0.0001). All subjects reported decreased use, which was well correlated with cotinine levels (spearman r=0.94, p=0.005). 71% of subjects quit smoking completely, while the quit rate was 57% at the end of one month.

Some animal work has indicated that the endogenous opioid [Berrendero et al., 2002] and dopamine systems [Mansvelder and McGehee, 2000] are directly involved in nicotine addiction. This also provide further evidence that there is a final common pathway for addiction [Gillman and Shevel, 1988; Gillman and Lichtigfeld, 1991b] but that PAN could exert its positive effects in ameliorating the nicotine withdrawal state and craving by acting on the endogenous opioid system to restore the homeostatic balance that has been disturbed during the pathogenesis of nicotine use.

Cannabis

Cannabis is the most common illegal substance of abuse in S.A. [Parry et al, 2002]. As a result, there has been a great call on treatment facilities in S.A. to treat patient's requiring acute withdrawal from this agent. Thus, since the early 1990's, all the SANCA facilities that treat acute withdrawal states with PAN have been using it to treat acute cannabis withdrawal states. All of these centres have reported good results.

Daynes and Gillman [1994] examined the effects of PAN on cannabis craving (see below for details in the section on craving).

In a later study, also single-blind, the combination of cannabis and methaqualone was also studied. The latter combination seems to be a problem mainly confined to S.A. [Gillman et al, 2006a]. In S.A. it is colloquially known as 'white pipes'.

A cohort consisting of 101 patients (98 male and 3 female; most of whom under the age of 30) treated consecutively were given 100% oxygen followed by carefully titrated PAN single-blind. A positive response was assumed if the patient improved by 50% or more on a rating instrument [Gillman et al, 2006a].

One case of the 101 was excluded from the analysis because their data was incomplete.

Of the 100 cases analysed, 43 patients improved by a minimum of 50% after oxygen alone. Despite the improvement in 37 of the 43, they were given 20 minutes of PAN with further amelioration. 6 of the 43 did not require PAN because their aggregate rating score was zero after oxygen alone. The improvement obtained by oxygen alone in 4 cases of the 37 was reversed by PAN, possibly because the dose was poorly titrated and was excessive [Gillman et al, 2006a]. In the other 2 cases of the 6, there was an improvement when PAN was added following O$_2$ by a minimum of 3 points. There was no further improvement following PAN in the 31 remaining cases of the 37. A total of 57 patients did not respond positively to oxygen alone but 44 of these did respond by a 50% or more improvement to PAN on their scores at baseline. 13 patients were recalcitrant either to oxygen or PAN.

In total 87 patients benefited either by breathing oxygen alone or oxygen followed by PAN. Thus, oxygen alone, or followed by PAN was therapeutic in 87% of patients. It would seem that this work indicates that PAN is useful for treating cannabis and cannabis/methaqualone abuse withdrawal states. Interestingly, naloxone and naloxonazine both opioid receptor anatagonists block the stimulating effects of heroin and cannabinoids on dopamine release in the nucleus accumbens [Tanda et al, 1997]. An observation that provides some basic experimental evidence that PAN, as an opioid, could act during withdrawal states to stimulate the μ-opioid receptor system which we have proposed is underactive during withdrawal states [Gillman and Lichtigfeld, 1983;1984; Lichtigfeld and Gillman, 1996]. It also gives support further support for the concept that there is a final common pathway in the pathogenesis of substance abuse [Gillman and Shevel, 1988; Gillman and Lichtigfeld, 1991b].

Polydrug Abuse

In 1991 my colleague and I suggested that PAN would be useful for treating polydrug abuse [Lichtigfeld and Gillman, 1991]. Soon after, PAN was used to successfully treat polysubstance abuse withdrawal states caused by a wide range of agents including alcohol, nicotine, cannabis, benzodiazepines, methaqualone, heroin and cocaine [Carey et al., 1991]. The latter physicians' private practice continued to use PAN for treating addictive withdrawal states from all forms of substance abuse and reported excellent results over many additional cases [Carey, unpublished observations].

Further support for the use of PAN for polydrug abuse comes from anecdotal reports from the centres in S.A. treating acute substance abuse withdrawal with PAN. Most of these centres do not have the resources to undertake routine testing for the substances that have been used by those admitted to their facilities. Nonetheless, their staff have established by careful history taking that their clients have admitted to have abused an array of agents, apart from the one that had forced their admission.

All these clinics have found that the PAN produces amelioration of these polydrug abusers' acute withdrawal states. The classical combination of dugs used are cannabis plus alcohol; alcohol plus sedative (usually a benzodiazepine); alcohol plus nicotine and other drug combinations. In such cases, careful observation of the patient is essential, particularly if they have been abusing benzodiazepines or other sedatives. The latter patients may require careful tapering of the benzodiazepine or other sedative, after the initial withdrawal state has been completed.

Anti-Craving Properties of PAN

Alcohol

In a study of 216 patients who were craving alcohol, PAN administered for 20 minutes abolished craving in 85.19%, it was reduced in 11.57% with 3.24% recalcitrant [Daynes and Gillman, 1994].

In a study conducted in Finland, PAN was found to useful in reducing craving between relapses in 20 alcoholic outpatients [Ojutkangas and Gillman, 1994].

In more recent work on rodents, the anticraving effects of PAN has as also been demonstrated [Kosobud et al, 2006] supporting the positive clinical findings.

All the above work indicates the potential for using PAN as an outpatient treatment for alcohol withdrawal, and its possible use for relapse prevention for outpatients, which merits further investigation.

Cannabis

In a study of 53 patients craving for cannabis, a 20 minute exposure to PAN reduced craving in 13.21% of patients, abolished it completely in 84.9% and had no effect in 1.89% [Daynes and Gillman, 1994].

Nicotine

Daynes and Gillman [1994] have studied the effects of a 20 minute exposure to PAN on tobacco craving. Of the 211 patients investigated, 82.46% had their craving abolished, 16.59% had their craving reduced and 0.95% were recalcitrant [Daynes and Gillman, 1994].

In an earlier study, of 35 heavy smokers, Gillman and Shevel [1988] found that the group aggregate score of craving was 316 (average per patient 9.02) before PAN. After 20 minutes of PAN this was reduced to 18 (average per patient 0.51).

It would seem that the anticraving effects of PAN for alcohol extend to nicotine and cannabis as well.

Thus, the anticraving effects of PAN may be a major factor in assisting the acute withdrawal state from alcohol, cannabis and nicotine and possibly other substances of abuse including cocaine, methaqualone and opioids [Kripke and Hechtman, 1972; Gillman and Lichtigfeld, 1985; Gillman et al 2006a;b].

Current Status of PAN for Substance Abuse Withdrawal

During our first trial [Lichtigfeld and Gillman,1982] we were very impressed with the speed and the lasting benefit of a single 20 minutes exposure of nitrous oxide given to chronic alcoholic patients during the acute withdrawal state. We also soon realized that the method of giving oxygen before the PAN, enabled approximately 50% to be detoxified with little or no other pharmaceutical intervention, thus maximizing the placebo response [Gillman and Lichtigfeld, 1986; 1990; 2002; 2004; 2006]. Indeed, PAN is the only pharmaceutical intervention for treating substance withdrawal that maximizes the placebo response.

PAN is also extremely safe. After all, clinical experience had shown that PAN is an agent with 'an impeccable safety record that has withstood the test of time' [Clark and Brunick, 2003;2008]. Thus the safety of the agent was not in question even in terms of withdrawal states because much lower doses of nitrous oxide are used for PAN than for anaesthesia. And thousands of alcoholic patients have received nitrous oxide during anaesthesia without any sequelae [Saidman and Hamilton, 1985; Zinn et al, 1985; Gillman, 1987; Everman and Koblin, 1991].

An added safety feature when using PAN for withdrawal, is that those patients who do not respond positively to oxygen or PAN can be placed on a sedative regimen within no more than 40 minutes from the beginning of gas administration [Gillman and Lichtigfeld,1990; 2002; 2004; 2006].

As mentioned earlier, we thought that the PAN therapy would catch on like wildfire because it was economic, safe and rapidly effective [Gillman and Lichtigfeld, 1990]. We were sadly disillusioned.

Almost 30 years after its first use, the PAN treatment although used by clinicians in S.A., Finland and the U.S.A. and possibly elsewhere, has failed to be widely used, despite its advantages and there being a great many publications confirming our findings [Kripke and Hechtman, 1972; Daynes, 1989; Carey et al, 1991; Ojutkangas, 1991;Christian, 1991; Myles, 1984; 1992; Bayrakdarian, 2000; Hall, 2005] and ourselves [Lichtigfeld and Gillman, 1982; Gillman and Lichtigfeld, 1985; 1986; 1990, 1991a; 2002; 2004d; 2006; 2007; Gillman et al, 2006a;b; 2007 Gillman and Shevel, 1988].

Thirty years later, health professionals excuse their disinterest, by saying that if PAN is so good, why is it not more widely used and why have there been so few studies published from institutions in the northern hemisphere.

My late colleague Fred Lichtigfeld and I, puzzled long and hard over this apparent paradox and eventually came up with possible reasons for this peculiar response to a valid and useful treatment that has many advantages over the addictive benzodiazepines for mild to moderate alcohol and other substance abuse withdrawal states [Gillman and Lichtigfeld, 1986; 1990; 2002; 2004d; 2006; Gillman et al, 2007].

We concluded that main obstacles were due to:

1. A credibility gap existing because the PAN treatment seemed on the surface to be too good to be true and this might have been aggravated by the fact that it was discovered by clinicians while researching outside an academic institution. Linked to this credibility gap was the difficulty of explaining to our colleagues, and particularly physicians, that PAN is not merely the use of any arbitrarily chosen subanaesthetic concentration of nitrous oxide in oxygen [Alho et al, 2002; 2003; Gillman and Lichtigfeld, 1990; 1997; 2002; 2004a;b;c;d; 2006; 2007] but rather a specific technique of administering and using nitrous oxide with specific custom-made, but readily available equipment. As discussed in some details in the introduction to this review, PAN is not merely the use of nitrous oxide. It is a specific technique in which the nitrous oxide is titrated in a specific manner to the individual clinical needs of each individual subject.

    In other words, PAN is unlike other pharmacological agents such as a tablet that are used at a specific dose and at a specific time within a multidosing schedule. Instead, PAN is a gaseous pharmaceutical agent usually utilized on one occasion but with a specific technique on custom-made equipment. Thus when PAN is used it is a pharmacological agent inextricably linked to the technique of administration; unlike most other pharmaceutical preparations and agents. Unlike PAN, tablets can usually be prescribed at an average dose and dosing schedule for an entire cohort.

In summary, the technique of using PAN is an integral and essential part of applying this gaseous agent which does not normally apply to non-gaseous medications such as tablets [Gillman and Lichtigfeld, 1990; 1997; 2002; 2004a;b;c;d, 2006], without which it is not PAN [Alho et al, 2002; 2003; Clark and Brunick, 1999; 2003; 2008; Clark et al, 2006; Gillman et al, 2007].

2. The lack of commercial support for research and travel to extend knowledge, research and the actual use of PAN.

I shall now deal with these apparent problems in some detail.

Credibility Gap

The credibility gap has been caused by a combination of factors.

First and foremost, there is a credibility gap because no other agent in medicine produces a lasting effect on withdrawal states within minutes. As mentioned above, PAN correctly given for 20 minutes, rapidly reverses the withdrawal state with lasting effect in 90% of inpatients in a period of less than an hour [Lichtigfeld and Gillman, 1982; Gillman and Lichtigfeld, 1990a].

The gold-standard medication, namely the benzodiazepines take some hours to days before the withdrawal state is reversed [Saitz et al., 1994; Gillman and Lichtigfeld, 2002; 2004d]. Furthermore the pharmacokinetics properties of nitrous oxide are well known. It has very evanescent effects, which for anaethesia, wear off within minutes. Any fair-minded but skeptical scientific observer would naturally be incredulous that an evanescent agent such as nitrous oxide, could have such a profound, rapid and lasting effect on a condition that usually takes hours to days to be reversed by the benzodiazepines.

There is also the linked problem (mentioned in the introduction), namely the inability of physicians, unlike dentists, to understand that PAN cannot be given at any arbitrarily chosen concentration of nitrous oxide.

Most physicians, when discussing nitrous oxide immediately think of anaesthesia and the domain of the anesthesiologists. Unfortunately very few anaesthesiologists that work with nitrous oxide understand the method of administration and indeed the concept of PAN. This is well illustrated by the work of Alho et al [2002; 2003]. The latter investigators chose a 60% inhaled concentration of nitrous oxide, judged by the anaesthetist in their team [personal communication, Darroch] as the target for the titration. Thus they did not titrate to the patients' clinical response but rather to their arbitrarily chosen target concentration. Alho et al [2002; 2003] used nitrous oxide as an isolated pharmacological agent. This indicates that they were unaware of the theoretical and scientific basis of the differences between PAN as a linked agent-technique as opposed to nitrous oxide used as an anesthetic agent [Gillman and Lichtigfeld, 2004a;b;c].

For these (and perhaps others unknown reasons), many of our colleagues simply did not believe us. This was problem enough, but some of them, particularly in academic circles, actually went out of their way to block the progress of the PAN method and spread misinformation, fear and even confusion about it [Gagiano, 1994; Emsley, 1994; Salaspuro and Alho, 1997; Metheun et al, 1997; Gillman and Lichtigfeld, 1997]. This, although they were clearly ignorant of how PAN was used. Their ignorance is encapsulated by their own writings and work on the subject [Gagiano, 1994; Emsley, 1994; Salaspuro and Alho, 1997; Metheun et al, 1997; Gillman and Lichtigfeld, 1997; Alho et al, 2002; 2003; 2004; Berglund et al, 2003]. That their opposition was biased [Gagiano, 1994; Emsley, 1994; Salaspuro and Alho, 1997; Metheun et al, 1997; Gillman and Lichtigfeld, 1997] is demonstrated by the fact that not a single one of these armchair critics ventured to come and see for themselves either in S.A. or Finland, before denigrating the use of PAN. An untenable attitude aggravated by the fact that centres using the gases were widely dispersed geographically in both countries.

It is of some importance to note that when the unsubstantiated criticisms levelled against PAN appeared in the South African Medical Journal (S.A.M.J.) [Gagiano, 1994; Emsley, 1994] so many practitioners wrote into the journal supporting the continued use of PAN for treating substance abuse withdrawal, that the editor published only a few representative examples [Daynes, 1994; Fourie, 1994, Keizan 1994; Gillman, 1994; Gillman and Lichtigfeld, 1994b]. In ending the correspondence, he did however mention that 'The SAMJ has received numerous testimonial letters of support for analgesic nitrous oxide from those who use this to treat alcohol addiction...' [Anonymous, 1994]. Notwithstanding, the letters from Gagiano, who at that stage was President of the Society of Psychiatrists of S.A. and Emsley the Vice-President, did a great deal of damage to the credibility of the PAN therapy both in S.A. and abroad. Indeed, Berglund et al [2001], in Sweden, denigrated the nitrous oxide treatment in a government supported technical document. The latter was compiled ostensibly to inform health professionals and others concerned with the treatment of substance abuse. Berglund et al [2001] used the brief Gagiano letter [1994] as the sole reference in their negative discussion of PAN. These workers neither mentioned the letters of support published simultaneously [Lichtigfeld, 1994; Gillman 1994; Fourie 1994, Keizan, 1994, Gillman and Lichtigfeld 1994, Daynes, 1994] nor any of the numerous published papers available, which showed positive results with PAN. In a subsequent review article Berglund et al, [2003] used the identical tactics to give a one-sided view of the evidence against the use of PAN. Other workers have followed this cue and also used the Gagiano letter [1994] to paint a skewed and negative picture of the use of PAN for substance abuse withdrawal states [Alho et al, 2004; Franck, 2004] indicating how damaging the letter has been and could still be. This propagation and misuse of skewed information from the scientific literature simultaneously illustrates the:

1. power and influence of prominent individuals in medical politics;
2. and the damage that such individuals can cause, if they use their positions of influence to purvey misinformation about treatments and other matters.

Unfortunately, this biased antagonism did not only apply to academics alone. A self-styled expert on substance abuse, who became a media favourite for quotes on the subject of substance abuse, also decided to attempt to use the media to destroy the PAN method. The individual concerned was a general medical practitioner who had no higher qualification in the field, nor scientific publications on the biology of substance abuse. His attack came, despite refusing to visit the facility where the therapy had been pioneered, four years before. He managed to find a journalist, to write a disparaging article, which was published in the largest circulation evening newspaper in S.A. i.e. 'The Star' [Openshaw, 1986]. Coincidentally, perhaps, the article was published while I was lecturing in the U.S.A. On my return to S.A., I was bombarded by journalists who believed that they were going to be able to release a juicy story on medical malpractice. I soon dampened their enthusiasm by directing them to the scientific publications on the therapy that had already appeared in prestigious medical journals [Gillman, 1986; Lichtigfeld and Gillman, 1982; 1983a;b; Gillman and Lichtigeld, 1980; 1983; 1984; 1985; 1986].

Needless to say, the media physician remained an implacable (and because of his excellent contacts with the media) also a powerful enemy of the PAN treatment. Not only did he try to start an unsuccessful media campaign against the treatment. He also applied a more insidious and destructive strategy by placing obstacles in the way of those wishing to learn more about PAN. When Ojutkangas asked for the writer's telephone number, so that he could get the information directly, he was told that I (Gillman) was too busy to be contacted and that the media expert would be the go-between. Ojutkangas heard nothing further and eventually, after loosing patience with the go-between, Ojutkangas himself phoned from Helsinki. [see below; Ojutkangas, 2005].

It is not difficult to understand that opposition by these high profile academics, regarded by most lay people and the media as being rational and fair-minded has had, and continues to have, very negative effects on the progress of the PAN method, by further widening the credibility gap. The progress of the PAN therapy could also have done without the enmity of a media favourite.

The only really open-minded interest came from clinicians who were faced, with treating this problem in their daily clinical practices [de Rooster, 1983; Myles, 1984; 1992; Carey et al, 1991; Christian, 1991; Ojutkangas, 1991; Fourie, 1994; Bayrakdarian, 2000; Ojutkangas, 2005].

The experience of Ojutkangas as reported at the World Congress of Biological Psychiatry in Vienna [Ojutkangas, 2005] is worth quoting, because it summarises the typical attitude of these armchair academics who have blocked the progress of PAN both in S.A. and Finland. Ojutkangas [2005] states:

'As a recovering alcoholic, with years of experience treating alcoholism, I was impressed, but highly sceptical when told that a single 20 min. exposure to PAN rapidly improves mild to moderate alcohol withdrawal states [AWS] with lasting effect'
'I later, witnessed the PAN treatment and realised this was a true breakthrough.'
'I tried to contact the pioneers, but was thwarted by the local self-styled SA addiction expert, who although obviously ignorant of PAN's use was nonetheless against it'

Ojutkangas [2005] goes on to say that after receiving the hands-on training he realised that without it, he would have been unlikely to reproduce the published work [Lichtigfeld and

Gillman, 1982; Gillman and Lichtigfeld, 1986; 1990]. This is in stark contrast with Alho et al [2002] who despite numerous warnings about the importance of hands-on training [Gillman and Lichtigfeld, 1990; Gillman and Lichtigfeld, 1997; Gillman, 2007] have suggested that my colleague and I have somehow hidden the technique from them by stating 'Gillman et al do not disclose in their publications the exact protocol for administering nitrous oxide that they have used in their studies.' [Alho et al, 2004]. As emphasised repeatedly throughout this chapter, a written description, no matter how good, cannot replace hands-on training, in order to titrate to the correct defined but subtle endpoint, where the patient is relaxed.

To illustrate not only their lack of knowledge about the technique of PAN, but also their unwillingness to make the least effort to understand or learn the technique the experience of some investigators in the U.S.A. is worth mentioning. These workers, who were truly interested in attempting to replicate our work with PAN [Gillman and Lichtigfeld; Gillman and Lichtigfeld, 2006] were able to reproduce our work [Bayrakdarian, 2000; Hall, 2005] by either following the description of the method in our papers [Gillman and Lichtigfeld, 1990] or by consulting one of the numerous textbooks on the technique [Langa, 1976; Bennet; 1978; Malamed, 1989; Clark and Brunick, 1999]. Nonetheless, it is most unusual for workers to be able to use the PAN method without hands-on training by a dentist or other practitioner familiar with the PAN technique, but clearly, it can be done, using the available literature.

Nonetheless, without exception, all the many hundreds of health professionals that I have trained have agreed that they would have had difficulty in reproducing the technique without brief hands-on training.

Ojutkangas [2005] also notes that the PAN therapy attracted heavy armchair criticism by Finnish academics:

'in Finland, as in SA, there was strong but unfounded armchair opposition to the use of PAN, culminating in a media conference, at which, an unscientific attack was made by certain academics. Unknown to them, Gillman was present and demolished their attack, resulting in the leader of the team storming out of the conference.' [Ojutkangas, 2005].

Ojutkangas was referring particularly to academics at the Helsinki University Medical School, namely Salaspuro, Alho and colleagues [Salaspuro and Alho, 1997; Metheun et al, 1997].

Similar attacks by Salaspuro, Alho and colleagues began to appear in the lay media in Finland [Tienhaara, 1995] well before their ill-fated attempt to use nitrous oxide [Alho et al, 2002; 2003]. Indeed, these attacks have continued unabated [Järvi, 2005; Gillman, 2007] (see below). This although Alho and colleagues have been informed many times in writing both by Gillman and Lichtigfeld [1997; 2004a;bc;d] and others Clark et al [2006], that the technique they used was incorrect (in terms of PAN) and therefore totally different to the technique used by those who have had positive results with PAN [Kripke and Hechtman, 1972; Daynes, 1989; Carey et al, 1991; Ojutkangas, 1991; Christian, 1991; Myles, 1984; 1992; Bayrakdarian, 2000] and ourselves [Lichtigfeld and Gillman, 1982; Gillman and Lichtigfeld, 1985; 1986; 1990, 1991a; 2002; 2004d; 2006; 2007; Gillman et al, 2006a;b; 2007 Gillman and Shevel, 1988].

Despite this, Alho, Salaspuro and colleagues refuse to admit (except in private; personal communication Darroch, 2006) that their negative findings with nitrous oxide may have been due to their using the wrong technique.

Indeed, unlike most scientists faced with reporting on work where they were unable to reproduce the work of others, they pointedly refuse to mention the possibility that methodological differences could have accounted for their negative findings reported in their published research [Alho et al, 2002; 2003; 2004]. This intransigent attitude remains even though these differences had been spelled out unequivocally before, during and after their work on nitrous oxide was published [Gillman and Lichtigfeld, 2004a;b;c; Gillman, 2007]. These workers continue to state that nitrous oxide for alcohol withdrawal is no better than placebo [Järvi, 2005; Salaspuro, 2006]. Indeed, Alho and colleagues, as done previously [Salaspuro and Alho, 1997] suggest that the use of PAN is not only ineffective but unethical for alcohol withdrawal [Lönnqvist et al, 2007].

These attacks continue unabated, so that in another typical attack by Alho and colleagues in a Finnish lay publication, I was forced to reply to them.

In my reply, I mentioned that Alho and colleagues had refused training although the standard textbook on the use of PAN regarded this as essential [Clark and Brunick, 1999] and that their dosage was approximately double the average dose usually used to treat alcohol withdrawal. Because Alho had submitted a draft of their paper to me before publication, I emailed him as follows [Gillman; 2007]:

'Any paper you submit for publication with your present results must explicitly include a statement in your discussion explaining that your technique was done without the necessary training [although it was offered] and that you may have not used the correct technique and that you were not sure what the therapeutic endpoint is. Without such a statement your results are tainted. To take your results and believe that these prove that the N2O does not work in withdrawal is like giving patient cyanide from a bottle marked aspirin and then when the patient dies, publishing a finding that aspirin causes fatalities!'

As mentioned earlier, Alho et al [2002; 2003; 2004] published despite this warning, without any statement indicating their method might have been different to that which produced positive results.

I then took them to task for continuing to purvey misinformation to the Finnish people by claiming that their 'faulty work' disproved the research that demonstrated that PAN was a useful treatment for alcohol withdrawal. In addition, I questioned why they had attacked the PAN therapy for almost 10 years before attempting a clinical trial [Gillman, 2007].

In addition, they falsified the lynchpin methodological reference [Alho et al, 2002] to justify the incorrect method they had used in their original papers [Alho et al, 2002; 2003; Gillman and Lichtigfeld, 2004a;b; Gillman, 2007]. Not satisfied with a single misquote, they went further and falsified another reference [Alho et al, 2004] in response to our rebuttal of their research findings [Gillman and Lichtigfeld, 2004a;b;c].

What I did not mention [Gillman, 2007] was the internal inconsistency in their paper. In their written description they state that 'each subject received the corresponding gas treatment during 30 min'[Alho et al, 2002], but in Figure 2 of the same paper, the graph shows that the time course was more than 40 minutes [Alho et al, 2002].

The resistance by Alho and colleagues seems to know no limits even though he and colleagues must by now be fully aware that they have used the nitrous oxide incorrectly in their quest to replicate our findings. To illustrate this point: in February 2008, Alho wrote to the Cochrane Collaboration indicating that if their papers [Alho et al, 2002; 2003] continued to be listed as excluded studies in a Cochrane Review on PAN [Gillman et al, 2007], this would somehow reduce the credibility of the entire Cochrane Collaboration. By now, the reasons for this exclusion from any Cochrane Review on PAN must be patently clear.

To put it beyond doubt, and succinctly, the work of Alho et al [2002; 2003] was excluded [Gillman et al, 2007] because they had chosen an arbitrary (and excessively high) single target concentration of nitrous oxide. They did use nitrous oxide but not PAN, because they did not titrate the concentration of nitrous oxide to each patient's individual clinical needs. The importance of individualising the dose of nitrous oxide is stated in the review as follows:

'There is no fixed concentration of nitrous oxide [N2O] or oxygen [O2] because each patient receives a carefully titrated amount of N2O and O2 sufficient only to ameliorate the patient's condition.' [Gillman et al, 2007]

To this day, I cannot explain the obdurate opposition of the various academics (and the S.A. media expert), who have for no apparent scientific reason opposed the use of PAN [Openshaw, 1986; Gagiano, 1994; Emsley, 1994; Salaspuro and Alho, 1997; Methuen et al, 1997; Alho et al, 2002; 2003; 2004; Salaspuro, 2006; Lönnqvist et al, 2007]. Indeed, they seem to be prepared to go out on a limb and stake their very reputations on their false belief that PAN is useless. This, despite the overwhelming published evidence [Kripke and Hechtman, 1972; Lichtigfeld and Gillman, 1982; Gillman and Lichtigfeld, 1985; 1986; 1990, 1991a; Daynes, 1989; Carey et al, 1991; Christian, 1991; Myles, 1984; 1992; Daynes; 1989; Daynes and Gillman, 1994; 1994; Bayrakdarian, 2000; Gillman and Shevel, 1988; Gillman et al, 2006a;b; Gillman et al, 2007; Carey et al, 1991; Ojutkangas, 1991; Ojutkangas and Gillman, 1994] that PAN does ameliorate withdrawal states when correctly used [Gillman et al, 2007].

These critics [Alho et al, 2002; 2003; 2004; Methuen et al, 1997; Alho et al, 2002; 2003; 2004; Salaspuro, 2006; Lönnqvist et al, 2007] seem intent on blocking the use of PAN and also preventing any further research into the technique.

This continued and intransigent resistance to the use of PAN is clearly unfounded scientifically, but is nevertheless a very large stumbling block to the further research and progress of the use of PAN for treating substance abuse withdrawal states.

Lack of Commercial Interest in PAN

As mentioned earlier, there has never been a commercial interest in the use of PAN for treating withdrawal states. After our first publication [Lichtigfeld and Gillman, 1982], we were advised that it was still possible to obtain a patent for nitrous oxide as a new use indication for nitrous oxide. We took no heed of this good advice and did not apply for such a patent.

Our decision not to patent this new use of nitrous oxide seems, in hindsight, to have been a grave blunder. Naively, we believed that the treatment we had discovered belonged to everyone and should not be used for personal enrichment. At that stage, we did not understand that had we patented this new indication, we would have been able to interest the gas manufacturers in supporting further research into PAN, not only by ourselves but by others investigators.

We had no conception at that stage, of the importance of commercial pharmaceutical interests for promoting any novel pharmaceutical agent or new indication of an existing agent. Only later, did we realize the importance of the almost unlimited funding available from a commercial sponsor, which allows and promotes research into the agent or new application of it. It also permits emissaries from universities and other institutions to travel throughout the world informing their peers at scientific meetings of the new product, through their researches on it. It is by these means that new treatments are publicized and gain acceptance for daily use in medical practice.

Such support has been notably lacking in regard to PAN. We have received paltry support from a gas company that manufactures nitrous oxide amounting to less than US$20 000 over 32 years i.e. less than US$750 per annum since we started our researches in 1976.

It is still my considered opinion that the lack of significant research funding which would have been readily available from a commercial interest has been a major handicap.

This lack of funding has conceivably lessened the interest of other workers to attempt to repeat our work on PAN. The only exception were the Finns, who were forced, after nearly 10 years of concerted attacks on PAN in the medical and lay media [Salaspuro and Alho, 1997; Methuen et al, 1997, Tienhaara, 1995] to undertake a study. It is noteworthy that these Finnish workers make no mention of their personal conflict of interest in terms of their heated opposition to the PAN therapy prior to their study that resulted in their publications on nitrous oxide [Alho et al, 2002; 2003; 2004]. This despite the fact that the Journal of Clinical Psychopharmacology specifically required such a statement at the time they submitted their work.

Perhaps unsurprisingly, in view of the above, their studies were defective and add nothing to the debate on the efficacy of PAN for treating withdrawal states [Gillman and Lichtigfeld, 20004;a;b;c;d; Gillman et al, 2007]. Nonetheless, their papers do contribute, in that it underlines the need for hands-on training, or at the very least, a thorough understanding of the theory of the technique, if clinicians wish to replicate our work [Gillman and Lichhtigfeld, 1990; 1997; 2002; 2006].

I have been forced to emphasise the work of Alho, Salaspuro and colleagues [Alho et al, 2002; 2003] and their incorrect use of nitrous oxide to treat alcohol withdrawal states because Alho and Salaspuro are prominent in the field of alcohol research. Thus their negative findings have important political impact in the field of alcohol research and add to the credibility problems. Those who do not know better, may regard their findings as the definitive proof that nitrous oxide is ineffective for treating alcohol withdrawal states or at the very least throw doubt on the work showing positive results. For example in a recent papers referring to the positive results reported [Gillman and Lichtigfeld, 1990; 1994b;

2002], Benturquia et al (2007) state 'However, these findings have not be confirmed by a recent clinical study comparing the effects of N$_2$O versus placebo' [Alho et al, 2003]. This, particularly as these workers [Alho et al, 2002; 2003], despite being appraised of their incorrect technique [Gillman and Lichtigfeld, 2004a;bc;c;d; Gillman et al, 2007] continue to propagate the idea that their work shows that nitrous oxide is no better than placebo for treating alcohol withdrawal states [Salaspuro, 2006; Lönnqvist et al, 2007].

Conclusion

What of the future? Hopefully those who read this paper and acknowledge the problems with the work of Alho et al [2002; 2003] will discount their work and attempt themselves, after receiving hands-on training, to replicate the use of PAN to treat substance abuse withdrawal states. But that is only one aspect of this fascinating opioid gas [Gillman and Lichtigfeld, 1994a; Gillman and Lichtigfeld, 2006]. The development of the endopepditases, which extend the biological half-life of the endogenous opioids [Roques et al, 1993; Coudoré-Civiale et al, 2001], could be used in combination with PAN to treat substance abuse states. It is also possible, that research will show that the synergism between the endopeptidases [Roques et al, 1993; Coudoré-Civiale et al, 2001], and PAN will produce enough analgesia to enable surgical anaesthesia to be obtained without unconsciousness.

Acknowledgements

I would like to acknowledge a debt of gratitude to the late Frederick J. Lichtigfeld, my scientific partner of many years, who passed away in 2005 ago and to whose memory this work is dedicated.

References

Abraini J.H., David H.N., Lemaire, M [2005]. Potentially neuroprotective and therapeutic properties of nitrous oxide and xenon. *Annals of the New York Academy of Sciences 1053*: 289-300.

Alho, H., Methuen, T., Paloheimo, M., Strid, N., Seppä, K., Tiainen, J., Salaspuro, M., Roine, R. [2002]. Long-term effects of and physiological responses to nitrous oxide gas treatment during alcohol withdrawal: a double-blind, placebo-controlled trial. *Alcoholism: Clinical and Experimental Research 26*: 1816-22.

Alho, H., Metheun, T., Paloheimo, M., Seppä, K., Strid, N., Apter-Kaseva, N., Tiainen, J., Salaspuro, M., Roine, R. [2003]. Nitrous oxide has no effect in the treatment of alcohol withdrawal syndrome: double-blind placebo-controlled randomised trial. *Journal of Clinical Psychopharmacology 23*: 211-14.

Alho, H., Metheun, T., Paloheimo, M., Strid, N., Seppä, K., Tiainen, J., Salaspuro, M., Roine, R. [2004]. Reply: Controlled technique demonstrates no benefit from nitrous oxide gas treatment on alcohol withdrawal. *Journal of Clinical Psychopharmacology 24*: 239-240.

Anonymous [1994]. Editorial note. *South African Medical Journal 84*: 708.

Baldessareni, R.J.[1996]. Psychosis and Anxiety In: J.G. Hardman, Limbird, L.E., Molinoff, P.B, Ruddon, R.W., A. Goodman-Gilman [Eds.], *Goodman and Gilman's The pharmacological Basis of Therapeutics*, [pp. 399-430], 9th Ed, New York: MacMillan.

Bayrakdarian, C. Effectiveness of nitrous Oxide [N$_2$0] in reducing cigarette smoking in subjects with nicotine dependence. *American Psychiatric Association Meeting [Abstract]* May 2000. p.2h.

Bennett, C.R. [1978]. *Conscious-sedation in dental practice*. St Louis: Mosby.

Benturquia N., Le Guen, S., Canestrelli, C., Lagente, V., Apiou, G., Roques, B.P., Noble, F. [2007]. Specific blockade of morphine- and cocaine-induced reinforcing effects in conditioned place preference by nitrous oxide in mice. *Neuroscience 149* :477-86.

Benturquia N, Le Marec T, Scherrmann JM, Noble F. *Neuroscience.* 2008 May 21. (Epub ahead of print).

Berglund, M., Andréasson, S., Franck, J, Fridell, M., Håkanson, I., Johansson, B.-A., Lindgren, A., Lindgren, B., Nicklasson, L., Rydberg, U., Salaspuro, M., Thelander, S., Andreasson, S., Ojehagen, A. [2001]. Lustgas in Behandling av alkohol-och narkotikaproblem [Translation: Nitrous oxide in treatment of alcohol and drug abuse] *SBU [Swedish Council of Technology Assessment in Health Care].August volume 1*: 994-95.

Berglund, M., Thelander, S., Salaspuro, M., Franck, J., Andreasson, S., Ojehagen, A. [2003] Treatment of alcohol abuse; an evidence-based review. *Alcohol: Clinical and Experimental Research 27*: 1645-1656.

Berrendero, F., Kieffer, B.L., Maldonado, R. [2002]. Attenuation of nicotine-induced antinociception, rewarding effects, and dependence in mu-opioid receptor knock-out mice. *Journal of Neuroscience 22*: 10935-40.

Carey, C., Clark, A., Saner, T. [1991]. Analgesic nitrous oxide for addictive withdrawal states in general practice. *South African Medical Journal 79*: 516.

Christian, M.K. [1991]. Analgesic nitrous oxide for management of addictive withdrawal: a successful implementation in a Third World alcohol rehabilitation programme. *36th International Institute on the Prevention and Treatment of Alcoholism [Paper]* Stockholm, June 1991.

Clark, M., Clark A., Campbell., S.A. [2006]. Technique for the administration of nitrous oxide/oxygen sedation to ensure psychotropic analgesic nitrous oxide [PAN] effects. *International Journal of Neuroscience 116*:871-877.

Clark, M., Brunick, A. [1999]. *Handbook of nitrous oxide and oxygen sedation*. 1st Edition, St Louis: Mosby.

Clark, M., Brunick, A. [2003]. *Handbook of nitrous oxide and oxygen sedation*. 2nd Edition, St Louis: Mosby.

Clark, M., Brunick, A. [2008]. *Handbook of nitrous oxide and oxygen sedation*. 3rd Edition, St Louis: Mosby.

Cohen, P.J.[1975]. Signs and stages of anesthesia. In: L.S. Goodman, A. Gilman, A.G. Gilman, G.E. Koelle [Eds.], *The pharmacological basis of therapeutics*, [pp. 60-65], New York: Macmillan.

Coudoré-Civiale, M.A., Méen, M., Fournié-Zaluski, M.-C., Boucher, M., Bernard P Roques, B.P., Eschalier. A. (2001). Enhancement of the effects of a complete inhibitor of enkephalin-catabolizing enzymes, RB 101, by a cholecystokinin-B receptor antagonist in diabetic rats. *British Journal of Pharmacology 133*: 179–185.

Daynes, G. [1989]. The initial management of alcoholism using oxygen and nitrous oxide: a transcultural study. *International Journal of Neuroscience 49*: 83-86.

Daynes, G. [1994]. Nitrous oxide for alcohol withdrawal. South African Medical Journal 84: 708.Daynes, G., Gillman, M.A. [1994]. Psychotropic analgesic nitrous oxide prevents craving after withdrawal for alcohol, cannabis and tobacco. *International Journal of Neuroscience 76*: 13-16.

De Rooster, [1983]. Die effektiwitiet van distikstofksied in die behandeling van die alkohol-onttrekingsindroom [Translation: The effectiveness of nitrous oxide in the treatment of the alcohol withdrawal state]. Thesis accepted in fulfilment of the requirements of M.A. [Clinical Psychology] at Rand Afrikaans University, South Africa.

Edwards, R. [1985]. Editorial. Anaesthesia and alcohol. *British Medical Journal 291*: 423-24.

Emsley, R.[1994]. Untitled. *South African Medical Journal 84*:516.

Everman, B.W., Koblin, D.D. [1991]. Again, chronic administration of ethanol, and acute exposure to nitrous oxide: effects on vitamin B_{12} and folate status in rats. *Mechanisms of Ageing and Development 62*: 229-243.

Fourie J. Distikstofoksied [Translation: Nitrous oxide]. [1994]. *South African Medical Journal 84*: 516.

Franck J. Expert response to Gillman/Alho. [2004]. *Alcoholism: Clinical and Experimental Research 28*: 1275.

Frost, E. A. M. [1985]. A history of nitrous oxide: In E.I. Eger 11 [Ed.], *Nitrous oxide/N2O* [pp. 1-22]. New York: Elsevier.

Gagiano, C.A. [1994]. Nitrous oxide for alcohol withdrawal and other psychiatric disorders. *South African Medical Journal 84*:359.

Gillman, M.A. [1985]. *Nitrous oxide as an opioid agonist: some experimental and clinical applications*. Thesis accepted in fulfilment of the requirements of DSc at Potchefstroom University for CHO, South Africa.

Gillman, M.A. [1986]. Nitrous oxide, an opioid addictive agent. *American Journal of Medicine 8l:* 97-l02.

Gillman, M. A. [1987]. Editorial. Haematological changes caused by nitrous oxide: cause for concern? *British Journal of Anaesthesia 59*: 143-146.

Gillman,M.A.[1992]. Nitrous oxide abuse in perspective. *Clinical Neuropharmacology 15*: 297-306.

Gillman, M.A [1994]. Analgesic nitrous oxide for addictive withdrawal. *South African Medical Journal 84*: 516.

Gillman, M. A. [1995]. Nitrous oxide has a very low abuse potential. *Addiction 90*: 439.

Gillman, M. A. [1996]. Envy as a retarding force in science. U.K. Aldershot: Avebury.

Gillman, M.A. [2006]. Psychotropic analgesic nitrous oxide for addictive withdrawal. *Chinese Journal of Drug Dependence 14*: 73-4.

Gillman, M.A. [2007]. Ilokaasum oikea käyttö auttaa [Translation: Laughing gas helps when used correctly]. *Suomen Kuvalehti 2*:57.

Gillman M.A. [2008]. Editorial: Tobacco cessation and nitrous oxide/oxygen sedation. *South African Dental Journal 63*: 66.

Gillman, M.A, Harker, N., Lichtigfeld, F.J. [2006a]. Combined cannabis/methaqualone withdrawal treated with psychotropic analgesic nitrous oxide. *International Journal of Neuroscience 116*: 859 - 869.

Gillman, M.A. Lichtigfeld, F.J. [1980]. Nitrous oxide and treatment of withdrawal symptoms. *Lancet 2*: 803.

Gillman, M.A., Lichtigfeld, F.J. [1983]. Receptor hypothesis of the alcohol withdrawal state. In Mandel, P., DeFeudis, F.V. [Eds.], *CNS Receptors from Molecular Pharmacology to Behaviour*. Raven Press: New York. pp.405-415.

Gillman, M.A., Lichtigfeld, F.J. [1984]. The opioid and anti-opioid system in addiction. *South African Medical Journal 66*: 592.

Gillman, M.A., Lichtigfeld, F.J. [1985]. Analgesic Nitrous Oxide : Adjunct to clonidine for opioid withdrawal. *American Journal of Psychiatry 142*: 784-785.

Gillman, M.A. Lichtigfeld, F.J. [1986]. Minimal sedation required with nitrous oxide-oxygen treatment of the alcohol withdrawal state. *British Journal of Psychiatry 148*: 604-606.

Gillman, M.A., Lichtigfeld, F.J. [1987]. Nitrous oxide analgesia is potentiated by low dose of naloxone: More possible evidence of a hyperalgesic opioid system. *South African Journal of Science 83*: 560-563.

Gillman, M.A., Lichtigfeld, F.J. [1990]. Analgesic nitrous oxide for alcohol withdrawal: a critical appraisal after 10 years' use. *Postgraduate Medical Journal 66*: 543-546.

Gillman, M.A., Lichtigfeld, F.J. [1991a]. Placebo and analgesic nitrous oxide for the alcohol withdrawal state. *British Journal of Psychiatry 159*: 672-675.

Gillman, M. A., Lichtigfeld, F. J. [1991b]. The opioid effects of analgesic [subanesthetic] nitrous oxide on the alcohol withdrawal state. *Annals of the New York Academy of Sciences 625*: 784-785.

Gillman, M. A., Lichtigfeld, F. J. [1994a]. Opioid properties of psychotropic analgesic nitrous oxide [laughing gas]. *Perspectives in Biology and Medicine 38*: 125-138.

Gillman, M. A., Lichtigfeld, F. J. [1994b]. The uses of analgesic nitrous oxide in neuropsychiatry. *South African Medical Journal 84*: 706.

Gillman, M.A., Lichtigfeld, F.J. [1997]. The current status of analgesic nitrous oxide for treating alcoholic withdrawal states. *Suomen Laakarilehti* [*Finnish Medical Journal*] *52*: 1055-58.

Gillman, M.A., Lichtigfeld, F.J. [2002]. Randomised double-blind trial of psychotropic analgesic nitrous oxide compared with diazepam for alcohol withdrawal state. *Journal of Substance Abuse Treatment 22*: 129-134.

Gillman, M.A., Lichtigfeld, F.J. [2004a]. An incorrect technique guarantees failure. *Alcoholism: Clinical and Experimental Research 28*: 1273-1274.

Gillman, M.A., Lichtigfeld, F.J. [2004b]. Further comments on the effects of nitrous oxide treatment on alcohol withdrawal. *Journal of Clinical Psychopharmacology 24*: 473-475.

Gillman, M.A., Lichtigfeld, F.J. [2004c]. Correct use of analgesic nitrous oxide for the alcohol withdrawal state essential. *Journal of Clinical Psychopharmacology 24*: 238-239.

Gillman, M.A., Lichtigfeld, F.J. [2004d]. Enlarged double-blind randomised trial of benzodiazepines against psychotropic analgesic nitrous oxide for alcohol withdrawal. *Addictive Behaviors 29*: 1183-1187.

Gillman MA, Lichtigfeld FJ. [2006]. Psychotropic analgesic nitrous oxide [PAN] as a probe of the endogenous opioid system in man and for treating substance abuse withdrawal In: L.A. Bennet [Ed.], *New Topics in Substance Abuse Treatment*, [pp. 1-72].New York: Nova Science.

Gillman, M.A., Lichtigfeld, F.J., Harker, N. [2006b]. Psychotropic analgesic nitrous oxide for acute cocaine withdrawal in man. *International Journal of Neuroscience 116*: 847-57.

Gillman, M.A., Lichtigfeld, F.J., Young, T. [2007]. Psychotropic analgesic nitrous oxide for alcoholic withdrawal states. [Review]. *The Cochrane Library, Issue* 2.

Gillman, M.A., Shevel, J. [1988]. Analgesic nitrous oxide and oxygen for acute withdrawal from cigarette smoking. *Proceedings of Drug and Alcohol Forum*, January 1988. pp. 66-74.

Glassman, A.H., Jackson, W.K., Walsh, B.T., Roose, S.P. [1984]. Cigarette craving, smoking withdrawal and clonidine. *Science 226*: 864-866.

Greenblatt, D.J., Shader, R.I. [1985]. Clinical pharmacokinetics of the benzodiazepines. In: D.E. Smith, D.R. Wesson (Eds.). *The benzodiazepines: current standards for medical practice*, (pp.43-58) Lancaster: MTP Press.

Hall, M. [2005] .Quitting smoking: A laughing matter with nitrous Oxide. http://maps.org/news-letters/v12n2/12223hal.html Accessed 2008-05-19.

Järvi, U. [2005]. Harva suuttuu, jos lääkäri kysyy alkoholinkäytöstä. [Translation: Very few become angry, if the doctor asks about alcohol use]. *Suomen Lääkärilehti [Finnish Medical Journal]* 60: 1646.

Kahn, R.S. [1983]. Treatment of alcoholic withdrawal states with oxygen and nitrous oxide. *South African Medical Journal 63*: 65-66.

Keizan, A. [1994]. Analgesic nitrous oxide is a very safe agent. *South African Medical Journal 84*: 516.

Kosobud, A. E. K., Kebabian, C.E., Rebec, G.V. [2006].Nitrous oxide acutely suppresses ethanol consumption in HAD and P rats. *International Journal of Neuroscience 116*: 835-45.

Kripke, B. J., Hechtman, H. B. [1972]. Nitrous oxide for pentazocine addiction and intractable pain. *Anesthesia and Analgesia 51*: 520-526.

Langa, H. [1976]. *Relative Analgesia in Dental Practice: Inhalation Analgesia with Nitrous Oxide*. Philadelphia: W B. Saunders.

Lichtigfeld, F.J. [1994]. Analgesic nitrous oxide for addictive withdrawal. *South African Medical Journal 84*: 513.

Lichtigfeld, F.J., Gillman, M.A. [1982]. The treatment of alcoholic withdrawal states with oxygen and nitrous oxide. *South African Medical Journal 61*: 349-351.

Lichtigfeld, F.J. Gillman, M.A. [1983a]. Treatment of alcoholic withdrawal states with oxygen and nitrous oxide. *Psychiatry Digest June*: 12-13.

Lichtigfeld, F.J., Gillman, M.A. [1983b]. The treatment of alcoholic withdrawal states with oxygen and nitrous oxide. *South African Medical Journal 63*: 66.

Lichtigfeld, F.J.,Gillman, M.A. [1989a]. The effect of placebo in the alcohol withdrawal state. *Alcohol and Alcoholism 24*: 109-112.

Lichtigfeld, F.J.,Gillman, M.A. [1989b]. Analgesic nitrous oxide for alcohol withdrawal is better than placebo. *International Journal of Neuroscience 49*:71-74.

Lichtigfeld, F.J.,Gillman, M.A. [1991]. Combination therapy with carbamazepine/ benzodiazepine for polydrug analgesic/depressant withdrawal. *Journal of substance Abuse Treatment 8*: 293-295.

Lichtigfeld, F.J.,Gillman, M.A. [1996]. Role of dopamine mesolimbic system in opioid action of psychotropic analgesic nitrous oxide [PAN] in alcohol and drug withdrawal. *Clinical Neuropharmacology 19*: 246-50.

Liu L. [1996]. Hand waving?, quoting van der Kolk B.A. *The Sciences 36*:13.

Lönnqvist, J., Alho, H., Aro, H., Eriksson, P., Isometsä, E., Kaprio, J., Kiianmaa, K.,Kuoppasalmi, K., Lillsunde, P., Marttunen, M., Partonen, T., Portman, M., Seppälä, T., Suvisaari, J. [2007]. *Kansanterveyslaitoksen Julkaisuja B 21/2007*:176. National Public Health Institute Department of Mental Health and Alcohol Research Background material for the international evaluation. Accessed 2008-05-20 www.ktl.fi/ attachments/suomi/julkaisut/julkaisusarja_b/2007/2007b21.pdf

Malamed, S.F. [1989]. *Sedation: A guide to patient management*, 2nd Edition. St Louis: Mosby.

Mansvelder, H.D., McGehee, D.S. [2000]. Long-term potentiation of excitatory inputs to brain reward areas by nicotine. *Neuron 27*: 349-57.

Marshall, B., Wollman, H. [1985].History and principles of anesthesiology, In: A. Goodman-Gilman, L.S. Goodman, T.W. Rall, F. Murad, [Eds.], *The pharmacological Basis of Therapeutics*, [pp. 260-275], 7th Ed, New York: MacMillan.

Mash, D.C., Staley, J.K. [1999]. D3 dopamine and kappa opioid receptor alterations in human brain of cocaine-overdose victims. *Annals of the New York Academy of Sciences 877*: 507-22.

Metheun, T., Poikolainen, K., Roine, R.P. [1997]. Alkoholin aiheuttamien vieroitusoireiden hoito-mika on ilokaasun asema ? [Translation: Treatment of alcohol withdrawal symptoms – status of nitrous oxide?] *Suomen Laakarilehti [Finnish Medical Journal] 52*: 989-992.

Myles, M.J. [1984].Treatment of the alcohol withdrawal state with nitrous oxide/oxygen. *South African Medical Journal 65*: 948.

Myles, M.J. [1992]. Managing alcohol withdrawal states with oxygen and nitrous oxide. *Nursing RSA 7*: 9-10.

Ojutkangas, R. [1991]. Psychotropic analgesic nitrous oxide: rapid safe therapy for addictive withdrawal. *Postgraduate Medical Journal 67*: 1027-1028.

Ojutkangas, R., Gillman, M.A.[1994]. Psychotropic analgesic nitrous oxide for treating alcohol withdrawal in an outpatient setting. *International Journal of Neuroscience 76*: 35-39.

Ojutkangas, R. [2005]. Pioneering PAN in Finland for withdrawal states: Success despite biased opposition. *World Journal of Biological Psychiatry 6 [Supplement 1]*:150-151.

Openshaw, J. [11 January 1986]. Call for probe into gas treatment. *The Star*: p.5.

Parry, C.D.H., Bhana, A., Pluddermann, A., Myers, B., Siegfried, N., Morojelle, N.K., Flisher, A.J., Kozell, N.J. [2002]. The South African Community Epidemiology Network on Drug Use [SACENDU]: description, findings [1997-1999] and policy implications. *Addiction 97*: 969-976.

Prince, V., Turpin, K.R. [2008]. Treatment of alcohol withdrawal syndrome with carbemazepine, gabapentin, and nitrous oxide. *American Journal of Health-System Pharmacy* 65: 1039-1047.<?xml:namespace prefix = o ns = "urn:schemas-microsoft-com:office:office"

Pfeiffer, C. C. [1987]. Mental illness and schizophrenia. <?xml:namespace prefix = st1 ns = "urn:schemas-microsoft-com:office:smarttags" />Wellingborough, UK: Thorsons, Prince, V., Turpin, K.R. [2008]. Treatment of alcohol withdrawal syndrome with carbemazepine, gabapentin, and nitrous oxide. *American Journal of Health-System Pharmacy* 65: 1039-1047.

Roques, B.P., Noble, F., Daugeâ , V., Fournieâ -Zaluski, M.C., Beaumont, A. (1993). Neutral endopeptidase 24-11: structure, inhibition and experimental and clinical pharmacology. *Pharmacology Reviews. 45*: 87-146.

Saidman, L.S., Hamilton, W.K. [1985]. We should continue using nitrous oxide: In E.I. Eger 11 [Ed.], *Nitrous oxide/N2O* [pp. 345-353]. New York: Elsevier.

Saitz, R., Mayo-Smith, M.F., Roberts, M.S., Redmond, H.A., Bernard, D.R., Calkins, D.R.[1994]. Individualized treatment for alcohol withdrawal. A randomised double-blind controlled trial. *Journal of the American Medical Association 272*: 519-523.

Salaspuro, M. [2006]. Slide 13, 9th international symposium on substance abuse treatment: Finnish Evidence Based guidelines for the Treatment of Alcohol and Drug Abusers. , University of Helsinki. Working group appointed by the Finnish Society of Addiction Medicine. Accessed 2008-05-20 http://www.nad.fi/sat2006/presentations/Salaspuro.ppt

Salaspuro, M.,Alho,H. [1997]. Lustgasbehandling och medicinska etikens gränser [Translation: Nitrous oxide treatment and the boundaries of medical ethics]. *Suomen Lääkärilehti [Finnish Medical Journal] 52*: 942-43.

Searll, A. [1989]. *It can't happen to me.* [pp.70-80]. Cape Town: Struik Publishers.

Skelly AM. [1998]. Dentistry. In: J.G. Whitwam, R.F. McCloy, [Eds.], *Principles and practice of sedation* [pp. 214-19], Oxford: Blackwell.

Smith, R.A, Beirne, O.R. [1985]. The use of nitrous oxide by dentists. In E.I. Eger 11 [Ed.], *Nitrous oxide/N2O* [pp. 282-304]. New York: Elsevier.

Tanda,G., Pontieri, F.E., Di Chiara, G. [1997] Cannabinoid and heroin activation of mesolimbic dopamine transmission by a common mu1 opioid receptor mechanism. *Science 276*: 2048- 2050.

Tienhaara, H. [29 January 1995]. Alkoholiprofessori ja menetelmän kehittäjä napit vastakkain. Ilokaasuhoidosta tuli iso riita [Alcohol professor and developer of treatment in argument]. *Iltalehti [Afternoon News]* p.1.

Zinn, S.E., Fairley, H.B., Glenn, J.D. [1985]. Liver function in patients with mild alcoholic hepatitis, after enflurane, nitrous oxide-narcotic, and spinal anesthesia. *Anesthesia and Analgesia 64*: 487-490.

In: Substance Withdrawal Syndrome
Editors: J. P. Rees and O. B. Woodhouse

ISBN 978-1-60692-951-3
© 2009 Nova Science Publishers, Inc.

Chapter II

Selective Serotonin Reuptake Inhibitors Withdrawal Syndromes: New Insights into Pathophysiology and Treatment

Elena Tomba, Emanuela Offidani and Giovanni A. Fava
Affective Disorders Program, Department of Psychology,
University of Bologna, Bologna, Italy

Abstract

There has been increasing awareness of the withdrawal syndromes which may occur with discontinuation of the selective serotonin reuptake inhibitors (SSRI). The literature that is surveyed indicates that they are frequent, may vary from one SSRI to another, occur with either abrupt or gradual disconfirmation, and are not necessarily reversible. These phenomena may be explained on the basis of the oppositional model of tolerance.

Continued drugs treatment may recruit processes that oppose the initial acute effect of a drug. When drug treatment ends, these processes may operate unopposed, at least for some time, induce withdrawal symptoms and increased vulnerability to relapse.

The model may provide an explanation also for other clinical findings in depression treatment: tolerance to the effects of antidepressants during long-term therapy, onset of resistance upon rechallenge with the same antidepressant drug, paradoxical effects of antidepressants in some patients, switching and cycle acceleration in bipolar disorder, very unfavourable long-term outcome of major depression treated by pharmacological means. The implications for treatment of depression are considerable.

The withdrawal syndrome following discontinuation of antidepressant treatment were soon recognized after the introduction of these drugs [1]. It has been described in literature as emerging upon abrupt discontinuation or intermittent non-compliance, as generally mild and short-lived, even though distressing [2]. Discontinuation symptoms have been reported with any type of antidepressant drugs [3], and particularly MAO inhibitors and SSRI [4-8].

For SSRI, a relative homogeneous drug class, differences among the pharmacokinetic properties such as elimination half-life and metabolism may be the most clinically relevant. Specifically, antidepressant discontinuation syndrome is more common in patients discontinuing agents with relatively short half-lives such as paroxetine than in those with longer half-lives such as fluoxetine [9].

One of the first potential explanations involved a cholinergic rebound, yet this hypothesis is unlikely to explain serotonergically mediated withdrawal syndromes of SSRI (10). The exact meaning of these syndromes is, however, unclear, as is their relationship with post treatment discontinuation recurrence risk. What we do not know is whether onset of withdrawal symptoms upon discontinuation of antidepressant drugs may be related to an increased vulnerability to depressive relapse and/or resistance upon reinstitution of drug treatment and/or loss of clinical effects during maintenance therapy. The issue has important clinical implications, since different antidepressant drugs may yield different rates of withdrawal syndromes [8].

What we know is that is that discontinuation of antidepressant drugs may trigger hypomania or mania [11, 12], despite adequate concomitant mood stabilizing treatment [13]. Further, mood shifts to euthymia or hypomania are not a rare event in a population withdrawn from medication because of a lack of efficacy [14]. Mood elevation may also occur with antidepressant drug decrease [15] and patients who failed to respond to mood stabilizers in combination with antidepressant drugs may improve upon discontinuation of the latter drugs [16]. These data suggest a relationship between antidepressant drug discontinuation and cycle acceleration in bipolar disorder (13). In unipolar depression, withdrawal phenomena may be associated with recurrence acceleration.

The importance of understanding and recognizing antidepressant withdrawal syndrome is threefold: 1. the syndrome is associated with significant psychosocial problems, work absenteeism and may on rare occasion be severe enough to require hospitalization [17]; 2. failure to recognize antidepressant discontinuation symptoms may results in medical and psychiatric misdiagnosis; 3. patients may be unwilling to use psychotropic medications in the future thereby increasing their vulnerability to future relapse of depression or anxiety disorders.

We will describe the characteristics of withdrawal syndromes, some of the pathophysiological explanations that have been suggested and we will outline a model, based on the concept of oppositional tolerance, which may provide an explanation for various clinical phenomena which may occur with antidepressant treatment of depression.

Characteristics of Discontinuation Syndromes

Earlier literature (up to the mid-nineties) has identified such syndromes as withdrawal reactions. More recent papers have used te term discontinuation syndromes; the reason for this switch in terminology is the fact that "discontinuation" lacks the negative psychological connotations that may be present with the term "withdrawal" and may be preferable for the pharmaceutical industry and marketing purposes. We will use the two terms interchangeably.

A broad range of somatic symptoms may emerge following antidepressant treatment discontinuation [1, 18,19]. The most commonly reported somatic symptoms include: headaches, dizziness, light-headedness, diminished appetite, fatigue, sweating, tremors, chills, sensory disturbances (paresthesias and tremors), sleep disturbance (vivid dreams and insomnia), somnolence, flulike symptoms and gastrointestinal physical symptoms (nausea and vomiting). Other less common somatic symptoms include myalgias, parkinsonism, balance difficulties and cardiac arrhythmias. Psychological symptoms may ensue, as well, such as agitation, anxiety, panic attacks, dysphoria, confusion and worsening of mood [18,19]. Discontinuation symptoms typically appear within three days of stopping antidepressant medication or initiating a medication taper. Untreated symptoms are usually mild and resolve spontaneously in one to two weeks. In some cases cases psychosis, catatonia or severe cognitive impairment are described [18,19].

Several methodological approaches have been used to determine the likelihood of experiencing discontinuation reactions with antidepressant. A common method involves the retrospective assessment of these symptoms in patients who are aware that their antidepressant has been discontinued. For example, Coupland [20] has reported the incidence of withdrawal symptoms on 171 patients who discontinued the treatment with clomipramine and different SSRI (fluoxetine, fluvoxamine, paroxetine and sertraline) using a retrospective charts. In these patients the most common symptoms were dizziness, lethargy, paresthesia, nausea, irritability and lowered mood. Further, symptoms occurred significantly more frequently in patients who had been treated either with one of the shorter half-life SSRI, fluvoxamine or paroxetine (17,2%) or with clomipramine (30,8%), than in patients taking on of the SSRI with longer half-life metabolites, sertraline or fluoxetine (1,5%). In another study [21], the UK database for spontaneous reports of suspected adverse drug reactions (ADRs) has been used to describe the reactions associated with the discontinuation of different SSRI. By March 1993 to July 1994, 430 reports were received. Particularly, withdrawal reactions with paroxetine constituted a greater proportion of the reports than with the other SSRI. An interesting finding is that these reactions tended to be more common in younger patients than in the elderly.

An alternative method is to assess the emergence of adverse events following the discontinuation of double-blind, placebo controlled antidepressant treatment. If the first approach may be affected by biases, since both the patients and clinicians know when treatment has been discontinued, the second method has the advantage of controlling this bias. However, both patients and clinicians are aware of the timing of the discontinuation and may be biased to report any symptoms.

The most rigorous methodological approach is probably blinding patients and clinicians to both the type of treatment and to the timing of the discontinuation. Many studies have used the Discontinuation-Emergent Signs and Symptoms scale (DESS) [8,22] to conduct a systematic assessment of the antidepressant discontinuation symptoms. DESS is a 43 item scale in which symptoms are classified as: new, old but worse, old but improved, old but unchanged and not present. This scale was originally developed by Massachusetts General Hospital investigators to allow for a systematic assessment of discontinuation reactions.

In a first trial [8] 242 patients, whose depression had remitted, were recruited while receiving maintenance therapy with open-label fluoxetine, sertraline or paroxetine for 4 to 24 months. Patients entered a 4-week study period during which they were randomly assigned to a 1-week (from 5 to 8 days), double-blind, placebo substitution period. Systematic assessment of discontinuation reactions was obtain with the 43-item DESS scale, the self-rated Symptom Questionnaire Somatic Symptom subscale [23], the 28-item, clinician-rated Hamilton Rating Scale for Depression (HAM-D-28) [24] and the clinician-rated Montgomery-Asberg Depression Rating Scale (MADRS) [25].

Following treatment interruption, mean increase in the number of DESS events were significant in the sertraline-treated (mean:5.7) and paroxetine-treated (mean: 7.8) patients but not in the fluoxetine-treated (mean:0.2) patients. When comparing across groups following treatment interruption, the mean number of DESS events was significantly higher in the sertraline and paroxetine groups than in the fluoxetine-treated patients, and the DESS events was also lower in the sertraline-treated patients than in the paroxetine treated patients. Further, mean increases in Symptom Questionnaire Somatic Symptom subscale, HAM-D-28, and MADRS scores were significant in the sertraline-treated (mean score changes: 2.3, 3.5 and 3.6 respectively) and paroxetine treated (mean score changes: 3.9, 5.6and 7.3) patients but not in the fluoxetine-treated patients.

When comparing across groups following treatment interruption, the number of events reported spontaneously by 10% or more of the patients was 4 for sertraline (dizziness, 18%; headache,18%; nervousness, 18%; and nausea, 11%), 8 for paroxetine (dizziness, 29%; nausea, 29%; insomnia, 19%; headache, 17%; abnormal dreams, 16%; nervousness, 16%; asthenia, 11%; and diarrhea, 11%) and 1 for fluoxetine (headache, 16%). This study supported the hypothesis that antidepressant with shorter half-lives such as paroxetine have a higher likelihood of discontinuation reactions than antidepressants with intermediate (sertraline) or long (fluoxetine) half-lives. The study also showed that spontaneous reports underestimate the occurrence of discontinuation reactions compared with the systematic inquiry approach with the 43-item DESS scale.

In a subsequent study, Michelson et al. [26] recruited patients with a history of depression successfully treated with fluoxetine, sertraline and paroxetine. At entry, patients had been taking medication continuously for at least 4 months but not more than 3 years, had no dose changes for the 2 months prior to study entry, were taking no other psychoactive medications, and had a score of 10 or less on the 21 item version of the HAD-D (HAM-D-21). Following the initial assessment, the study consisted of two 5-days periods separated by at least 2 weeks but not more than 4 weeks. Under double-blind, order-randomized conditions, all subjects underwent placebo substitution during one 5-day period and continued treatment with their usual SSRI during the next 5-day period. Subjects continued treatment with the SSRI at all other times. Patients completed a 17 item adverse event scale daily for 5 days following the study entry and during the two blinded periods, with the items queried based on the DESS. Each item was rated from 0 to 3 (absent, mild, moderate and severe) and scores were reported as the change from the most symptomatic of the 5 days immediately following study entry. At the baseline and at the end of each 5-day period, the HAM-D-21, the State Anxiety Inventory (SAI), and a self-rated assessment of social and occupational functioning during the previous 4 days were administered. The study showed that placebo substitution, but not continued active medication, was associated with statistically significant increases in total numbers of solicited adverse events for patients treated with paroxetine by the end of the fourth day. Increases in symptoms for patients treated with paroxetine became statistically significant as early as the time of the second dose of placebo. Mean severity worsened by the end of the fourth day of placebo substitution for 13 of the 17 items on the solicited adverse events scale among patients treated with paroxetine, for 3 of 17 among patients treated with sertraline. Also at the end of the placebo substitution period, patients taking paroxetine, but not those taking fluoxetine or sertraline, demonstrated statistically significant increases in HAM-D-21 and SAI scores compared with patients who continued taking the active drug.

A final study [27] assed the relative risk of emergence of adverse events on venlafaxine versus escitalopram discontinuation with the 43 item version of DESS scale. Following a 8 week, randomised, double-blind study comparing the efficacy and tolerability of escitalopram (10-20 mg/day; N=148) to that of venlafaxine extended release (75-150 mg/day; N=145) in primary care patients with MDD, at the end of the 1 week run-out period (week 9), a total of 23 symptoms were reported on the DESS, with an incidence ≥ 10% in either treatment group: 5 symptoms in the escitalopram group and 23 symptoms in the venlafaxine group. Of these, a total of 11 symptoms occurred with statistically significantly higher incidence in the venlafaxine group than in the escitalopram group.

Withdrawal reactions were also reported in patients with major depressive disorders (MDD) treated with duloxetine, the most recent drug from the pharmacological family of serotonin (5-HT) and norepinephrine reuptake inhibitors [28]. Data were obtained from 9 clinical trials assessing the efficacy and safety of duloxetine on MDD. In all studies, duloxetine was abruptly discontinued, followed by a lead-out phase of 1 or 2 weeks to allow for the collection of withdrawal symptoms at a set time after the discontinuation of duloxetine or placebo. Significantly more duloxetine treated patients (44.3%) reported al least 1 discontinuation symptoms than placebo treated patients (22.9%), with dizziness being the most common symptom. In term of duration of these symptoms, following duloxetine discontinuation, 46.3% had resolved prior to final contact with study patients and the remaining 53.7% were unresolved.

A SSRI withdrawal-like syndrome has been also described in neonates exposed to maternal antidepressant use during pregnancy. Typical postnatal reactions, such as insomnia, irritability and myoclonus are suggestive of adult SSRI discontinuation symptoms [1, 29]. However, other features, including respiratory distress and seizures differ from adult reactions. Recently Haddad [30] proposed that some reactions may be related to serotonin toxicity. Still the majority of these reactions are likely to be related to discontinuation effect, since they appear to occur at higher frequency with short half-life antidepressant such as paroxetine.

In fact a further study [31] showed a greater incidence of perinatal complications in infants exposed to paroxetine in the third trimester compared with those who were never exposed. Two recent studies have also described withdrawal reactions following SSRI discontinuation on patients with anxiety disorders and are worth mentioning here for their implications.

In the first study Baldwin et al. [32] have analysed different randomised control trials to address not only whether antidepressant of the same classes differ in their discontinuation symptoms, but also whether symptoms differ between depression and anxiety. Data came from two comparative studies of escitalopram in major depressive disorder (MDD) (one vs. venlafaxine XR and one vs. paroxetine), two studies in social anxiety disorder (SAD) (one of which used paroxetine as the active reference) and one study in generalised anxiety disorder (GAD), using paroxetine as an active reference [total number of patients: escitalopram (n=1051); paroxetine (n=336); venlafaxine (n=124); placebo (n=239)]. All studies used the DESS checklist to assess the presence of discontinuation symptoms. The results confirmed that all three antidepressants showed more discontinuations symptoms compared to placebo (p<0.001). There was a significantly lower increase in total DESS score 1 week after discontinuation in the escitalopram groups than in the venlafaxine XR and paroxetine groups in the MDD trials. Also paroxetine showed significantly greater discontinuation symptoms than escitalopram in SAD (p<0.05) and GAD (p<0.001). No differences between major depression, SAD, and GAD studies were detected when the change in total DESS scores were compared.

In an investigation by Fava et al. (10) the prevalence and features of discontinuation syndromes ensuing with gradual tapering of selective serotonin reuptake inhibitors (SSRI) in patients with panic disorder and agoraphobia has been explored. Specifically the aim of the study was to report on discontinuation syndromes ensuing in optimal clinical conditions: remission of panic disorder upon behavioral exposure, slow tapering, adequate patient education about the transient and benign nature of potential symptoms, availability of the treating physician, exclusion of patients with previous mood disorder. 26 consecutive outpatients who fulfilled the DSM-IV criteria for panic disorder with agoraphobia while taking SSRI and were treated in an Affective Disorders Program over a period of 5 years were recruited in the study. The patients diagnoses were established by a psychiatrist and a clinical psychologist independently using the Schedule for Affective Disorders and Schizophrenia [33]. Patients with co-occurring mood disorder and /or social phobia and/or obsessive-compulsive disorder were excluded.

After initial diagnostic evaluations, all patients were treated according to a standardized behavioral protocol by experienced psychiatrists. Therapy was based on behavioral exposure homework only and feedback from the therapist without therapist-aided exposure (34). Treatment consisted of 12 sessions; each session lasted 30 minutes, once every two weeks. Twenty patients completed treatment and 20 were panic free from both major and minor panic at the time of the post-treatment evaluation and were rated as "much better" according to a global scale of improvement [35]. Comorbidity wad assessed at the end of behavioral treatment, to minimize state-trait contaminations, using again the SADS [33]. A global assessment of the severity of panic and depressed mood concerned with the pre-treatment status was made using two 1-7 point scales of the Clinical Interview for Depression [36]. The two scales consist of specific anchor points and were found to yield a sensitive measurement of change upon behavioral treatment in panic disorder [39]. Upon entering the study, the 20 patients were taking the antidepressant drugs, since at least 6 months. Twelve patients were taking benzodiazepines. In the course of behavioral treatment, according to a standardized protocol [36], benzodiazepines were tapered and, whenever possible, discontinued. In patients who had trouble tapering their benzodiazepines (mostly alprazolam and lorazepam) the psychiatrist prescribed clonazepam in substitution. Aside from these cases, the treating physician did not prescribe any new psychotropic drugs. At the end of treatment, 7 patients were still taking benzodiazepines even though at much lower dosages. These dosages were kept unchanged during the study period.

Tapering of antidepressant drugs was performed at the slowest possible pace (50 mg every other week for fluvoxamine and sertraline, 10 mg every other week for paroxetine, fluoxetine and citalopram, with 10 mg every other day in the last segment).

After 15 days from discontinuation all patients were assessed with the Discontinuation-Emergent Signs and Symptoms (DESS) check-list [8]. This allowed a comprehensive collection of all manifestations of discontinuation syndrome since some may become evident only in the second week. Patients were classified as experiencing "discontinuation syndrome" if the number of DESS check-list events reported increased by four or from the beginning to the end of the treatment interruption period. Patients were reassessed after 1 month and 12 months. None of the 20 patients refused follow-up assessments, which consisted of an update of clinical state, including persistence of discontinuation symptoms, any potential treatment contacts or use of medications, and occurrence of any relapse of panic disorder or onset of a new psychiatric disorder, using again the SADS [33]. Patients were instructed to call if any new symptoms appeared and were guaranteed further treatment if necessary also during the follow-up.

Nine of the 20 patients (45%) experienced a discontinuation syndrome according to specific criteria [37]. All discontinuation syndromes subsided within a month in all but 3 patients (27%). These three patients all had been taking paroxetine and displayed alternation of worsened mood, fatigue and emotional lability with trouble sleeping, irritability and hyperactivity, meeting the DSM-IV criteria for cyclothymic disorder except for duration. The first patient (32 F), who had been taking paroxetine 20 mg/day for 18 months, after 3 months of persistence of symptoms was prescribed clonazepam 0.5 mg b.i.d.. She improved considerably. Subsequent attempts to discontinue clonazepam were, however, unsuccessful, for re-emergence of symptoms. The second patient (58 M) had been taking paroxetine 20 mg/day for 84 months. Clonazepam up to 1 mg t.i.d did not yield any improvement. Fluvoxamine (initially 50 mg/day, then 100 mg) was also of little help (6 week trial). Symptoms subsided when paroxetine 10 mg was started again. The third patient (39 M) had been taking paroxetine 20 mg for 96 months. Clonazepam up to 1 mg t.i.d. was of modest help. He was offered paroxetine again but refused. Symptoms persisted unchanged for the duration of the observation period. None of these patients had previous or family history of bipolar disorder or cyclothymia.

During the one-year follow-up one patient taking citalopram who had discontinuation syndrome also had a relapse of panic disorder. She was offered a new course of treatment based on exposure and became panic free at the end of such treatment. Another patient who had been treated with paroxetine and had a discontinuation syndrome developed a major depressive disorder, which responded to treatment with paroxetine 20 mg/day.

The naturalistic design represents the major methodological limitation of the study since it does not allow the control of variables how it happens in randomized control trials. Discontinuation syndromes cannot be compared among patients treated with different types of SSRI. However, discontinuation syndromes were common in patients taking SSRI. Particularly, in 3 patients who had been taking paroxetine for a long time symptoms persisted and had cyclothymic features, despite lack of previous bipolar spectrum symptoms. Re-institution of paroxetine in one case, and administration of clonazepam in another were effective in improving symptoms. This latter drug was used, since it was reported to improve depressive symptoms emerging during the treatment of panic disorder with fluvoxamine [38]. In another patient treated with paroxetine, a major depressive disorder ensued during the one-year follow-up.

These findings are consistent with the onset of manic and hypomanic symptoms after antidepressant drug discontinuation [39] and with the onset of panic symptoms one month following abrupt paroxetine discontinuation (40) In this latter case, symptoms were unresponsive to citalopram and abated only when paroxetine was resumed, as was found to be the case in one of our patients.

To explain the occurrence of withdrawal symptoms several hypotheses have been formulated.

Previous reports highlighted that, in the presence of 5-HT$_{1A}$ autoreceptor desensitization [41], after the discontinuation of SSRI, the firing rate of 5-HT could rebound or increase significantly. Thus, an enhanced level of endogenous 5-HT, previously produced by reuptake inhibition, would no longer keep the firing rate of 5-HT neurons within the normal range after an SSRI discontinuation. This may lead to an excess of synaptic 5-HT in the projection areas. Nevertheless, this situation is unconvincing, because, on one hand, 48 hours after the interruption of 14-days treatment with a 5-HT$_{1A}$ agonist, the 5-HT$_{1A}$ autoreceptor is still desensitized, the exogenous 5-HT$_{1A}$ agonist in no longer present, and the firing rate of 5-HT neurons is within the normal range [42]. On the other hand, after long term administration of SSRI post-synaptic 5-HT receptors are desensitized as well. Hence, the down regulation of postsynaptic 5-HT receptors usually counteracts this upward trend in 5-HT transmission.

In the same vein, it has been supposed that restoration of 5-HT reuptake activity following discontinuation of SSRI in combination with this down-regulation of postsynaptic 5-HT receptors, could lead to an acute hyposerotoninergic state [43,44]. Subsequently, a decrease in the 5-HT synaptic level would account for the manifestation of discontinuation symptoms.

Different hypotheses involved the modulatory role of serotonin on the firing activity of norepinephrine neurons, in the occurrence of antidepressant withdrawal syndrome. Specifically, long term administration of SSRI leads to a progressive decrease in firing activity of norepinephrine (NE) neurons in the locus ceruleus [45,46]. This decrease is caused by an enhanced inhibitory 5-HT tone on NE neurons [47]. Consequently, it was hypothesised that, after the abrupt lifting of this inhibitory tone on NE neurons, there is a hyperadrenergic state that contributes to some discontinuation symptoms such as restlessness, headache and weakness. However, it is unlike that a rebound noradrenergic action would to contribute to the discontinuation symptoms associated with the tricyclics, because cessation of the nontricyclics but potent NE reuptake inhibitors reboxetine and atomoxetine have not been related to such problems [48,49].

In contrast, most tricyclics are relatively potent antagonist of the cholinergic muscarinic receptors [50]. In this contest, it would be possible that the more frequently reported occurrence of discontinuation symptoms with paroxetine that the other SSRI could be attributed in part to its moderate affinity for muscarinic receptors [50].

Also, a recent hypothesis [51] suggested a NMDA receptor involvement in imipramine withdrawal effects. In fact, the increase in N-methyl-D-aspartate (NMDA) receptor density reported after antidepressant withdrawal would appear to be a sign of a primary increase in glutamatergic tone subsequent to removal of inhibitory effect of the antidepressant. The reversal of the resulting behavioral and neurochemical effects of imipramine withdrawal with the glutamate receptor antagonist dizocilpine (MK801) supports a role for prior NMDA receptor activation [52].

The Oppositional Tolerance Model

Even though several authors provided many acceptable hypotheses to explain the emergence of withdrawal syndrome, none of these afford a comprehensive account for different phenomena induced by antidepressant drugs, such as, tolerance, resistance, dependence and withdrawal symptoms.

To understand the possible implications of these phenomena we must refer to the oppositional tolerance model. This model has been introduced by Fava in 1995 and subsequently elaborated in 2003 [53,54]. According to this model continued drug treatment may recruit process that oppose the initial acute effects of a drug or of receptor alterations. Use of antidepressant drugs may also propel the illness to a more malignant and treatment-unresponsive course. When drug treatment ends, oppositional processes may operate for some time, resulting in appearance of withdrawal symptoms and increase vulnerability to relapse. As Baldessarini sustains [55] the assumption that such physiologic processes will readjust after a withdrawal phase is not supported by current awareness in the field of drug dependence.

The model also provides illustration for a number of clinical phenomena in addition to withdrawal syndrome. For example, a number of clinical observations scattered in the psychiatric literature provide a potential ground for postulating - at least in some patients – that antidepressant drugs may worsen the course of depression. Many of these data derive from uncontrolled clinical observations and bear limited implications if they are considered on their own, but achieve meaning and raise important questions if they are examined in the light of a unifying hypothesis.

Long-Term Outcome of Major Depression Treated by Pharmacological Means

There is evidence that casts some doubt on the ability of antidepressant drugs to favorably affect the course of depressive illness, despite their recognized ability to treat the depressive episode. Viguera et al. [56] analyzed 27 studies with variable length of antidepressant treatment which reported follow-up upon drug discontinuation. Duration of drug treatment did not seem to affect long-term prognosis once the drug was discontinued.

Whether you treat a depressed patient for 3 months or 3 years, it does not matter when you stop the drugs. There was a significant trend which suggested that the longer is the drug treatment, the higher is the likelihood of relapse [56]. In a subsequent analysis [57], including one more study [58], risk of postdiscontinuation relapse was nearly significantly greater after long treatment following recovery from an index episode of major depression (rho= 0.37; p= 0.052). In a naturalistic prospective study [59], low-doses of antidepressants appeared to be less beneficial than either higher doses or clinical management without antidepressant drugs. The latter two treatments yielded almost identical outcome. An observational study of 236 unipolar patients, who had received antidepressants during recovery and were followed for an affective recurrence for up to 5 years, showed that the rate of recurrence for patients with fewer than five previous episodes was not affected by medication after the initial 8 months [60]. Patients who had experienced more than several recurrences were at a greater risk of recurrence and continued to benefit from any level of medication during the first year after recovery [60]. A large double-blind placebo controlled study [61] on the optimal duration of antidepressant treatment found a significant protective effect of fluoxetine compared to placebo as to relapse rate after 24 weeks of treatment (26% for fluoxetine and 48% for placebo), but not after 62 weeks (11% for fluoxetine and 16% for placebo). Both studies indicate that antidepressant drugs generally fail to protect after 6 months of treatment but do not imply that antidepressant drugs may worsen the natural course of depression. Further, in naturalistic studies [59, 60] we cannot be sure about the compliance of patients.

Stassen et al. [60] found that the time course of improvement among responders to amitriptyline, oxaprotiline and placebo was independent of the treatment modality, and thus identical in all three groups. Once triggered, the time course of recovery from illness became identical to the spontaneous remission observed under placebo. Antidepressants, therefore, may not change the pattern of the natural course of recovery from depression, but simply speed the recovery and change the boundary between "responders" and "non-responders" [62]. Baldwin [63] observed that, after drug treatment, about one quarter of patients with major depression in later life remain symptom-free, one third experience at least one relapse but with further recovery, and the remainder have residual symptoms. In about 10% of all cases, depressive symptoms remain severe and intractable. These proportions appear to have altered little since antidepressant drugs became available [63].

The literature thus indicates that antidepressant drugs are effective in preventing recurrences while they are administered [64], and do not yield a protective effect once they are discontinued. The correlation between duration of antidepressant drug treatment and likelihood of relapse upon discontinuation may suggest that it is not simply a matter of failure to protest, but that a neurobiologic mechanism increasing vulnerability may be triggered.

Paradoxical Effects of Antidepressant Drugs

In 1968 Di Mascio et al. [65] studied the effects of imipramine on individuals varying in levels of depression, using a double-blind placebo controlled procedure. They found an increase in depression levels after the use of imipramine in the subjects with the lowest scores of depression. A few years later, Van Scheyen [66] performed a naturalistic follow-up study of 56 female and 28 male patients with recurrent vital depression. At a time when antidepressant drugs were not as widely prescribed as today, he observed that systematic treatment with tricyclic antidepressants proved to be associated with an increase in the total number of recurrences, which attained statistical significance in female patients. Van Scheyen wondered "whether such an increased number of depressive phases would not be regarded as a side effect or paradoxical effect which, after protracted therapy, is produced by the tricyclic antidepressants so far most commonly used" [66]. Patients, however, were not randomized to treatment with antidepressant drugs or not and this observation may have reflected the more severe characteristics of illness of those patients who were judged to be in need of antidepressant drugs. More recently, in the course of randomized double-blind cross-over study comparing the effects of reboxetine and sertraline in a group of healthy volunteers [67], two subjects reported becoming depressed and other two suicidal.

Similar observations have been made with treatment of anxiety disorders by antidepressant drugs. Commenting on the development of endogenous depression in patients with panic disorder treated with therapeutic doses of antidepressants, Aronson [68] suggested the possibility that antidepressant medications may unmask a depressive diathesis. Fux et al. [38] observed the emergence of depressive symptoms in 7 of 80 patients (9%) during treatment of panic disorder by fluvoxamine. These patients had no history of mood disorder, and no symptoms of depression were present before the treatment with fluvoxamine. The symptoms abated when fluvoxamine was discontinued and tricyclic antidepressants or clonazepam were prescribed and reappeared when fluoxetine was administered. Fux et al. [38] suggest the possibility of a vulnerability among some of panic disorder patients to a noradrenergic - serotonergic imbalance caused by SSRI. The question that arises is whether such paradoxical phenomena may only affect a few individuals or are manifestations of a subtle, but general effect. The results of a recent randomized controlled trial comparing cognitive behavioral therapy (CBT), imipramine, or their combination for panic disorder [69] would point to the latter possibility as to panic disorder. Six months after treatment discontinuation, response rates were 41% for CBT plus placebo, against 26% for CBT combined with imipramine. A relationship between use of antidepressant drugs and increased relapse risk of panic disorder has been reported by other investigators [70-72] and depression was found to occur also during the follow-up of patients receiving tricyclic antidepressants for panic disorder [73]. Another intriguing phenomenon involves the concept of therapeutic window, which was originally applied to nortriptyline [74], but was subsequently described with SSRI [75-79]. The possibility of paradoxical or no effects occurring above a certain dosage would be in line with the phenomena described with patients with affective disorders and healthy controls.

In any event, these effects appear to occur in a very limited percentage of patients treated with antidepressants.

Antidepressant-Induced Switching in Bipolar Disorder

The occurrence of mania upon treatment with antidepressant drugs in depressed patients is a relatively old clinical observation. A switch into mania is frequent in patients with bipolar disorder, even though they are treated with a mood stabilizer. Post et al. have estimated that antidepressants may double the incidence of a switch (50% of cases) compared to placebo (25%). Such incidence may be even higher in rapid cycling bipolar disorder [80]. Angst, in a study that reviewed the experience over six decades in his clinic [81], presented evidence that can be interpreted as consistent with drug-induced cycling as distinct from spontaneous cycling. In the early eighties, Kukopulos et al. [82, 83] observed how treatment by antidepressant drugs may contribute to changes of course from unipolar to bipolar illness, and to an increased frequence of cyclicity. Cycle acceleration has been subsequently confirmed by other investigators [80]. Kukopulos et al. [82, 83] deserve credit in raising the issue that antidepressant-induced mania may not simply be a temporary and fully reversible phenomenon, but trigger complex biochemical mechanisms of illness deterioration. A case of tricyclic-induced mania in a 60-year old woman, with a long-standing history of unipolar depression (that was followed by rapid cycling refractory to lithium), illustrates the hormonal implications of such mechanisms [84].

Despite initial denial, the view that use of antidepressant drugs may worsen the course of bipolar disorder has achieved wide currency [80]. The possibility, however, that antidepressant drugs may induce episode acceleration in unipolar depression has not been adequately studied. Goodwin [85] has illustrated how this could occur. If both depressive and manic episodes tend naturally to evolve toward remission (either into a euthymic phase or into an episode of opposite polarity) and antidepressant drugs accelerate this natural tendency, drug treatment may accelerate the next sequence in the natural course (i.e., the onset of a manic episode instead of euthymia). "If the natural sequence of recurrent unipolar illness goes from depression to recovery and then eventually to the next episode, treatments that accelerate recovery of the index depression could also accelerate the onset of the next episode" [85].

Tolerance to Antidepressant Drugs

The return of depressive symptoms during maintenance antidepressant treatment was found to occur in 9 to 57% in published trials [86]. Possible explanations include pharmacological tolerance, loss of placebo effect, increase in disease severity, change in disease pathogenesis, the accumulation of a detrimental metabolite, unrecognized rapid cycling, and prophylactic inefficacy [86].

Several clinical observations point to the existence of tolerance phenomena during antidepressant treatment [57, 87]. Some data point to dispositional (pharmacokinetic) tolerance, which reduces the concentration of a drug or its duration. For instance, patients who relapsed while on fluoxetine treatment (20 mg/d) responded to an increased dosage of the same drug (40 mg/d) [88]. Other studies, however, suggest the likelihood of pharmacodynamic processes which change sensitivity to the drug. Mann [89] observed loss of antidepressant effect with long-term monoamine oxidase inhibitor treatment without loss of monoamine oxidase inhibition. Lieb and Balter [90] described the development of tolerance to antidepressant effects which was refractory to dosage increase. The effectiveness of drug increase for relapse during maintenance treatment of major depression was assessed in a recent study concerned with fluoxetine administered as 20 mg daily or 90 mg weekly dose [58]. Patients on fluoxetine 20 mg/day had their dose increased to 40 mg/day and those on 90 mg weekly dose to 90 mg twice a week. 57% of patients of 40 mg daily group and 72% of enteric-coated 90 mg twice weekly group responded to the dose increase. One patient out of five who initially responded to dose increase relapsed again during the 25 week trial [58]. It is conceivable that this percentage would have increased with continuation of the trial as was found to be the case in recurrent depression [91]. These data, therefore, strongly point to pharmacodynamic tolerance.

One should pay attention, however, also to the percentage of patients who do not display a loss of therapeutic effect during maintenance treatment (for instance to the 82% of patients who stay well during the 3-year Pittsburgh Maintenance Study, against the 18% of patients who relapsed while being on full-dose imipramine) [92]. The phenomena subsumed under the rubric of tolerance in mood disorder bear strong resemblances with progressive loss of effects which have been observed with both antidepressant and antianxiety drugs in anxiety disorders [93]. These phenomena have also been defined as fading (progressive decrease of therapeutic effects refractory to dosage increase, after non immediate symptomatic improvement) [94].

Resistance to Antidepressant Drugs

There is considerable confusion about the term resistance in mood disorder. An important distinction is whether they are applied to depressive illness (an episode which does not respond to drugs or psychotherapy) or to antidepressant drug therapy (a drug which resulted in clinical response is no longer effective when it is started again after a drug free period). The former use is the one which is prevalent, but also the latter is worthy of clinical attention.

In 1984, Lieb and Balter (90) described the resistance of some patients to antidepressant drugs that had previously been effective. Change to another antidepressant drug yielded clinical benefits, but was followed by refractoriness as well. Ten years later, similar phenomena were described and related to long-term low-dose antidepressant treatment [95]. Lieb and Balter defined this resistance as tachyphylaxis (the increasing tolerance to a drug that develops following repeated administration). In bipolar disorder, it has repeatedly been observed [96- 98], that patients who responded well to lithium do not always regain the same degree of initial responsiveness with lithium reinstitution. This, however, may also indicate the progression of the illness and not a drug-related phenomenon. Indeed, a large, naturalistic follow-up of patients with affective disorders failed to provide evidence that lithium discontinuation results in treatment resistance when lithium is resumed [99]. In a 6 year outcome study of unipolar depression [100], patients who relapsed while drug-free were prescribed the same antidepressant that was effective in the initial episode. Resistance occurred in 4% of cases. Friedman et al. [101] observed onset of resistance after reinstitution of desipramine treatment in 1 of 12 patients with dysthymia who had relapsed after being switched to placebo. Donaldson [102] described three patients with major depression who relapsed while being on phenelzine and developed a severe chronic depression that was refractory to other treatments. The phenomenon of resistance was analyzed in a study on 122 patients who, after initially responding to fluoxetine, were assigned to placebo. About half of patients relapsed. Thirty-eight percent of patients either did not respond or initially responded but again relapsed after re-initiation of medication [103]. Similar results were obtained after discontinuation of SSRI in obsessive-compulsive disorder [104].

The few data available thus indicate that when drug treatment is reinstituted the patient may not respond to the same antidepressant which improved depressive symptoms the first time. The prevalence of this resistance that ensues varies. Patients who respond to reinstitution of the same antidepressant drug may display a subsequent loss of therapeutic effect [103]. This suggests that resistance and loss of clinical effects may be related and share a common mechanism. Episodes which are simply defined as responding poorly to antidepressant drugs [105] may underlie the phenomena described here (previous successful response to antidepressant drugs). This issue is currently neglected, but it is worthy of research attention.

The Sequenced Treatment Alternatives to Relieve Depression Study (STAR*D)

The main confirmation of the oppositional tolerance model has came from the Sequenced Treatment Alternatives to Relieve Depression Study (STAR*D) [106]. The aim of the trial was to apply the best pharmacological strategies for obtaining remission in major depression. A sample of 3671 patients was treated with citalopram in an open fashion: only 36,8% of patients were remitted. The rate was low and difficult to attribute to specific effects of citalopram, since a variety of non-specific therapeutic ingredients, as in the other major trials [107-109], were used. Those who did not recover were submitted to four sequential steps involving switching, augmentation and combination strategies, based on available literature. Because of the type of randomization that was chosen, the role of cognitive therapy could not be established, since the patients who opted for it were too few. The results were rather disappointing. The cumulative rate of remission after 4 sequential steps was 67% [106]. However, when sustained recovery (taking into account relapse rates while on treatment) was considered, the cumulative rate was 43% [110]. This means that the strenuous efforts after step one (open treatment with citalopram) yielded an additional 6% of sustained recovery (Table 1). This indicates the failure of current pharmacological strategies in determining lasting remission in depressed patients.

Even though each step of the trial was carefully conceived to increase the likelihood of response in patients who did not remit, remission rates decreased after each treatment step [106]. In the follow-up phase, participants were strongly advised to continue the previously effective medication at the doses used in acute treatment. Rates of relapse increased after each treatment step in patients who achieved remission (Table 1). As Nelson noted [110], it is particularly worrisome that in steps 3 and 4, in addition to low remission rates, nearly half of those remitting relapsed. Further, intolerance (dropouts for any reason during the first 4 weeks, or side effects afterwards) increased after each treatment step (Table 1). Finally, the lack of differences between treatments at the various levels, such as the fact that a second

SSRI (sertraline) was just as effective as drug with a different mechanism (bupropion) or a "dual-action" agent (venlafaxine), "leaves us without a road map to guide treatment selection" [110].

Table 1. Remission, relapse and intolerance in the STAR*D trial [107]

	Remission	Relapse	Intolerance
Step 1	36.8%	33.5%	16.3%
Step 2	30.6%	47.4%	11.5%
Step 3	13.7%	42.9%	25.6%
Step 4	13.0%	50.0%	34.1%

The indications from the STAR*D findings are pretty clear: pharmacological manipulations, either by switching or augmentation (steps 1 and 2) may propel depressive illness into a refractory phase, characterized by low remission, high relapse and high intolerance (steps 3 and 4). The underlying mechanism is that of oppositional tolerance (53). Not all antidepressant drugs are likely to induce oppositional tolerance to the same extent. For instance, dual reuptake inhibitors seem to incur lower rates of loss of clinical effect than SSRIs [111]. Maurizio Fava and John Rush, the leading investigators of the STAR*D trial, have advocated a novel approach to improve practice involving the use of augmentation or combination strategies at the outset of initial treatment to enhance the chances of remission through synergy and/or a broader spectrum of action [112]. It possible that the mechanism of oppositional tolerance may be triggered by use of subsequent pharmacological manipulations, as in STAR*D, while effective initial treatment may yield lasting remission and neurotrasmittor stabilization. But it is also possible that augmentation or combination strategies at the onset may trigger oppositional tolerance regardless of the timing of intervention. This appears to be a key issue in the research agenda concerned with pharmacological treatment of depression [113].

Pathophysiological Interactions

What type of oppositional processes can be recruited and/or sensitised by antidepressant drugs is an open question. Nevertheless, several hypotheses may be formulated.

Interaction between Different Types of Serotonin Receptors

There is an increasing awareness of the complex mutual inhibitory effects of different serotonin receptors, particularly, 5-HT1 and 5-HT2 receptors [114]. Berendsen has suggested that an important function of antidepressants is to restore a disturbed balance between 5-HT1A, 5-HT1B and 5-HT2 receptors. It is, therefore, conceivable that a therapeutic action of antidepressant drugs may, under certain conditions, trigger changes in post-receptor signal transduction, in intra-neuronal signalling pathways, or in neuronal architecture that are likely to affect the balance of serotonin receptors. Indeed, there is a preclinical evidence of the auto-regulation of serotonin and its potential effect on neuro-genesis [115].

Interactions between Different Neurotransmitters

In the same vain, there is increasing awareness of the complex mutual inhibitory effects of different neurotransmitter systems that may be affected in depression [114]. In fact, earlier studies have demonstrated that major depression is accompanied by alterations in the serine/glycine ratio as well glutamate [116, 117]. Elevated levels of nitrogen oxide metabolites have also been observed in patients with depression [51]. Antidepressant drugs may yield changes in connections or sensitivity to neurotransmitters indirectly related to the specific actions.

Interaction between Neurotransmitter Balance and the Hypothalamic-Pituitary-Adrenal Axis

Neurophysiologist have used the term sensitization, as oppose to habituation, to refer to the long-lasting increment in response occurring on repeated presentation of a stimulus that reliably elicits a response and its initial presentation [118]. Psychostimulants such as amphetamine and cocaine have been found to induce sensitization. Antidepressant therapy may also induce time-dependent sensitization [119]. The hypothalamic-pituitary-adrenal (HPA) axis, through an action on corticotropin releasing factor neurons, can modulate both sensitization and tolerance [120]. By facilitating 5-HT1 receptor-mediated neurotransmission, 5-HT2 postsynaptic down regulation, a putative final common pathway of the activation of different antidepressants, may also induce an activation of the HPA axis. This activation, in turn, may affect serotoninergic receptor functioning [121].

Cross-Sensitization with Behavioral and Cognitive Phenomena

There are considerable evidences of cross sensitization between psychoactive drugs and environmental stressor and such cross-sensitization may be HPA mediated [122]. Inappropriate antidepressant withdrawal associated with stress may engender neurochemical imbalances in glutamate and GABA, as well as alter the expression of critical cellular resilience proteins. The ensuing actions of raised glutamate and Nitric Oxide (NO) on synaptic plasticity and cellular aspects may change neuronal and synaptic structure in such a way that prior antidepressant response is altered. This response could lay the foundation for relapse, requirement for higher dose and future treatment resistance [51].

Conclusions

There are no feasible alternatives to treating major depressive episodes with antidepressant drugs and potential adverse phenomena are overshadowed by this clinical consideration. However, appraisal of these withdrawal syndromes may yield important insights into the modalities of such practice, and in preventing recurrences with long-term antidepressant drug therapy. At present, the oppositional tolerance model applied to antidepressant drugs may provide room for a number of clinical phenomena which would otherwise lack explanation. Antidepressant drugs were developed and found to be effective in the treatment of major depressive episodes, but, in recent years, we should be aware that we are stretching their original indications (123). Their use has been prolonged and extended to maintenance and prevention of relapse, anxiety disorders and demoralization. In clinical medicine, however, treatments that are effective in the acute phase of illness are not necessarily the most suitable for post-acute and residual phase of maintenance [124].

When we prolong treatment over 6-9 months, we may thus recruit different phenomena, such as tolerance, episode acceleration, sensitization and paradoxical effects [113]. Some individuals, either for genetic or for the combination of psychopathological and psychosocial factors may be particularly vulnerable to the persistence of discontinuation effects after antidepressant treatment. This highlights the importance of studying specific subgroups of patients when evaluating psychiatric treatment [125, 24].

A very serious clinical problem arises when antidepressant withdrawal symptoms are misidentified as signs of impending relapse, as it may occur in busy clinical settings or as a result of pharmaceutical propaganda. Antidepressant drugs are then promptly reinstituted, yielding the misleading impression that it was indeed a relapse. This strategy actually only postpones and aggravates the problem. An example is offered by a patient who had been successfully treated for an episode of major depression with venlafaxine 75mg by a young psychiatrist working in a mental health center. After one year of treatment the drug was tapered and discontinued. A few days after discontinuation, the patient experienced acute anxiety, insomnia, and various somatic symptoms. The psychiatrist told her it was a depressive relapse and that the drug had to be re-instituted. The patient was, however, doubtful ("I did not feel depressed") and so was her primary care physician who asked for an urgent consultation. The withdrawal nature of the symptoms was evident. The consultant called the psychiatrist, who refused to entertain this possibility ("I never heard of these withdrawal reactions during my residency training and attending meetings") and was not interested in reading literature that was offered.

In the setting of anxiety disorders, withdrawal reactions from antidepressant drugs may have other important clinical indications. First of all the perception that benzodiazepine can lead to dependence and may avoided by use of antidepressant drugs is not supported by research evidence. Also SSRI and related drugs such venlafaxine and duloxetine may cause problems upon discontinuation. Further, the likelihood of relapse upon discontinuation is even higher than in depression. The findings may thus call for a more caution use of antidepressant drugs in the setting of anxiety disturbances.

References

[1]   Kramer JC, Klein DF, Fink M. Withdrawal symptoms following discontinuation of imipramine therapy. *Am J Psychiatry* 1961; 118: 549-550.

[2]   Schatzberg AF, Zajecka J. Serotonin reuptake inhibitor discontinuation syndrome: a hypothetical definition. *J Clin Psychiatry* 1997; 58: 5-10.

[3]   Disalver SC. Heterocyclic antidepressant, monoamine oxidase inhibitor and neuroleptic withdrawal phenomena. *Progr Neuropsychopharmacol Biol Psychiatry* 1990; 14: 137-161.

[4]   Lejoyeux M, Adès J, Mourad I, et al. Antidepressant withdrawal syndrome. *CNS Drugs* 1996; 5: 278-292.

[5]   Zajecka J, Tracy KA, Mitchell S. Discontinuation symptoms after treatment with serotonin reuptake inhibitors. *J Clin Psychiatry* 1997; 58: 291-297.

[6]   Medawar C. The antidepressant web. *Int J Risk Safety Med* 1997; 10: 75-126.

[7]   Oliver JS, Burrows GD, Norman TR. Discontinuation syndromes with selective serotonin reuptake inhibitors. *CNS Drugs* 1999; 12:171-177.

[8]   Rosenbaum JF, Fava M, Hoog SL, et al. Selective serotonin reuptake inhibitor discontinuation syndrome: a randomized clinical trial. *Biol Psychiatry* 1998; 44: 77-87.

[9]   Judge R, Parry MG, Quail D, Jacobson JG. Discontinuation symptoms: comparison of brief interruption in fluoxetine and paroxetine treatment. *Int Clin Psychopharmacol* 2002; 17: 217-225.

[10]   Fava GA, Bernardi M, Tomba E, Rafanelli C. Effects of gradual discontinuation of selective serotonin reuptake inhibitors in panic disorder with agoraphobia. *Int J Neuropsychopharmacol* 2007; 10:835-838.

[11]   Mirin SM, Schatzberg AF, Creasey DE. Hypomania and mania after withdrawal of tricyclic antidepressants. *Am. J Psychiatry* 1981; 138: 87-89.

[12]   Landry P, Roy L. Withdrawal hypomania associated with paroxetine. *J Clin Psychopharmacol* 1997; 17: 60-61.

[13]   Goldstein TR, Frye MA, Denicoff KD, et al. Antidepressant discontinuation-related mania. *J Clin Psychiatry* 1999; 60: 563-567.

[14]   McGrath PJ, Stewart JW, Tricamo E, et al. Paradoxical mood shifts to euthymia or hypomania upon withdrawal of antidepressant agents. *J Clin Psychopharmacol* 1993; 13: 224-225.

[15]   Corral M, Sivertz K, Jones BD. Transient mood elevation associated with antidepressant drug decrease. *Can J Psychiatry* 1987; 32: 764-767.

[16]   Sharma V. Loss of response to antidepressants and subsequent refractoriness. *J Affect Disord* 2001; 64: 99-106.

[17]   Lejoyeux M, Rodiere-Rein C, Ades J. Withdrawal syndrome from antidepressive drugs. Report of 5 cases (In French). *Encephale* 1992; 18: 251-255.

[18]   Therrien F, Markowitz JS. Selective serotonin reuptake inhibitors and withdrawal symptoms: a review of literature. *Hum Psychopharmacology* 1997; 12: 309-323.

[19]   Haddad PM. Newer antidepressants and discontinuation syndrome. *J Clin Psychiatry* 1997; 58. 17-21.

[20] Coupland NJ, Bell CJ, Potokar JP. Serotonin reuptake inhibitor withdrawal. *J Clin Pharmacol* 1996; 16: 356-362.

[21] Price JS, Waller PC, Wood SM, Mackay AVP. A comparison of the post marketing safety of four selective serotonin reuptake inhibitors including the investigation of symptoms occurring on withdrawal. *Br J Clin. Pharmacol* 1996; 42:757-763.

[22] Fava M. Prospective studies of adverse events related to antidepressant discontinuation. *J Clin Psychiatry* 2006;67(suppl 4):14-21.

[23] Kellner R. A symptom Questionnaire. *J Clin Psychiatry* 1987; 48: 268-274.

[24] Hamilton M. A rating scale for depression. *J Neurol Neurosug Psychiatry* 1960; 23:56-62.

[25] Montgomery SA, Asberg M. A new depression scale designed to be sensitive to change. *Br J Psychiatry* 1979; 134:382-389.

[26] Michelson D, Fava M, Amsterdam J. Interruption of selective serotonin reuptake inhibitor treatment: double-blind, placebo controlled trial. *Br J Psychiatry* 2000; 176: 363-368.

[27] Montgomery SA, Huusom AK, Bothmer J. A randomised study comparing escitalopram with venlafaxine XR in primary care patients with major depressive disorder. *Neuropsychobiol* 2004; 50: 57-64.

[28] Perahia DG, Kajdasz DK, Desaiah D, Haddad PM. Symptoms following abrupt discontinuation of duloxetine treatment in patients with major depressive disorder. *J Affect Disord* 2005;89:207-212.

[29] Haddad PM. Antidepressant discontinuation syndromes. *Drug Saf* 2001; 24:183-197.

[30] Haddad PM, Pal BR, Clarke P. Neonatal symptoms following maternal paroxetine treatment: serotonin toxicity or paroxetine discontinuation syndrome? *J Psychopharmacol* 2005; 19:554-557.

[31] Costei AM, Kozer E, Ho T. Perinatal outcomes following third trimester exposure to paroxetine. *Arch Pediatr Adolesc Med* 2002; 156: 1129-1132.

[32] Baldwin DS, Montgomery SA, Nil R, Lader M. Discontinuation symptoms in depression and anxiety disorders. *Int. J. Neuropsychopharmacol.* 2007; 10:73-84.

[33] Endicott J, Spitzer RL. A diagnostic interview: the Schedule for Affective Disorders and Schizophrenia. *Arch Gen Psychiatry* 1978;*35, 837-844.*

[34] Fava GA, Rafanelli C, Grandi S, Conti S, Ruini C, Mangelli L, Belluardo P. Long-term outcome of panic disorder with agoraphobia treated by exposure. *Psychol Med* 2001; *31, 891-898.*

[35] Kellner R. Improvement criteria in drug trials with neurotic patients. Part 2. *Psychol Med* 1972; 2, 73-80.

[36] Paykel ES. The clinical interview for depression. *J Affect Disord* 1995; 9, 85-96.

[37] Fava GA, Grandi S, Belluardo P, Savron G, Raffi AR, Conti S, Saviotti FM. Benzodiapines and anxiety sensitivity in panic disorder. *Prog Neuropsychopharmacol Biol Psychiatry* 1994. 18, 1163-1168.

[38] Fux M, Taub M, Zohar J. Emergence of depressive symptoms during treatment for panic disorder with specific 5-hydroxytryptophan reuptake inhibitors. *Acta Psychiatr Scand* 1993;88: 235-237.

[39] Andrade C. Antidepressant-withdrawal mania. *J Clin Psychiatry* 2004; 65 ,987-993.

[40] Montgomery SA, Dunbar G. Paroxetine is better than placebo in relapse prevention and the prophylaxis of recurrent depression. *Int Clin Psychopharmacol* 1993;8, 189-195.

[41] Chaput Y, de Montigny C, Blier P. Effects of selective 5-HT reuptake blocker, citalopram, on the sensitivity of 5-HT autoreceptors: electrophysiological studies in the rat brain. *Naunyn Schmiedebergs Arch Pharmacol* 1986; 333:342-348.

[42] Blier P, de Montigny C. Modification of 5-HT neurons properties by sustained administration of 5-HT$_{1A}$ agonist gepirone: electrophysiological studies in the rat brain. *Synapse* 1987; 1:470-480.

[43] Schatzberg AF, Blier P, Delgado PL, Fava M, Haddad PM, Shelton RC. Antiderpessant discontinuation syndrome: Consensus panel recommendation for clinical management and additional research. *J Clin Psychiatry* 2006; 67:27-30.

[44] Blier P, Tremblay P. Physiologic mechanisms underlying the antidepressant discontinuation syndrome. *J Clin Psychiatry* 2006; 67:8-13.

[45] Szabo ST, de Montigny C, Blier P. Modulation of noradrenergic neuronal firing by selective serotonin reuptake blockers. *Br J Pharmacol* 1999; 126:568-571.

[46] Seager MA, Huff KD, Barth VN. Fluoxetine administration potentiates the effect of olanzapine on locus ceruleus neuronal activity. *Biol Psychiatry* 2004;55:1103-1109.

[47] Szabo ST, Blier P. Functional and pharmacological characterization of the modulatory role of serotonin on the firing activity of locus ceruleus norepinephrine neurons. *Brain Res* 2001; 922:9-20.

[48] Mucci M. Reboxetine: a review of antidepressant tolerability. *J Psychopharmacol* 1997; 11:S33-S37.

[49] Wernicke JF, Adler L, Spencer T et al. Changes in symptoms and adverse events after discontinuation of atomoxetine in children and adults with attention deficit/hyperactivity disorder: a prospective, placebo-controlled assessment. *J Clin Psychopharmacol.* 2004; 24:30-35.

[50] Owens MJ, Morgan WN, Plott SJ, et al. Neurotransitter receptor and transporter binding profile of antidepressants and their metabolites. *J Pharmnacol Exp Ther* 1997; 283:1305-1322.

[51] Harvey BH, McEwen BS, Stein DJ. Neurobiology of antidepressant withdrawal: Implications for the longitudinal outcome of depression. *Biol Psychiatr* 2003; 54:1105-1117.

[52] Harvey BH, Jonker LP, Brand L, Heenop M, Stein DJ. NMDA receptor involvement in imipramine withdrawal associated effects on swim stress, GABA levels and NMDA receptor binding in rat hippocampus. *Life Sci* 2002; 71:43-54.

[53] Fava GA. Can long term treatment with antidepressant drugs worsen the course of depression? *J Clin Psychiatry* 2003; 64. 123-133.

[54] Fava GA. Do antidepressant and anxiety drugs increase chronicity in affective disorders? *Psychother Psychosom* 1995; 63: 137-141.

[55] Baldessarini RJ. Risk and implications of interrupting maintenance psychotropic drug therapy. *Psychother Psychosom* 1995; 63: 137-141.

[56] Viguera AC, Baldessarini RJ, Friedberg J. Discontinuing antidepressant treatment in major depression. *Harvard Rev Psychiatry* 1998;5:293-306.

[57] Baldessarini RJ, Ghaemi SN, Viguera AC. Tolerance in antidepressant treatment. *Psychother Psychosom* 2002; 71: 177-179.

[58] Schmidt ME, Fava M, Zhang S, et al. Treatment approaches to major depressive disorder relapse. Part I: dose increase. *Psychother Psychosom* 2002; 71: 190-194.

[59] Brugha TS, Bebbington PE, MacCarthy B, et al. Antidepressants may not assist recovery in practice. *Acta Psychiatr Scand* 1992; 86: 5-11.

[60] Dawson R, Lavori PW, Coryell WN, et al. Maintenance strategies for unipolar depression. *J Affect Disord* 1998; 49: 31-44.

[61] Remherr FW, Amsterdam JD, Quitkin FM, et al. Optimal length of continuation therapy in depression. *Ann J Psychiatry* 1998; 155: 1247-1253.

[62] Stassen HH, Delini. Stula A, Angst J. Time course of improvement under antidepressant treatment. *Eur Neuropsychopharmacol* 1993;3:127-135.

[63] Baldwin RC. Antidepressants in geriatric depression: what difference have they made? *Int Psychogeriatrics* 1995; 7: 55-68.

[64] Kupfer DJ. Maintenance treatment in recurrent depression. *Br J Psychiatry* 1992; 161: 309-316.

[65] Di Mascio A, Meyer RE, Stifler L. Effects of imipramine on individuals varying in level of depression. *Am J Psychiatry* 1968; 127 (Supp.): 55-58.

[66] Van Scheyen JD. Recurrent vital depressions. *Psychiatr Neurol Neurochir* 1973; 76: 93-112.

[67] Healy D. Emergence of antidepressant induced suicidality. *Prim Care Psychiatry* 2000;6:23-28.

[68] Aronson TA. Treatment emergent depression with antidepressants in panic disorder. *Comp Psychiatry* 1989; 30: 267-271.

[69] Barlow DH, Gorman JM, Shear KM, et al. Cognitive-behavioral therapy, imipramine, or their combination for panic disorder. *JAMA* 2000;285:2529-2536.

[70] Brown TA, Barlow DH. Long-term outcome in cognitive behavioral treatment of panic disorder. *J. Consult Clin. Psychol.* 1995;63:754-765.

[71] Otto MW, Pollack MH, Sabatino SA. Maintenance of remission following cognitive behavior therapy for panic disorder. *Behav Therapy* 1996;27:473-482.

[72] Fava GA, Rafanelli C, Grandi S, et al. Long-term outcome of panic disorder with agoraphobia treated by exposure. *Psychol Med* 2001; 31: 891-898.

[73] Noyes R, Garvey HJ, Cook BL. Follow-up study of patients with panic disorder and agoraphobia with panic attacks treated with tricyclic antidepressants. *J Affect Disord* 1989;16:249-257.

[74] Molnar G, Gupta RN. Plasma levels and tricyclic antidepressant therapy. Biopharm *Drug Disposition* 1980; 1: 283-305.

[75] Cain JW. Poor response to fluoxetine. *J Clin Psychiatry* 1992; 53: 272-277.

[76] Fichtner CG, Jobe TH, Braun BG. Possible therapeutic window for serotonin reuptake inhibitors. *J Clin Psychiatry* 1994; 55: 36-37.

[77] Pitchot W, Gonzales-Moreno A, Ansseau M. Therapeutic window for 5-HT reuptake inhibitors. *Lancet* 1992; 339: 684.

[78] Fichtner CG, Jobe TH, Braun BG. Does fluoxetine have a therapeutic window? *Lancet* 1991; 338: 520-521.

[79] Benazzi F. A therapeutic window with citalopram in a case of depression. *Pharmacopsychiatry* 1996; 29: 42.

[80] Post RM, Denicoff KD, Leverich GS, et al. Drug-induced switching in bipolar disorder. *CNS Drugs* 1997; 8: 352-365.

[81] Angst J. Switch from depression to mania. A record study of decades between 1920 and 1982. *Psychopathology* 1985; 18: 140-155.

[82] Kukopulos A, Reginaldi D, Laddomada P, et al. Course of the manic-depressive cycle and changes caused by treatments. *Pharmakopsychiat* 1980; 13: 156-167.

[83] Kukopulos A, Caliari B, Tundo A, et al. Rapid cyclers, temperament, and antidepressants. *Comp Psychiatry* 1983; 24: 249-258.

[84] Perini GI, Fava GA, Morphy MA, et al. The metyrapone test in affective disorders and schizophrenia. Changes upon treatment. *J. Affect Disord* 1984;7:265-272.

[85] Goodwin FK. The biology of recurrence. *J. Clin. Psychiatry* 1989; 50 (12, Suppl.): 40-44.

[86] Byrne SE, Rothschild AJ. Loss of antidepressant efficacy during maintenance therapy. *J Clin Psychiatry* 1998; 59: 279-288.

[87] Cohen BM, Baldessarini RJ. Tolerance to therapeutic effects of antidepressants. *Am J Psychiatry* 1985; 142: 489-490.

[88] Fava M, Rappe SM, Pava JA, et al. Relapse in patients on long-term fluoxetine treatment: response to increased fluoxetine dose. *J. Clin. Psychiatry* 1995; 56: 52-55.

[89] Mann JJ. Loss of antidepressant effect with long term monoamine oxidase inhibition. *J. Clin. Psychopharmacol.* 1983; 3: 363-366.

[90] Lieb J, Balter A. Antidepressant tachyphylaxis. *Med. Hypotheses* 1984; 15: 279-291.

[91] Franchini L, Rossini S, Bongiorno F, et al. Will a second prophylactic treatment with a higher dosage of the same antidepressant either prevent or delay new depressive episodes? *Psychiatry Res* 2000; 96: 81-85.

[92] Frank E, Kupfer DJ, Perel JM, et al. Three-year outcomes for maintenance therapies in recurrent depression. *Arch Gen Psychiatry* 1990; 47: 1093-1099.

[93] Marks IM. Behavioral and drug treatments of phobic and obsessive-compulsive disorders. *Psychother Psychosom.* 1986; 46: 35-44.

[94] Fava GA. Fading of therapeutic effects of alprazolam in agoraphobia. *Progr. Neuropsychopharmacol Biol. Psychiatry* 1988; 12: 109-112.

[95] Fava GA. Do antidepressant and antianxiety drugs increase chronicity in affective disorders? *Psychother Psychosom* 1994; 61: 125-131.

[96] Post RM, Leverich GS, Altschuler L, et al. Lithium discontinuation-induced refractoriness. *Am J Psychiatry* 1992; 149: 1727-1729.

[97] Maj M, Pirozzi R, Magliano L. Non response to reinstituted lithium prophylaxis in previously responsive bipolar patients. *Am J Psychiatry* 1995; 152: 1810-1811.

[98] Faedda GL, Tondo L, Baldessarini RJ, et al. Outcome after rapid vs gradual discontinuation of lithium treatment in bipolar disorders. *Arch Gen Psychiatry* 1993; 50: 448-455.

[99] Coryell W, Solomon D, Leon AC, et al. Lithium discontinuation and subsequent effectiveness. *Am. J Psychiatry* 1998; 895-898.

[100] Fava GA, Rafanelli C, Grandi S, et al. Six-year outcome for cognitive behavioral treatment of residual symptoms in major depression. *Am. J Psychiatry* 1998; 155: 1443-1445.

[101] Friedman RA, Mitchell J, Kocsis JH. Retreatment for relapse following desipramine discontinuation in dysthymia. *Am. J Psychiatry* 1995; 152: 926-928.

[102] Donaldson SR. Tolerance to phenelzine and subsequent refractory depression. *J Clin Psychiatry* 1989; 50: 33-35.

[103] Fava M, Schmidt ME, Zhang S, et al. Treatment approaches to major depressive disorder relapse. Part II. Re-initiation of antidepressant treatment. *Psychother Psychosom* 2002; 71: 195-199.

[104] Maina G, Albert U, Bogetto F. Relapses after discontinuation of drug associated with increased resistance to treatment in obsessive-compulsive disorder. *Int Clin Psychopharmacol* 2001; 16: 33-38.

[105] Fava M, Davidson KG. Definition and epidemiology of treatment - resistant depression. *Psychiat Clin N Am* 1996; 19: 179-200.

[106] Rush AJ, Trivedi MH, Wisniewski SR, et al. Acute and longer-term outcomes in depressed outpatients requiring one or several treatment steps. *Am J Psychiatry* 2006;163:1905-1917.

[107] Fava M, Evins AE, Dorer DJ, Schoenfeld DD. The problem of the placebo response in clinical trials for psychiatric disorders. *Psychother Psychosom* 2003;72:115-127.

[108] Vieta E, Carnè X. The use of placebo in clinical trials on bipolar disorder. *Psychother Psychosom* 2005; 74:10-16.

[109] Gaudiano BA, Herbert JD. Methodological issues in clinical trials of antidepressant medications. *Psychother Psychosom.* 2005;74:17-25.

[110] Nelson JC. The STAR*D study: a four course meal that leaves us wanting more. *Am J Psychiatry* 2006;163:1864-1866.

[111] Posternak MA, Zimmerman M. Dual reuptake inhibitors incur lower rates of tachyphylaxis than selective serotonin reuptake inhibitors. *J Clin Psychiatry* 2005;66:704-707.

[112] Fava M, Rush AJ. Current states of augmentation and combination treatments for major depressive disorder. *Psychother Psychosom* 2006;75:139-153.

[113] Fava GA, Tomba E, Grandi S. The road to recovery from depression: don't drive today with the yesterday's map. *Psychother Psychosom* 2007;75:139-153.

[114] Leonard BE. Serotonin receptors and therir function in sleep, anxiety disorders and depression. *Psychother Psychosom* 1996;65:66-75.

[115] Barker MW, Croll RP. Modulation of in vivo neuronal sprouting by serotonin in the adult CNS of the snail. *Cell Mulecular Neurobiol* 1996; 16:561-576.

[116] Altamura C, Maes M, Dai J, Meltzer HY. Plasma concentration of excitatory amino acids, serine, glycine, taurine and histidine in major depression. *Eur Neuropsychopharmacol* 1995; 5: 71-75.

[117] Suzuki E, Yagi G, Nakaki T, Kamba S, Asai M. Elevated plasma nitrate levels in depressive states. *J Affect Disord* 2001; 63:221-224.

[118] Antelman SM, Gershon S. Clinical application of time dependent sensitization to antidepressant therapy. *Prog. Neuropsychopharmacol Biol Psychiatr* 1998; 22:65-78.

[119] Ritzmann RF, Colbern DL, Zimmermann EG. Neurohypophyseal hormones in tolerance and physical dependence. *Pharmacol Ther* 1984; 23:281-312.

[120] Van Praag HM. Faulty cortisol-serotonin interplay. *Psychoatr Res* 1996; 65:143-157.

[121] Stewart J, Badiani A. Tolerance and sensitization to the behavioral effects of drugs. *Behav Pharmacol* 1993; 4: 289-312.

[122] Editorial sparks debate on effects of psychoactive drugs. *Psychiatric News*, May 20,1994.

[123] Otto MW, Nierenberg AA. Assay sensitivity, failed trials, and the conduct of science. *Psychother Psychoso.* 2002; 71: 241-243.

[124] Fava GA. The concept of recovery in affective disorders. *Psychother Psychosom* 1996;65:2-13.

[125] Benazzi F. Suicidal ideation and depressive mixed states. *Psychother Psychosom* 2005; 74, 61-62.

In: Substance Withdrawal Syndrome
Editors: J. P. Rees and O. B. Woodhouse

ISBN 978-1-60692-951-3
© 2009 Nova Science Publishers, Inc.

Chapter III

Benzodiazepine Withdrawal Syndrome and Strategies for Discontinuing Benzodiazepine Use: Appropriate Treatment with SSRIs and SNRIs

Mutsuhiro Nakao*, Kyoko Nomura and Takeaki Takeuchi
Department of Hygiene and Public Health,
Teikyo University School of Medicine and Division of Psychosomatic Medicine,
Teikyo University Hospital, Tokyo, Japan

Abstract

Although benzodiazepines are among the most commonly prescribed medications, owing to their roles in multiple areas of therapeutic action as anxiolytics, sedative hypnotics, anticonvulsants and muscle relaxants, they are also highly addictive. Long-term use can lead to dependency, rebound anxiety, memory impairment, and withdrawal. Excessive prescription of benzodiazepines has emerged as a major clinical issue in Japan. The number of people taking these medications has been increasing, and the costs associated with benzodiazepine use are substantial. In our recent study, we showed that a minimal dose of a selective serotonin reuptake inhibitor (SSRI) increased the success rate of a benzodiazepine discontinuation program among chronic benzodiazepine users, without association with major depression. Ten subjects (45.5%) in the SSRI-assisted benzodiazepine-reduction group (n = 22) succeeded in becoming benzodiazepine-free after completing the program, whereas only four (17.4%) in the simple benzodiazepine-reduction group (n = 23) succeeded. SSRI use significantly predicted the success of becoming benzodiazepine-free (P = 0.023), controlling for the effects of age, sex, duration of benzodiazepine use, and baseline scores on the Hamilton Rating Scales for Depression and Anxiety. However, the SSRI itself might cause a withdrawal syndrome;

---
* Address for reprints: Mutsuhiro Nakao, M.D. Department of Hygiene and Public Health, Teikyo University School of Medicine, 2-11-1, Itabashi, Tokyo 173-8605, Japan, Tel: +81-3-3964-1058 Ext 2175; Fax: +81-3-3964-1058; E-mail: mnakao@med.teikyo-u.ac.jp

indeed, one participant who received a minimal dose of SSRI suffered from SSRI withdrawal syndrome after changing to a tricyclic antidepressant. Benzodiazepines are much more frequently prescribed in Japanese hospitals and clinics than SSRIs and serotonin and noradrenaline reuptake inhibitors (SNRIs), especially among physicians practicing internal medicine. For example, among the 644,444 prescriptions emanating from our university hospital in 1 year, 76,563 (11.9%) ordered benzodiazepines and 10,627 (1.6%) ordered SSRIs and SNRIs. Although future studies should collect multi-institutional data, the dissemination of relevant medical knowledge to internists and primary care physicians about the clinical issues accompanying benzodiazepine use and the suggested alternative medications, such as SSRIs, represents one public health approach to this imbalance between benzodiazepine and SSRI/SNRI prescriptions. In this paper, we discuss the difficulties attending benzodiazepine withdrawal and the appropriate use of benzodiazepines, SSRIs, or SNRIs, as demonstrated in our clinical studies.

Introduction

Although benzodiazepines are among the most commonly prescribed medications because of their diverse therapeutic roles (i.e., they are prescribed as anxiolytics, sedative hypnotics, anticonvulsants, and muscle relaxants), long-term use can lead to dependency, rebound anxiety, memory impairment, and withdrawal [1]. Currently, selective serotonin reuptake inhibitors (SSRIs) and serotonin and noradrenaline reuptake inhibitors (SNRIs) are suggested as first-line treatments for depression [2] and for various anxiety disorders, including panic disorders [3]. For example, the Royal College of Psychiatrists [4] recommended that the prescription of benzodiazepines be limited to cases of depression characterized by severe irritability.

A substantial proportion of chronic benzodiazepine users, in both psychiatric departments and internal medicine and other hospital departments, suffer from depression [5,6]. Although a single prescription of benzodiazepines may be unsuitable or inadequate for patients with depression, benzodiazepine prescriptions could be supplanted or reduced in the absence of severe depression, since their long-term use carries risks for dependency, rebound anxiety, memory impairment, and withdrawal [7,8]. Many clinicians, especially primary care physicians, have experienced the difficulty of reducing benzodiazepine prescriptions for chronic users. Benzodiazepines are associated with a characteristic discontinuation syndrome consisting of three types of symptoms: recurrence, rebound, and withdrawal [9]. Recurrence represents a gradual return of the original symptoms at their pretreatment intensity. Rebound represents a rapid return of the original symptoms, but in more severe form than before treatment. Withdrawal refers to symptoms that were not present before treatment, and that follow abrupt discontinuation [1]. New symptoms observed during benzodiazepine withdrawal include dysphoria, depersonalization, appetite loss, headaches, muscle aches and twitches, nausea, tremor, and sleep and perceptual disturbances such as metallic tastes, paresthesias, and hypersensitivity to light, sound, touch, and smell [9].

According to the Diagnostic and Statistical Manual of Mental Disorders, Fourth Edition, Text Revision (DSM-IV-TR) [10], the essential feature of sedative, hypnotic, or anxiolytic withdrawal is the presence of a characteristic syndrome that develops after a marked decrease in or cessation of intake after several weeks or more of regular use (Table 1).

Table 1. The DSM-IV-TR criteria for sedative, hypnotic, or anxiolytic withdrawal [10]

A. Cessation of (or reduction in) sedative, hypnotic, or anxiolytic use that has been heavy and prolonged.

B. Two (or more) of the following, developing within several hours to a few days after Criterion A:
   (1) autonomic hyperactivity (e.g., sweating or pulse rate greater than 100)
   (2) increased hand tremor
   (3) insomnia
   (4) nausea or vomiting
   (5) transient visual, tactile, or auditory hallucinations or delusions
   (6) psychomotor agitation
   (7) anxiety
   (8) grand mal seizure

C. The symptoms in Criterion B cause clinically significant distress or impairment in social, occupational, or other important areas of functioning.

D. The symptoms are not due to a general medical condition and are not better accounted for by another mental disorder.

Specify if:

With perceptual disturbances

The time course of the withdrawal syndrome is generally predicted by the half-life of benzodiazepine medications; these typically last approximately 10 hours or less (e.g., lorazepam, oxazepam, and temazepam), and produce withdrawal symptoms within 6 to 8 hours of decreasing blood levels.

Such symptoms tend to peak in intensity on the second day and improve markedly by the fourth or fifth day. Withdrawal from benzodiazepines with longer half-lives (e.g., diazepam) may be characterized by symptoms that are delayed for more than a week, peak in intensity during the second week, and decrease markedly during the third or fourth week. Additional longer-term symptoms, at a much lower levels of intensity, may persist for several months.

Several psychometric evaluations of benzodiazepine withdrawal symptoms have been developed, including the Clinical Institute Withdrawal Assessment—Benzodiazepines [11], Physician Withdrawal Checklist [12], and Benzodiazepine Withdrawal Symptom Questionnaire [13]. For example, items on the Benzodiazepine Withdrawal Symptom Questionnaire are shown in Table 2.

According to a previous study on a benzodiazepine discontinuation program [14], reliability coefficients during the program fell between 0.84 and 0.88, and test–retest correlations fell between 0.75 and 0.88 during withdrawal. It is important to assess benzodiazepine withdrawal symptoms as objectively as possible in order to establish a standardized benzodiazepine discontinuation program that can be applied in daily clinical practice.

Table 2. Twenty items on the Benzodiazepine withdrawal symptom questionnaire [13]

1. Feeling unreal 2. Very sensitive to noise 3. Very sensitive to light 4. Very sensitive to smell 5. Very sensitive to touch 6. Peculiar taste in mouth 7. Pains in muscle 8. Muscle twitching 9. Shaking or trembling 10. Pins and needles 11. Dizziness 12. Feeling faint 13. Feeling sick 14. Feeling depressed 15. Sore eyes 16. Feeling of things moving 17. Hallucinations 18. Inability to control movements 19. Loss of memory 20. Loss of appetite

Benzodiazepine Issues in Japan

Excessive prescription of benzodiazepines represents an important clinical and economic issue in Japan. Annual sales of etizolam, the most commonly prescribed benzodiazepine in Japan, totaled approximately $100 million in 2007, equaling the sales of diltiazepam, a commonly used calcium channel blocker [15].

The Japanese people are known to have high thresholds for visiting psychiatric clinics [16], and approximately 60–70% of patients with depression visit internal medicine clinics rather than psychiatry clinics at their first presentation [17]. For example, our recent study found that the prevalence of the DSM-IV diagnosis of major depression was 32% among chronic benzodiazepine users visiting internal medicine clinics [18]. Five years have elapsed since two SSRIs (fluvoxamine and paroxetine) and one SNRI (milnacipran) were approved for use in Japan. Therefore, it is reasonable to assume that some internists may overprescribe benzodiazepines for patients who may potentially have depression when they could be prescribing SSRIs, SNRIs, or other antidepressants [19]. Although the data are not optimally current [20], note that the number of prescriptions for anxiolytic benzodiazepines in response to neurotic disorders was estimated to be higher in Japan (15–18 million prescriptions per year) than in the United States (8–10 million) between 2000 and 2002, even though the number of prescriptions for antidepressants for such disorders was much higher in the United States (9–12 million) than in Japan (1.8–2.1 million) during the same period.

The Teikyo University Hospital has recently installed a computer ordering system that has enabled us to count the number of drug prescriptions in the hospital. Thus, using these data, we identified the trends characterizing the benzodiazepine prescription practices of various medical specialists. In addition, benzodiazepine prescriptions were compared with prescriptions for SSRIs, SNRIs, and other antidepressants in terms of the department membership of the prescribing physicians in order to examine the reasoning behind prescribing benzodiazepines, especially among nonpsychiatrists [6,19].

Study 1: Benzodiazepine Prescription in a Hospital

The university hospital, located in the Tokyo metropolitan area, is visited by approximately 600,000 outpatients per year. For purposes of analysis, 21 departments within the hospital were categorized into five groups according to the relationship of each department to a psychological speciality. The departments included internal medicine (general internal medicine and the renal disease center), surgery (general surgery, brain surgery, cardiac surgery, orthopedics, plastic surgery, obstetrics and gynecology, ophthalmology, otorhinolaryngology, dermatology, urology, oral surgery, and anesthesia), neurology (neurology), psychiatry (general psychiatry and psychosomatic medicine), and other groups (pediatrics, rehabilitation, radiology, and emergency medicine). The study was approved by the university ethics committee and was conducted between September 1, 2002 and August 31, 2003.

In total, 20 types of benzodiazepines are registered for prescription in Japan. These consist of 11 anxiolytic benzodiazepines (alprazolam, bromazepam, clotiazepam, cloxazolam, diazepam, ethyl loflazepate, etizolam, lorazepam, medazepam, oxazolam, and tofisopam) and nine hypnotic benzodiazepines (brotizolam, estazolam, flunitrazepam, flurazepam, lormetazepam, nitrazepam, quazepam, rilmazafone hydrochloride, and triazolam). Although etizolam was approved as both an anxiolytic and a hypnotic benzodiazepine by the Japanese Ministry of Health, Labor and Welfare, etizolam was classified as an anxiolytic benzodiazepine for analysis in this study. Two SSRIs and one SNRI were registered for prescription in the target hospital.

The data were analyzed using the SAS Statistical Package [21]. A ratio of the number of anxiolytic benzodiazepines prescribed (excluding hypnotic benzodiazepines) relative to that of SSRIs and SNRIs prescribed (B/S ratio) was calculated to estimate the number of outpatients who could potentially change from treatment with benzodiazepines to treatment with SSRIs or SNRIs. The B/S ratio was compared among the departments. We excluded prescriptions for anxiolytic benzodiazepines, made only once as a hypnotic or a premedication agent, because such a situation lacks the potential for addiction.

Results showed that prescriptions for benzodiazepines, and for SSRIs or SNRIs, comprised 11.9 and 1.6% of the total number of prescriptions, respectively (Table 3). Among 76,563 benzodiazepine prescriptions, 31,630 (41.3%) were ordered for men. The mean age (standard deviation) of patients prescribed benzodiazepines was 55.4 ($\pm$17.8) years.

The total number of outpatients who received prescriptions for anxiolytic benzodiazepines was 4,454. Among the total sample of outpatients, 2,503 (56.2%) received anxiolytic benzodiazepines four or more times, and 317 (7.1%), 782 (17.6%), and 852 (19.1%) received anxiolytic benzodiazepines three times, twice, and once, respectively. Excluding the data from the 852 outpatients receiving anxiolytic benzodiazepines once, the B/S ratio for all hospital departments was 3.71. The internal medicine department had the highest B/S ratio, five times that of the psychiatry department (Figure 1).

Implications of study 1

Benzodiazepine prescription varied greatly among different departments. Specifically, the numbers of anxiolytic benzodiazepine and SSRI (SNRI) prescriptions written by the internal medicine group were about half and one-tenth less than the numbers written by the psychiatry group, respectively, resulting in a large difference in the B/S ratio between the internal medicine and psychiatry departments.

Table 3. Annual prescriptions of benzodiazepines, SSRIs, and a SNRI in departments of a Japanese university hospital

Department group (annual prescription)	Benzodiazepine, n (%)		Antidepressants, n (%)	
	All	Anxiolytics	All	SSRIs and a SNRI
Internal medicine (n = 256,368)	20,495 (27)	9,975 (25)	2,737 (10)	767 (7)
Surgery and related (n = 180,911)	8,932 (12)	4,574 (12)	2,599 (10)	606 (6)
Neurology (n = 23,816)	2,812 (4)	1,627 (4)	695 (3)	337 (3)
Psychiatry (n = 129,538)	43,268 (56)	22,518 (57)	20,046 (75)	8,715 (82)
Others (n = 53,811)	1,056 (1)	769 (2)	542 (2)	202 (2)
Total (n = 644,444)	76,563 (100)	39,463 (100)	26,619 (100)	10,627 (100)

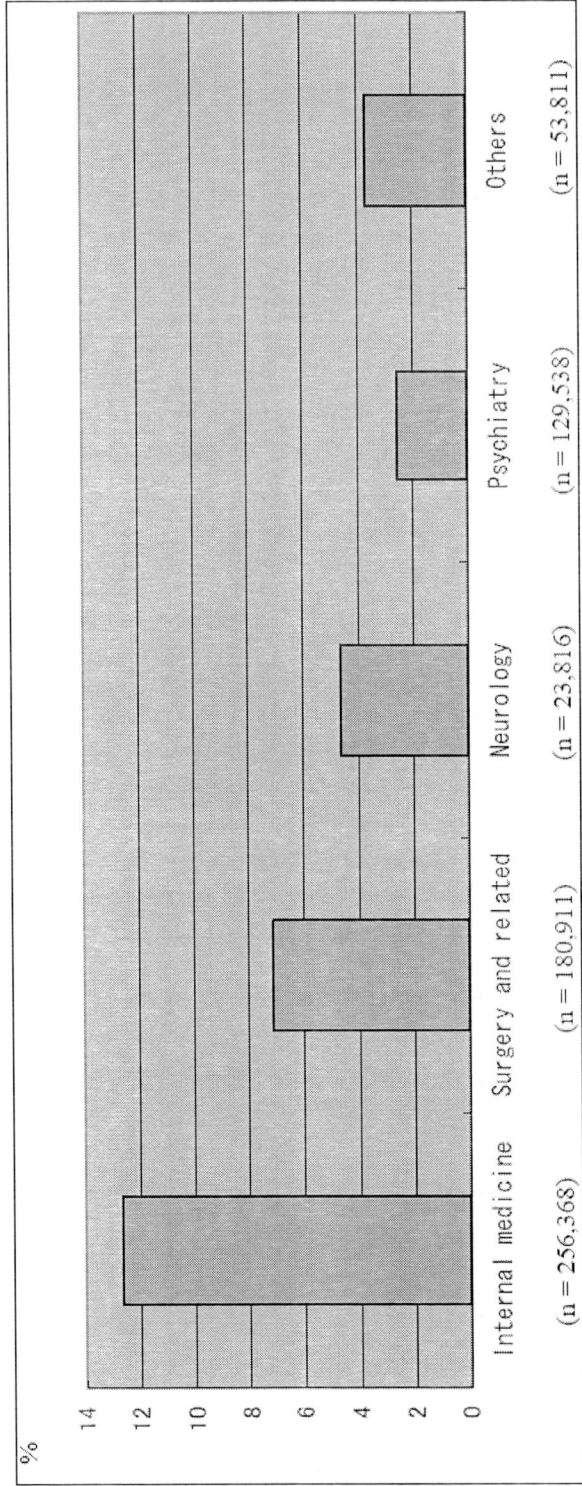

Figure 1. Prescription ratios of anxiolytic benzodiazepines to SSRIs or a SNRI (B/S ratio) in departments of a Japanese university hospital.

Although our results were based on data obtained from a single hospital, they suggest that a substantial proportion of outpatients who visited internists might have been treated inappropriately with benzodiazepines.

This study is limited by the possibility that prescriptions for anxiolytic benzodiazepines as premedications or as myorelaxing agents might have been included in the prescriptions emanating from the surgery and internal medicine departments. Although this point should be kept in mind when interpreting our results, we nevertheless controlled for this by excluding those prescriptions for anxiolytic benzodiazepines that were given only once. Second, we could not compare our data with those obtained from other medical institutions in Japan because this study represents the first of its type in Japan. Further studies of other Japanese institutions and of hospitals in other countries are required before any generalizations of our conclusions can be offered. Finally, since relevant diagnostic information was unavailable in our computer system, we used the number of prescriptions for antidepressants to determine the prevalence of depression-related conditions. However, the possibility still exists that visits to the internal medicine department were precipitated by psychological problems other than depression, whereas only patients with severe depression visited the psychiatry department [22–24]. Future studies should provide more definitive diagnostic information.

We reanalyzed the diagnostic information for all inpatients at the same hospital in order to address this diagnostic issue. The study population included 21,489 adult inpatients, aged 18 years or older, admitted between April 1, 2005 and December 31, 2006. We analyzed the first of the two ICD-10 diagnoses recorded by the attending physicians. Patients were divided into two groups according to benzodiazepine use: the benzodiazepine (+) group consisted of patients who had been treated with benzodiazepines during hospitalization, and the benzodiazepine (–) consisted of patients who had not received benzodiazepine treatment during hospitalization. Benzodiazepine treatment was most common among patients diagnosed with chronic renal failure (N18, 31.3%), followed by heart failure (I50, 29.3%), acute myocardial infarction (I21, 28.9%), malignant neoplasm of the liver and intrahepatic bile ducts (C22, 28.0%), postprocedural disorders of the nervous system (G97, 28.0%), malignant neoplasm of the bronchus and lung (C34, 27.7%), non-insulin-dependent diabetes mellitus (E11, 25.0%), and malignant neoplasm of the bladder (C67, 22.2%) (Table 4).

In summary, although future studies are still required to determine more precisely the causes of the high B/S ratio in Japanese hospitals, education of internists and primary care physicians about the use of SSRIs and SNRIs would seem to represent a promising public health strategy for preventing excessive prescription of benzodiazepines in Japan.

Strategies for Benzodiazepine Withdrawal

The results of study 1 suggest that the use of benzodiazepines is quite common among internal medicine and other nonpsychiatric practitioners. It is essential to educate clinicians not only about appropriate prescription protocols for benzodiazepines, but also about appropriate titrating protocols for chronic benzodiazepine users. Although several studies [25–27] have shown that tricyclic antidepressants and other psychotropic agents have some effectiveness in the treatment of benzodiazepine withdrawal, the advisability of using SSRIs for treating benzodiazepine withdrawal remains ambiguous.

Table 4. Prevalence of benzodiazepine prescriptions in 21,489 inpatients

Variables	N	% of Benzodiazepine (+)
Age, years		
18–44	5,023	14.0
45–64	6,028	19.8
65–74	5,355	22.7
75	5,083	23.0
Sex		
Men	11,844	18.6
Women	9,645	21.6
Major departments		
General internal medicine	6,811	23.7
General surgery	3,394	24.1
Ophthalmology	2,139	6.5
Urology	1,760	13.8
Obstetrics and gynecology	1,532	10.8
Orthopedics	1,378	26.3
Otorhinolaryngology	1,371	19.3
Neurosurgery	901	20.3
Emergency medicine	752	14.2
Neurology	520	35.8
Major ICD-10 diseases		
Neoplasms (C00-D48)	5,321	23.3
Circulatory diseases (I00-I99)	3,221	22.2
Eye diseases (H00-H59)	2,094	7.0
Digestive diseases (K00-K93)	1,883	18.0
Respiratory diseases (J00-J99)	1,188	18.6
Genitourinary diseases (N00-N99)	1,141	17.5
Nervous system diseases (G00-G99)	931	27.3
Musculoskeletal diseases (M00-M99)	859	28.6
Obstetrical diseases (O00-O99)	791	5.9
Endocrine diseases (E00-E90)	699	24.0

The Dutch Chronic Benzodiazepine Working Group [28] studied chronic benzodiazepine users diagnosed with major depression who attended a benzodiazepine discontinuation program in the primary care setting. They reported that the use of paroxetine, an SSRI, was of limited value in discontinuing chronic benzodiazepine use [28]. The absence of a positive relationship between SSRI treatment and benzodiazepine tapering could derive from the sample consisting of patients with major depression who had been treated previously with SSRI. If nondepressed patients had attended a benzodiazepine discontinuation program that included SSRI treatment from the beginning of the intervention, different results might emerge.

Thus, we hypothesized that a minimal dose of paroxetine would increase the success rate of a benzodiazepine discontinuation program attended by chronic benzodiazepine users without diagnoses of major depression. To test this hypothesis, outpatients without diagnoses of major depression were randomly assigned to one of three groups: the first group attended a standardized benzodiazepine discontinuation program that included treatment with paroxetine, a comparable group attended the program but were not treated with paroxetine, and a control group did not attend the program or receive paroxetine [18,29].

Study 2: Benzodiazepine Withdrawal Using SSRI

The sample included 97 outpatients (63 women and 34 men) who were consecutively treated at the Internal Medicine Clinic at Teikyo University Hospital in Tokyo. None of the patients had been treated with SSRI, and none was currently undergoing psychiatric treatment. The subject selection criteria were as follows: 20 to 70 years of age; stable medical conditions and drug regimens (i.e., no changes in the latter for more than 3 months); use of either alprazolam, bromazepam, etizolam, or lorazepam for at least 3 months prior to visiting the clinic; and ability to participate in an 8-week intervention (or control). The four benzodiazepines listed in criterion 3 were selected because of their widespread use in the hospital, and because as high-potency benzodiazepines with short durations of action, they are more likely to cause benzodiazepine abuse and dependency. The content of the study, including written information on the study protocol, was explained to all candidate participants; only those who provided written consent were included in the study. The study protocol was approved by the university ethics committee. A total of 101 patients met the criteria but four (4.0%) did not visit the clinic on their appointed day, and thus 97 patients were evaluated according to the study protocol.

Structured clinical interviews for DSM-IV Axis I disorders (SCID-I) were conducted to identify major depression [30] and comorbid anxiety disorders [30,31]. The Hamilton Rating Scale for Depression (HAM-D), as well as the Hamilton Rating Scale for Anxiety (HAM-A), were administered to all patients after the interview [32,33] to confirm the severity of depression and anxiety. Quality of life was assessed by the 36-item Short-Form Health Survey (SF-36), which is a self-report questionnaire consisting of eight subscales representing physical functioning, physical roles, body pain, general health perceptions, vitality, social functioning, emotional roles, and mental health [34].

Following the SCID-I assessments, 31 outpatients (32%) diagnosed with major depression were excluded; the remaining 66 were selected to participate in the study. The clinical characteristics of outpatients with and without major depression are shown in Table 5. The nondepressed group was composed of 44 women (67%) and were diagnosed according to ICD-10 criteria by the internal medicine clinic with hypertension (n = 15), diabetes mellitus (n = 10), premature ventricular contraction (n = 5), angina pectoris (n = 5), hyperlipidemia (n = 4), and other (n = 27). Participants without major depression were randomly assigned to one of three groups: the SSRI-assisted benzodiazepine-reduction group [10–20 mg of paroxetine, SSRI (+) group], the simple benzodiazepine-reduction group [no paroxetine, SSRI (–) group], or the no benzodiazepine-reduction group (control group). The SSRI (–) group did not receive a placebo.

Table 5. Comparisons between 31 chronic benzodiazepine users with major depression and 66 without depression

	Major depression (+)	Non-depressed (–)	P values[a]
Age, years	56.9 (9.9)	58.5 (8.4)	0.411
Disease period, months	96.7 (77.8)	132.0 (79.9)	0.044
Benzodiazepine use period, months	62.3 (35.9)	72.4 (49.4)	0.311
Hamilton Depression Scale, scores	19.5 (7.0)	7.4 (5.8)	<0.001
Hamilton Anxiety Scale, scores	15.9 (9.3)	6.9 (8.3)	<0.001
Short-Form-36 (SF-36), scores			
Physical functioning	69.7 (32.5)	79.5 (26.1)	0.115
Role, physical	65.6 (35.2)	75.9 (35.0)	0.181
Bodily pain	57.8 (31.4)	79.2 (23.4)	<0.001
General health perception	27.7 (20.0)	39.1 (20.9)	0.013
Vitality	38.4 (18.7)	56.7 (17.1)	<0.001
Social functioning	66.7 (31.2)	72.1 (26.7)	0.381
Role, emotional	48.1 (44.6)	68.5 (40.0)	0.026
Mental health	54.2 (19.7)	69.1 (18.3)	<0.001

[a] Student's *t*-test (two-tailed) was used for group comparisons.

The control group was included to examine whether those in the two treatment groups showed greater exacerbations of depression and anxiety than those without treatment. Both the HAM-D and the HAM-A, as well as the Benzodiazepine Withdrawal Symptom Questionnaire [13] consisting of 20 items with a 5-point scale, were administered at weeks 0 (baseline), 1, 2, 4, and 8 to subjects in the two benzodiazepine-reduction groups.

Subjects in the two benzodiazepine-reduction groups participated in an 8-week program involving gradual benzodiazepine discontinuation. This program represented a modified version of the program used in a previous Dutch study [28] (Table 6). The period of benzodiazepine tapering was prolonged to 8 weeks to minimize the number of participants dropping out due to rapid withdrawal.

Table 6. Benzodiazepine discontinuation program

Stage 0:	No benzodiazepine tapering
Stage 1:	Benzodiazepine tapering by 25%
Stage 2:	Benzodiazepine tapering by 50%
Stage 3:	Benzodiazepine tapering by 75%
Stage 4:	Free of benzodiazepine

Baseline   Start tapering off from Stage 1

Week 1	Continue Stage 1 when judged successful or go back to Stage 0 when unsuccessful
	(Go to Stage 0 or <u>1</u>)
Week 2	Step up by one stage when judged successful or stay in the same stage
	(Go to Stage 0, 1, or <u>2</u>)
Week 4	Step up by one stage when judged successful or stay in the same stage
	(Go to Stage 0, 1, 2, or <u>3</u>)
Week 8	Step up by one stage when judged successful or stay in the same stage
	(Go to Stage 0, 1, 2, 3, or <u>4</u>)

Underlined step indicates that benzodiazepine discontinuation is completely successful.

Table 7. Comparisons of benzodiazepine reduction during the study period

	Intervention period				
Classification of reduction, n (%)	Baseline	1 week	2 weeks	4 weeks	8 weeks[a]
SSRI[b] (+) group (n = 22):					
Stage 0 (full dose of benzodiazepine)	22 (100)	7 (31.8)	2 (9.1)	1 (4.6)	1 (4.6)
Stage 1 (25% taper)	-	15 (68.2)	7 (31.8)	2 (9.1)	0 (0)
Stage 2 (50% taper)	-	-	13 (59.0)	7 (31.8)	3 (13.6)
Stage 3 (75% taper)	-	-	-	12 (54.5)	8 (36.4)
Stage 4 (benzodiazepine free)	-	-	-	-	10 (45.5)
SSRI (–) group (n = 23):					
Stage 0 (full dose of benzodiazepine)	23 (100)	4 (17.4)	4 (17.4)	2 (8.7)	1 (4.4)
Stage 1 (25% taper)	-	19 (82.6)	7 (30.4)	7 (30.4)	4 (17.4)
Stage 2 (50% taper)	-	-	12 (52.2)	9 (39.1)	10 (43.5)
Stage 3 (75% taper)	-	-	-	5 (21.7)	4 (17.4)
Stage 4 (benzodiazepine free)	-	-	-	-	4 (17.4)

[a] P = 0.003 compared to the SSRI (–) group (Wilcoxon's rank-sum test).
[b] SSRI, selective serotonin reuptake inhibitor.

Upon increases of more than 10% in any of the scores on the Benzodiazepine Withdrawal Scale, HAM-D, or HAM-A, subjects were interviewed in detail by the research physician and held at their current taper level. Reduction in benzodiazepine use for more than 5 days per week was regarded as successful tapering-off; this definition allowed participants to revert to previous benzodiazepine doses during 2 days per week. Patients regarded as successful moved through the stages at the appropriate pace (i.e., those classified as stage one at the 1-week assessment moved to stage two at 2 weeks, to stage three at 4 weeks, and to stage four at 8 weeks). All the patients in the SSRI (+) group started with 10 mg of paroxetine at the beginning of the program. If subjects failed to move to the next stage at the two consecutive assessments, they were asked to increase their dose of paroxetine by 10 mg (this increased dose was given only to those who agreed). During the entire 8-week study protocol, each participant was consistently assessed by one of three research physicians who specialized in both psychiatry and internal medicine and practiced under the continuous supervision of a physician-in-charge. After completion of the program, each participant was returned to the care of the physician-in-charge, with the exception of those choosing to continue treatment with the research physicians.

All analyses were performed using the SAS statistical package [22]. A P value of <0.05 was set as the threshold for significance. Wilcoxon's rank-sum test was used to compare the progress between the two benzodiazepine-reduction groups after completion of the 8-week program with regard to benzodiazepine tapering, across steps 0–4, in relation to the effects of paroxetine. Following this, a multiple logistic regression analysis was conducted to examine the independent effects of SSRI assistance [SSRI (+) group or SSRI (–) group] on achieving benzodiazepine-free status after program completion, controlling for the effects of age, sex, length of treatment at the internal medicine clinic, duration of benzodiazepine use, and HAM-D and HAM-A scores at baseline. The degree of change between baseline and 8-week assessment in the scores on the three questionnaires (HAM-D, HAM-A, and Benzodiazepine Withdrawal Symptom Questionnaire) was estimated; one-way analysis of variance was used for group comparisons.

The sample consisted of 22 of the 66 nondepressed patients in the SSRI (+) group, 23 in the SSRI (–) group, and 21 in the control group. The results of the benzodiazepine discontinuation program within the two benzodiazepine-reduction groups are shown in Table 7. At the 1-week assessment, seven patients in the SSRI (+) group had not followed the drug regimen for tapering benzodiazepine use; three of these failed to follow the regimen due to the side effects of paroxetine (two experienced nausea and one experienced headaches). As a result, one patient did not reduce benzodiazepine intake or take the 10-mg dose of paroxetine during the program; this participant was placed at stage 0 in all of the assessments. Of the remaining 21 patients in the SSRI (+) group, 15 continued at 10 mg of paroxetine during the program, four were given 10 mg for the first 2 weeks and 20 mg for the remaining 6 weeks, and two were given 10 mg for the first 4 weeks and 20 mg for the final 4 weeks. At baseline, 4-week, and 8-week assessments, no significant differences were observed in the scores on the Benzodiazepine Withdrawal Symptom Questionnaire, the HAM-D scores, and HAM-A scores among the three groups (Table 8).

Table 8. Group comparison of changes in withdrawal symptoms, depression, and anxiety in those without major depression

Means (standard deviations)	Benzodiazepine reduction groups		No benzodiazepine reduction	
	SSRI (+) (n = 22)	SSRI (–) (n = 23)	controls (n = 21)	P values[a]
Benzodiazepine Withdrawal Symptom Scale, scores				
Baseline	26.4 (3.7)	24.1 (3.5)	25.7 (7.4)	-
Differences, 4 weeks	–2.3 (3.2)	1.1 (3.9)	–0.6 (4.7)	N.S.
Differences, 8 weeks	–2.7 (3.4)	0.4 (3.9)	–2.0 (2.4)	N.S.
Hamilton Rating Scale for Depression, scores				
Baseline	8.8 (6.8)	5.6 (3.4)	7.9 (6.6)	-
Differences, 4 weeks	–2.7 (6.2)	1.0 (3.3)	8.4 (8.0)	N.S.
Differences, 8 weeks	–2.3 (5.2)	0.9 (3.2)	8.7 (7.2)	N.S.
Hamilton Rating Scale for Anxiety, scores				
Baseline	10.1 (9.2)	7.7 (6.8)	9.0 (9.1)	-
Differences, 4 weeks	–1.6 (4.3)	4.3 (5.3)	3.8 (9.9)	N.S.
Differences, 8 weeks	–0.5 (9.7)	4.7 (6.2)	–0.7 (6.4)	N.S.

[a] Analysis of variance was used for group comparisons. N.S. means "not significant (P > 0.05)."

At the 8-week assessment, 45% of the patients in the SSRI (+) group were successful, as compared to 17% in the SSRI (–) group. The results of multiple logistic regression analysis indicated that the use of SSRIs significantly contributed to the success of becoming benzodiazepine-free after program completion [odds ratio (95% confidence intervals): 6.09 (1.14–32.49), P = 0.023], controlling for the effects of age, sex, duration of benzodiazepine use, length of treatment at the internal medicine clinic, and HAM-D and HAM-A scores at baseline.

Implications of Study 2

We conducted a standardized benzodiazepine discontinuation program among patients without major depression. The proportion of patients (45%) who discontinued benzodiazepine use was significantly higher in the SSRI (+) group than in the SSRI (–) group. These results are noteworthy because the previous Dutch study [28] concluded that paroxetine is of limited value in gradual benzodiazepine withdrawal during a benzodiazepine discontinuation program. Our findings are additionally noteworthy because the higher success rates in the SSRI (+) group were achieved in the absence of deterioration in the scores obtained by this group on the Benzodiazepine Withdrawal Symptom Questionnaire, and the HAM-D, and HAM-A, as compared to those obtained by the SSRI (–) group.

In this study, major depression was observed in 32.0% of the chronic benzodiazepine users treated by the internists. This incidence of major depression appears to be high in comparison with that found in two of our previous studies (both n > 1,000). The latter reported that the prevalence of major depression, as assessed through the same DSM-IV interviews, was 4.0–4.5% in a sample of Japanese patients visiting a psychosomatic medicine clinic [35,36] and 2.5–3.0% in a sample of Japanese workers [37,38]. Affective and cognitive symptoms of depression may not be readily observable, at least in some cases, during visits to internal medicine clinics [39,40], and it may be difficult for internists to identify "masked depression" [41].

This study has limitations deriving from its design as a non-blinded randomized controlled trial, and thus the data must be interpreted with caution. We avoided adopting a sham treatment using placebo tablets of paroxetine because of ethical considerations [42]. Although we obtained promising findings based on daily clinical practice, the nature of the non-blinded study design requires future research to consider the possible effects of variability in both physician factors (e.g., the fluency of instructions for treatment) and patient factors (e.g., the willingness to accept instructions) [43].

In summary, we showed that a minimal dosage of paroxetine might facilitate the discontinuation of chronic benzodiazepine use among outpatients visiting an internal medicine clinic. Confirmation of these results at other institutions, taking into account the factors not controlled in the present study, represents an important next step for research in this area. A follow-up study is also required to confirm the long-term anxiolytic effect of SSRIs after the successful completion of a benzodiazepine discontinuation program.

The Possibility of SSRI Withdrawal Syndrome

On the basis of the results of study 2, we suggest that SSRI treatment might facilitate benzodiazepine withdrawal. SSRIs have been available in the Japanese pharmaceutical market for nearly 10 years, and this class of medications now plays a central role in pharmacotherapy for depression. However, we must remain alert to the possibility that SSRIs themselves can cause a withdrawal syndrome [44–47].

For example, a 26 year-old Japanese man diagnosed with depression suffered from agitated and irritable symptoms, especially in response to noise, 3 to 4 days after his medication was changed from paroxetine 10 mg (duration of 4 months) to amitriptyline 50 mg for financial reasons [48]. At first, SSRI discontinuation syndrome was not diagnosed because the clinical symptoms were masked by symptoms associated with depression (e.g., irritability, nausea, and headache). Although the impulsiveness and agitation soon disappeared, this patient remained highly confused and annoyed by the sudden onset of the syndrome and came to distrust the physician responsible for this treatment. He canceled his appointments to see this physician, and the physician–patient relationship deteriorated. Symptoms of the SSRI discontinuation syndrome were hypothesized to have exacerbated the patient's anxiety and depression, generating distrust of the physician. The latter attempted to maintain a supportive attitude and explain the nature of the SSRI discontinuation syndrome. At the same time, the underlying depressive state was ameliorated and the patient started keeping medical appointments.

Critical appraisals of epidemiological studies on SSRI discontinuation syndrome have shown that the syndrome is self-limiting and abates after a relatively short duration [49–56] (Table 9). Furthermore, no evidence of a statistically significant relationship between SSRI discontinuation syndrome and suicidal ideation or dose at the time of discontinuation has been established. The aforementioned case implies that a physician planning to terminate or reduce SSRI use should provide adequate information about any possible adverse effects before implementing any changes. By so doing, the physician–patient relationship might be maintained or reinforced, contributing to continued treatment.

Table 9. Characteristics of eight published epidemiological studies on SSRI withdrawal syndrome

Author	Year	Study design	Drugs	Subjects	Mean age (years)	Female (%)	Treatment period before withdrawal	Withdrawal methods	Methods
Black et al. [49]	1993	Multicenter, double-blind clinical trial	Fluvoxamine (n = 14; 300 mg/d)	Panic disorder, Depressive disorder	34	57	8 months	Abruptly withdrawn	CAS[a], CGI[b]
Oehrberg et al. [50]	1995	Randomized double-blind, placebo-controlled trial	Paroxetine (n = 55; 20–60 mg/d) Placebo (n = 52)	Panic disorder	38	76	12 weeks	Abruptly switched to placebo	Panic disorder attack frequency and any adverse events description
Coupland et al. [51]	1996	Retrospective descriptive study	Clomipramine, Fluvoxamine, Paroxetine, Sertraline, Fluoxetine (n = 352)	Panic disorder, social phobia, obsessive-compulsive disorder, depressive disorder,	42	53	12-37 weeks	NA	Chart review
Zajecka et al. [52]	1998	Multicenter, randomized double-blind placebo	Fluoxetine (n = 299; 20 mg/d) Placebo (n = 96)	Depressive disorder	40	69	12 weeks	Abruptly swiched to placebo	Any adverse events frequency and description
Rosenbaum et al. [53]	1998	Multicenter, randomized double-blind placebo controlled trial	Fluoxetine (n = 81; 25 mg/d) Sertraline (n = 79; 75 mg/d) Paroxetine (n = 82; 22 mg/d)	Unipolar depressive disorder	44	77	11 months	Interrupted with placebo substitution for 5–8 days	HRSD-21[c], MADRS[d], Self-assessment scores
Michelson et al [54]	2000	Randomized double-blind, placebo-controlled trial	Fluoxetine (n = 37; 20–60 mg/d) Sertraline (n = 34; 50–150 mg/d) Paroxetine (n = 36; 20–60 mg/d)	Depressive disorder	39	72	4 months–3 years	Interrupted with placebo substitution for 5 days	HRSD-21[c], SAI score[e], Self-assessment scores
Judge et al. [55]	2002	Multicenter, randomized double-blind, placebo-controlled trial	Fluoxetine (n = 75; 20–60 mg/d) Paroxetine (n = 75; 20–50 mg/d)	Unipolar depressive disorder	44	77	4 months–2 years	Interrupted with placebo substitution for 3–5 days	HRSD-21[c], MADRS[d], DESS[f], CGI[g]
Bogetto et al. [56]	2002	Interventional study	Fluoxetine(n = 52; 28 mg/d) Paroxetine(n = 45; 31 mg/d)	Dythmic disorder	46	59	8 weeks	Gradual and non-gradual discontinuation	HRSD-17[c], MADRS[d], Symptom checklist

[a] The Clinical Anxiety Scale.
[b] Clinical Global Impression ratings.
[c] Hamilton Depression Rating Scale.
[d] Montgomery–Asberg Depression Rating Scale.
[e] State Anxiety Inventory; Discontinuation, Emergent Signs and Symptoms.
[g] Clinical Global Impressions—Severity Scale.

Conclusions

Excessive prescription of benzodiazepines represents an important clinical issue in Japan and other countries. The number of people taking benzodiazepines has been increasing, and the costs associated with benzodiazepine use are substantial. In our recent study, we showed that a minimal dose of SSRI increased the success rate of a benzodiazepine discontinuation program among chronic benzodiazepine users. However, SSRIs themselves may cause a withdrawal syndrome. The rationales for prescribing benzodiazepines should be thoroughly discussed in educational programs directed at physicians working in hospitals and clinics. Moreover, actual prescription practices require careful and continuous monitoring.

References

[1]   Chouinard G. Issues in the clinical use of benzodiazepines: Potency, withdrawal, and rebound. *J. Clin. Psychiatry* 65(Suppl 5):7–12, 2004.

[2]   Crismon ML, Trivedi M, Pigott TA, et al. The Texas Medication Algorithm Project: Report of the Texas Consensus Conference Panel on Medication Treatment of Major Depressive Disorder. *J. Clin. Psychiatry* 60:142–156, 1999.

[3]   Mendes HA, Lima MS, Hotopf MH. Serotonin reuptake inhibitors and new generation antidepressants for panic disorder. Cochrane Database of Systematic Reviews 2, 2004.

[4]   The Royal College of Psychiatrists. Benzodiazepines: Risks, benefits or dependence: A re-evaluation. London, UK: The Royal College of Psychiatrists Council Report CR59 January 1997.

[5]   Valenstein M, Taylor KK, Austin K. Benzodiazepine use among depressed patients treated in mental health settings. *Am. J. Psychiatry* 161:654–661, 2004.

[6]   Nakao M, Takeuchi T, Yano E. Prescription of benzodiazepines in comparison with SSRIs and SNRIs for outpatients attending a Japanese university hospital. *Int. J. Clin. Pharmacol. Ther.* 45:30–35, 2007.

[7]   Rickels K, Case WG, Schweizer E, et al. Benzodiazepine dependence: Management of discontinuation. *Psychopharmacol Bull* 26:63–68, 1990.

[8]   Moller HJ. Effectiveness and safety of benzodiazepines. *J. Clin. Psychopharmacol* 19:2S–11S, 1999.

[9]   Nelson J, Chouinard G. Guidelines for the clinical use of benzodiazepines: Pharmacokinetics, dependency, rebound and withdrawal. Canadian Society for Clinical Pharmacology. *Can. J. Clin. Pharmacol.* 6:69–83, 1999.

[10]   American Psychiatric Association. *Diagnostic and statistical manual of mental disorders, Text revision*. American Psychiatric Press, Washington, DC, 2000.

[11]   Busto UE, Sykora K, Sellers EM. A clinical scale to assess benzodiazepine withdrawal. *J. Clin. Psychopharmacol* 9:412–416, 1989.

[12]   Schweizer E, Rickels K, Case WG, et al. Long-term therapeutic use of benzodiazepines I: Effect of abrupt taper. *Arch Gen Psychiatry* 47:899–907, 1990.

[13]   Tyrer P, Murphy S, Riley P. The Benzodiazepine Withdrawal Symptom Questionnaire. *J. Affect Disord.* 19:53–61, 1990.

[14] Couvee JE, Zitman FG. The Benzodiazepine Withdrawal Symptom Questionnaire: Psychometric evaluation during a discontinuation program in depressed chronic benzodiazepine users in general practice. *Addiction* 97:337–345, 2002.

[15] Anasako R, Usami M, Tamashiro M, et al. Medical rankings 2007. *Month Med Info Expr* 35:52–54, 2007. [in Japanese]

[16] Nakao M, Kuboki T. Treatment guidelines of depression for internists: Advantages and disadvantages of SSRIs. *Mod. Phys.* 22:2002–2009, 2002. [in Japanese]

[17] Miki O. Depression in primary care. *Update Psychiatry* 1:157–164, 1996. [in Japanese]

[18] Nakao M, Takeuchi T, Nomura K, et al. Clinical application of paroxetine for tapering benzodiazepine use in non-major-depressive outpatients visiting internal medicine clinics. *Psychiat Clin. Neurosci.* 60:605–610, 2006.

[19] Nakao M, Takeuchi T, Yano E. Excessive prescriptions of benzodiazepines by nonpsychiatrists in a Japanese hospital: Prescription-based data analysis using a computer-ordering system. *J. Psychosom. Res.* 58:S39, 2005.

[20] Murasaki M. History and prospects of development of anxiolytics in Japan. *Clin Psychopharmacol* 6:671–688, 2003. [in Japanese]

[21] SAS Institute Inc. *SAS Institute SAS/STAT user's guide, Release 8.01 edition*. Cary, NC: SAS Institute Inc., 1999.

[22] Ormel J, VonKorff M, Ustun TB, et al. Common mental disorders and disability across cultures: Results from the WHO Collaborative Study on Psychological Problems in General Health Care. *JAMA* 272:1741–1748, 1994.

[23] Tanaka E. Clinically significant pharmacokinetic drug interactions with benzodiazepines. *J. Clin. Pharm. Ther.* 24:347–355, 1999.

[24] Nakao M, Yamanaka G, Kuboki T. Major depression and somatic symptoms in a mind/body medicine clinic. *Psychopathology* 34:230–235, 2001.

[25] Tyrer P, Ferguson B, Hallstrom C, et al. A controlled trial of dothiepin and placebo in treating benzodiazepine withdrawal symptoms. *Br. J. Psychiatry* 168:457–461, 1996.

[26] Sontheimer DL, Ables AZ. Is imipramine or buspirone treatment effective in patients wishing to discontinue long-term benzodiazepine use? *J. Fam. Pract* 50:203, 2001.

[27] Rickels K, Schweizer E, Garcia-Espana F, et al. Trazodone and valproate in patients discontinuing long-term benzodiazepine therapy: Effects on withdrawal symptoms and taper outcome. *Psychopharmacology* 141:1–5, 1999.

[28] Zitman FG, Couvee JE. Chronic benzodiazepine use in general practice patients with depression: An evaluation of controlled treatment and taper-off: Report on behalf of the Dutch Chronic Benzodiazepine Working Group. *Br. J. Psychiatry* 178:317–324, 2001.

[29] Nakao M, Takeuchi T, Nomura K, et al. Clinical application of selective serotonin reuptake inhibitors for chronic benzodiazepine users at an internal medicine clinic. *Ther. Res.* 27:2001–2009, 2006.

[30] First MB, Spitzer RL, Gibbon M, et al. *User's guide for the structured clinical interview for DSM-IV axis I disorders.* American Psychiatric Press, Washington, DC, 1997.

[31] Sansone RA, Hendricks CM, Gaither GA, et al. Prevalence of anxiety symptoms among a sample of outpatients in an internal medicine clinic: A pilot study. *Depress Anxiety* 19:133–136, 2004.

[32] Hamilton M. A rating scale for depression. *J. Neurol. Neurosurg Psychiatry* 23:56–62, 1960.

[33] Hamilton M. The assessment of anxiety states by rating. *Br. J. Med. Psychol* 32:50–55, 1959.

[34] Ware JE, Sherbourne CD. The MOS 36-item short-form health survey (SF-36) I: Conceptual framework and item selection. *Med. Care* 30:473–480, 1992.

[35] Nakao M, Nomura S, Yamanaka G, et al. Assessment of patients by DSM-III-R and DSM-IV in a Japanese psychosomatic clinic. *Psychother Psychosom* 67:43–49, 1998.

[36] Nakao M, Yamanaka G, Kuboki T. Major depression and somatic symptoms in a mind/body medicine clinic. *Psychopathology* 34:230–235, 2001.

[37] Nakao M, Yano E. Reporting of somatic symptoms as a screening marker for detecting major depression in a population of Japanese white-collar workers. *J. Clin. Epidemiol.* 56:1021–1026, 2003.

[38] Nakao M, Yano E. Somatic symptoms for predicting depression: One-year follow-up study in annual health examinations. *Psychiat. Clin. Neurosci.* 60:219–225, 2006.

[39] Nakao M, Barsky AJ, Kumano H, et al. Relationship between somatosensory amplification and alexithymia in a Japanese psychosomatic clinic. *Psychosomatics* 43:55–60, 2002.

[40] Brown C, Schulberg HC. Diagnosis and treatment of depression in primary medical care practice: The application of research findings to clinical practice. *J. Clin. Psychol.* 54:303–314, 1998.

[41] Stoudemire A, Linfors E, Kahn M, et al. Masked depression in a combined medical-psychiatric unit. *Psychosomatics* 26:221–228, 1985.

[42] Rothman KJ, Michels KB. The continuing unethical use of placebo controls. *N. Engl. J. Med.* 331:394–398, 1994.

[43] Bull SA, Hu XH, Hunkeler EM, et al. Discontinuation of use and switching of antidepressants: Influence of patient–physician communication. *JAMA* 288:1403–1409, 2002.

[44] Frost L, Lal S. Shock-like sensations after discontinuation of selective serotonin reuptake inhibitors. *Am. J. Psychiatry* 152:810, 1995.

[45] Zajecka J, Tracy KA, Mitchell S. Discontinuation symptoms after treatment with serotonin reuptake inhibitors: A literature review. *J. Clin. Psychiatry* 58:291–297, 1997.

[46] Nuss S, Kincaid CR. Serotonin discontinuation syndrome: Does it really exist? *WV Med J* 96:405–407, 2000.

[47] Black DW, Shea C, Dursun S. Selective serotonin reuptake inhibitor discontinuation syndrome: Proposed diagnostic criteria. *J. Psychiatry Neurosci.* 25:255–261, 2000.

[48] Nomura K, Nakao M, Takeuchi T, et al. A case report of SSRI discontinuation syndrome caused by a termination of paroxetine 10mg resulting in difficult diagnosis and treatment. *Jpn. J. Psychosom. Med.* 47:41–47, 2007. [in Japanese]

[49] Black DW, Wesner R, Gabel J. The abrupt discontinuation of fluvoxamine in patients with panic disorder. *J. Clin. Psychiatry* 54:146–149, 1993.

[50] Oehrberg S, Christiansen PE, Behnke K, et al. Paroxetine in the treatment of panic disorder: A randomised, double-blind, placebo-controlled study. *Br. J. Psychiatry* 167:374–379, 1995.

[51] Coupland NJ, Bell CJ, Potokar JP. Serotonin reuptake inhibitor discontinuation. *J. Clin. Psychopharmacol.* 16:356–362, 1996.

[52] Zajecka J, Fawcett J, Amsterdam J, et al. Safety of abrupt discontinuation of fluoxetine: A randomized, placebo-controlled study. *J. Clin. Psychopharmacol.* 18:193–197, 1998.

[53] Rosenbaum JF, Fava M, Hoog SL, et al. Selective serotonin reuptake inhibitor discontinuation syndrome: A randomized clinical trial. *Biol Psychiatry* 44:77–87, 1998.

[54] Michelson D, Fava M, Amsterdam J, et al. Interruption of selective serotonin reuptake inhibitor treatment: Double-blind, placebo-controlled trial. *Br. J. Psychiatry* 176:363–368, 2000.

[55] Judge R, Parry MG, Quail D, et al. Discontinuation symptoms: Comparison of brief interruption in fluoxetine and paroxetine treatment. *Int. Clin. Psychopharmacol* 17:217–225, 2002.

[56] Bogetto F, Bellino S, Revello RB, et al. Discontinuation syndrome in dysthymic patients treated with selective serotonin reuptake inhibitors: A clinical investigation. *CNS Drugs* 16:273–283, 2002.

In: Substance Withdrawal Syndrome
Editors: J. P. Rees and O. B. Woodhouse

ISBN 978-1-60692-951-3
© 2009 Nova Science Publishers, Inc.

Chapter IV

Carisoprodol Withdrawal Syndrome

Roy R. Reeves, Randy S. Burke and Mark E. Ladner

Mental Health Service, G.V. (Sonny) Montgomery VA Medical Center, Jackson,
MS Department of Psychiatry, University of Mississippi School of Medicine

Abstract

Carisoprodol (N-isopropyl-2 methyl-2-propyl-1,3-propanediol dicarbamate; N-isopropylmeprobamate) is a commonly prescribed centrally acting skeletal muscle relaxant. The drug is structurally similar to meprobamate, a Schedule IV controlled substance at the Federal level with known risk for causing addiction. In fact, carisoprodol is metabolized to hydroxycarisoprodol, hydroxymeprobamate, and meprobamate, with meprobamate being the primary active metabolite. The abuse potential of meprobamate is equal to, if not greater than, that of benzodiazepines. With meprobamate having this degree of abuse potential, one might expect a risk of misuse of carisoprodol. A number of reports suggest this to be a valid concern. Carisoprodol has been abused (usually in amounts much larger than the recommended daily dose of 350 mg three or four times daily) for its sedative and relaxant effects, has been used to augment or alter the effects of other drugs (e.g., to increase the sedating effects of benzodiazepines or help calm persons after cocaine use), and has been combined with other prescribed medications (e.g., tramadol) to produce euphoric effects. It appears to be somewhat less difficult to obtain prescriptions for carisoprodol than for controlled substances. Carisoprodol abuse has increased significantly during the past decade, particularly in the southern US.

Because of the abuse potential of the drug, withdrawal symptoms might be expected to occur with cessation of intake of large doses of carisoprodol. As the misuse of carisoprodol has increased, descriptions of a carisoprodol withdrawal syndrome have begun to emerge. Symptoms typically encountered during this withdrawal syndrome include anxiety, tremulousness, jitteriness, and muscle twitching. Psychotic symptoms such as hallucinations occur in some patients. These symptoms are similar to those previously described during meprobamate withdrawal. Because of these similarities, symptoms occurring during carisoprodol withdrawal may be postulated to be due to withdrawal from accumulations of meprobamate present as a result of taking excessive amounts of carisoprodol.

Carisoprodol is metabolized to a controlled substance, has clear evidence of abuse potential and increasing incidence of abuse, and has shown evidence of a withdrawal syndrome with abrupt cessation from intake of large amounts of the drug. Carisoprodol has been assigned a Schedule IV controlled substance status in several states. These facts have caused some to conclude that it is time for carisoprodol to become a controlled substance at the Federal level. This article will discuss the abuse potential of carisoprodol and recent descriptions of a carisoprodol withdrawal syndrome, and will explore the clinical implications of these occurrences.

Introduction

Carisoprodol (N-isopropyl-2 methyl-2-propyl-1,3-propanediol dicarbamate; N-isopropylmeprobamate) is a commonly prescribed centrally acting skeletal muscle relaxant available in the United States since its approval by the Food and Drug Administration (FDA) in 1959. The drug is currently marketed in the US as Soma (MedPointe Healthcare, Inc., Somerset, New Jersey) and in the United Kingdom as Carisoma (Forest Laboratories UK Limited, Kent, United Kingdom) (Reeves, Hammer, and Pendarvis, 2007). It is manufactured in Guadalajara, Mexico under the name Somacid (Davis, 2004). In the past carisoprodol has also been distributed in the US under the names Rela and Soridol (Littrell, Hayes, and Stillner, 1993). Carisoprodol is widely used in primary care settings for the treatment of musculoskeletal conditions associated with paravertebral muscle spasms and back pain.

As the chemical nomenclature suggests, carisoprodol is structurally related to meprobamate, a Schedule IV controlled substance at the Federal level with known risk for causing addiction. In fact carisoprodol is a congener of meprobamate; the primary active metabolite of carisprodol *is* meprobamate. Research has demonstated the abuse potential of meprobamate to be equal to, if not greater than, the abuse potential of benzodiazepines (Roache and Griffiths, 1987). Thus it is not unreasonable to suspect that carisoprodol is likely to have abuse potential. In addition, because a withdrawal syndrome may occur with cessation from intake of meprobamate, a withdrawal syndrome might be anticipated to occur with cessation of intake of large amounts of carisoprodol. This article will discuss the basic pharmacology of carisoprodol, review the literature on the potential for carisoprodol to be a substance of abuse, present recent evidence of the occurrence of a carisoprodol withdrawal syndrome, and touch upon the possible need for cariosprodol to be classified as a controlled substance at the Federal level.

Pharmacological Properites and Metabolism of Carisoprodol

Carisoprodol is available as tablets containing 350 mg tablets of the medication. The recommended dosage is one tablet three to four times daily. The drug begins to act within 30 minutes of oral ingestion and has a half life of approximately 1.5 hours (Bramness, Skurveit, and Morland, 2004). Drowsiness, dizziness, and orthostatic hypotension are the most prominent side effects of carisoprodol. Clinical impairment and symptoms of intoxication have been shown to occur in some patients when combined serum concentrations of carisoprodol and meprobamate exceeded 10 mg/L, a level still within the normal therapeutic range (Logan, Case and Gordon, 2000).

Carisoprodol undergoes transformation in the liver to three primary metabolites: hydroxycarisoprodol, hydroxymeprobamate, and meprobamate. These metabolites are excreted in the urine (Littrell, Hayes, and Stillner, 1993). The pharmacologically active metabolite is meprobamate which has a half life of approximately 11 hours, but this may be prolonged to up to 48 hours with chronic usage (Meyer and Straughn, 1977). The exact mechanism of action of carisoprodol is unknown, but the drug is thought to act by producing muscle relaxation by blocking intraneuronal activity and suppressing the transmission of polysynaptic neurons in the spinal cord and descending reticular system of the brain (Del Castilo and Nelson, 1960). Thus the effect of the drug has been postulated to occur more as a result of CNS actions resulting in sedation, rather than from direct skeletal muscle relaxation (Littrell, Hayes, and Stillner, 1993). There appears to be cross tolerance to carisoprodol in animals dependent on barbiturates and there is evidence that meprobamate has barbiturate like activating activity at $GABA_A$ receptors (Logan, Case and Gordon, 2000). How much of the clinical effect observed in a patient taking carisoprodol is due to carisoprodol itself, and how much is contributed by the meprobamate metabolite is not clear.

Abuse Potential of Carisoprodol

Early Case Reports of Carisoprodol Abuse

As early as 1978, a report of the abuse of carisoprodol appeared in the literature (Morse and Chua, 1978). The case involved a woman, previously addicted to other drugs, who became dependent on cariosprodol. This description of carisoprodol misuse was followed by a number of others, suggesting that the drug probably had abuse potential. Initial case reports included that of a patient who tried to obtain carisoprodol prescriptions for the drug from several different physicians (Elder, 1991) and the description of a group of four patients who regularly obtained quantities of carisoprodol and then used the drug in excessive amounts to achieve mind altering effects (Rust, Hatch and Gums, 1993). An article by physicians in India presented details about a group of patients who attempted to use carisoprodol as a substitute for opiates (Sikdar et al, 1993). Another patient was discovered to have abused the drug after obtaining it through a veterinarian mail order service (Luehr, Meyerle and Larson, 1990). Legal action was taken against one patient on a criminal charge of forging prescriptions to obtain carisoprodol (Littrell, Sage, and Miller, 1993). In 1997 a series of three additional cases were described, one involving a patient used carisoprodol to calm himself after abusing cocaine, one involving a young woman who appeared to use large amounts of carisoprodol as a substitute for more potent illicit drugs, and one involving a patient who became dependent on carisoprodol as a sleep aid (Reeves, Pinkofsky, and Carter, 1997).

Other Aspects of Carisoprodol Abuse

Carisoprodol has been used to alter the effect of some illicit drugs. The medication has been taken along with sedatives such as benzodiazepines or alcohol to increase the effect of these drugs. Cocaine abusers have used carisoprodol to curb the stimulant effect they may experience following cocaine usage (Reeves, Carter, and Pinkofsky, 1999). Abuse of combinations of carisoprodol and tramadol has occurred with abusers describing a euphoric and relaxing effect as the result of taking the two drugs together. Patients abusing the combination stated that it was much easier to obtain prescriptions for carisoprodol and tramadol than for controlled substances such as benzodiazepines (Reeves and Liberto, 2001).

Bailey and Briggs (2002) evaluated the characteristics of a series of 19 patients during a six month period who were found to be positive for carisoprodol on urine drug screens. The typical user in this series was a white man or woman (with equal frequency) of age in the early 40s who abused carisoprodol or used it for medical purposes (with equal frequency). Clinical histories suggested that in seven cases the drug was abused or implicated in a suicide attempt or gesture. The authors concluded that carisoprodol and its metabolite, meprobamate, should be included in comprehensive drug screening. Reeves and colleagues (1999) surveyed a group of 40 patients taking carisoprodol for three or more months. Among those who had a history of substance abuse (N = 20), 40% admitted using the drug in larger than prescribed amounts; 30% reported using it for an effect other than for which prescribed; 10% reported using it to augment the effect of another drug; 5% reported using it to counteract the effect of another medication; 20% reported attempting to obtained extra carisoprodol by prescription; and 10% reported using obtaining carisoprodol by means other than a legal prescription. A survey of 100 physicians conducted as part of the same study revealed that 95% of respondents were aware that meprobamate was a controlled substance, but only 39% felt that carisoprodol had abuse potential and only 18% were aware that it is metabolized to a controlled substance. The authors concluded that the abuse potential of carisoprodol was underestimated by a significant proportion of physicians.

Evidence of Increasing Abuse of Carisprodol

The diversion and abuse of carisoprodol have increased significantly over the last several years. Information from the Drug Abuse Warning Network (DAWN) database reveals that the numbers of emergency department episodes involving carisoprodol were 6,569 in 1994, 7,771 in 1995, 11,239 in 2001, 10,094 in 2002, 17,366 in 2004, and 19,513 in 2005 (Deparment of Health and Human Services, 2002 and 2006), representing an almost 300% increase from 1994 to 2005. According to the National Survey on Drug Use and Health (NSDUH), data collected from 2002- 2005 indicate that the occurrence of misuse of carisoprodol was approximately equal to that of clonazepam during that period (Office of Applied Studies of the Substance Abuse and Mental Health Services, 2006). In the US, the street value of Soma® is estimated to be $1 to $5 per 350 mg tablet (Davis, 2004).

Problems related to cariosprodol misuse became particularly noticeable in the southern US in the early 1990s. In 1991, 71,000 doses of the drug were found to be missing in

Mississippi (Ukens, 1992). Two pharmacists were fined and put on probation. Investigation found that some patients might have been illicitly taking as much as 20 or more carisoprodol tablets daily. The Mississippi pharmacy board issued a warning regarding the increase of carisoprodol abuse (Ukens, 1992). The director of the Louisiana pharmacy board also felt that carisoprodol had demonstrated abuse potential in his state, noting that theft or loss of controlled substances there often also involved missing carisoprodol (Ukens, 1992). In Alabama a few pharmacists were brought before their licensing boards for personal misuse of the drug (Ukens, 1992). A retrospective study of cases of deceased persons examined at the Jefferson County (Alabama) Medical Examiner Office from January 1, 1986 to October 31, 1997 revealed that carisoprodol was present in 24 cases. The study concluded that carisoprodol was "probably responsible, in part, for those deaths" (Davis and Alexander, 1998).

Carisoprodol abuse outside the US followed by importation into this country may also be a problem. Carisoprodol manufactured in Guadalajara and sold under the name Somacid has been reported to be easily obtained in Mexico. Several thousand pills supposedly may be purchased at a time. Mexican pharmacies workers near the US border have said they may fill carisoprodol orders several times per week for American teenagers, and have been doing so for years (Davis, 2004). In their review of facts to determine whether the drug should be a controlled substance in Florida, legislators found that, according to the Los Angeles Police Department, carisoprodol is the pharmaceutical drug most frequently encountered at the US-Mexico border crossing (Florida State Legislature, 2002a).

A particularly distressing report (Reeves, Henderson, and Ladner, 2007) recently suggested that cariosprodol may indeed be becoming a popular substance of abuse. A 28-year-old male from Meridian, Mississippi with a history of bipolar disorder and polysubstance abuse, was admitted to a psychiatric unit. He had been abusing alcohol, cocaine and marijuana, and apparently had been trafficking in drugs to support his own habit. In addition he also admitted frequent misuse of prescription medications such as hydrocodone and alprazolam which he purchased from other individuals or attempted to obtain by prescription from local physicians. He noted that when he could not obtain prescriptions for these controlled substances he could often get a physician to prescribe carisoprodol, which is not a controlled substance in Mississippi. He preferred alprazolam but when it was not available he would take up to 20 to 30 carisoprodol tablets per day with a resulting feeling of relaxation. He could achieve what he described as a feeling of deep restfulness by combining carisoprodol with alcohol or a benzodiazepine He also admitted taking carisoprodol with large doses of olanzapine, an antipsychotic agent with sedating side effects in some individuals, to produce a feeling of being "zoned out".

According to this patient, carisoprodol could be purchased and sold for about $3 per tablet in eastern Mississippi. He described it as a popular drug among polysubstance abusers, particularly when benzodiazepines were desired but not available. He felt that a large dose of carisprodol could, to some degree, provide somewhat of a substitute for benzodiazepines, particularly if the drug were combined with alcohol or another substance with sedating properties. He considered the perceived relative ease of obtaining a carisoprodol prescription a favorable attribute of the drug, and related that the fact that carisoprodol was not a controlled substance in Mississippi actually resulted in substance abusers from western

Alabama driving to the Meridian area (located near the Mississippi-Alabama border) to obtain prescriptions for the drug. Consequently the street value of carisoprodol was higher in Alabama than in Mississippi (sometimes as much as $4 to $5 per tablet). Carisoprodol is a Schedule IV controlled substance in Alabama and, according to the patient, much more difficult to obtain there.

Carisoprodol Withdrawal Syndrome

Evidence of Withdrawal Symptoms from Early Case Reports

During the initial years of cariosprodol marketing, a withdrawal syndrome was not recognized. Based on evidence from animal studies and human clinical trials, the Physician's Desk Reference (Medical Economics Company, 2005) stated that "in dogs, no withdrawal symptoms have been described after abrupt cessation of carisoprodol from dosages as high as 1g/kg/day". However it was also noted that in a study of abrupt cessation of carisoprodol in humans at dosages of 100 mg/kg/day (approximately five times the recommended daily dosage), some subjects did have withdrawal symptoms such as abdominal cramps, insomnia, chills, headache, and nausea. Delirium and convulsions did not occur in any of the subjects in that study.

A review of several of the case studies reporting carisoprodol abuse contained elements suggests that some of the patients had at lease some degree of withdrawal symptoms when they decreased or stopped carisoprodol intake. In one of the earliest descriptions of cariosprodol abuse, a 44-year-old patient who reported taking 30 to 50 tablets per day had anxiety, tremulousness, and craving when he tried to stop taking the drug (Moore and Chua, 1978). A woman who took as many as 13 tablets at bedtime reported abstinence anxiety and tremors during the daytime. These complaints resolved with the ingestion of additional carisoprodol tablets (Luehr, Meyerle, and Larson, 1990). In the report of carisoprodol abuse from India, 69% of patients were described as experiencing withdrawal symptoms, including body aches, anxiety, restlessness, and insomnia (Sikdar et al, 1993). In a study involving prisoners in Norway (Wyller, Korsmo, and Gadeholt, 1991), carisoprodol was gradually withdrawn from patients who had been taking 700 to 2100 mg/day for at least 9 months. Most of them reported anxiety, insomnia, irritability, cranial and muscular pain, and vegetative symptoms. Reeves and colleagues (1997) described withdrawal symptoms in two patients following cessation of doses of carisoprodol as low as four to eight tablets daily, including irritability, back pain, headache, and dysphoria. In 2003 (Reeves and Parker) similar but more severe symptoms were described in five patients who abruptly stopped daily intake of 2,100 to 4,200 mg of carisoprodol. These patients also demonstrated a statistically significant increase in the number of somatic dysfunctions (an osteopathic measure representing the degree of restrictions of spinal motion) over a period of several days following cessation of carisoprodol. The authors suggested that the increase in the number of somatic dysfunctions observed following cessation of intake of the drug was evidence for the existence of a carisoprodol withdrawal syndrome.

Cases of Carisoprodol Withdrawal Syndrome

A patient with what was believed to be a full blown carisoprodol withdrawal syndrome was described in 2004 (Reeves, Beddingfield, and Mack). The case involved a 43-year-old man who had been abusing hydrocodone until he could no longer obtain prescriptions for it. However, he could obtain prescriptions for carisoprodol and took up to 30 or more carisoprodol tablets (10,500 mg or more) as a substitute daily for several weeks. Then, suspecting abuse, his physicians refused to write any more prescriptions for carisoprodol, so the patient was forced to abruptly stop taking the drug. Within 48 hours of cessation he developed anxiety, tremors, muscle twitching, insomnia, auditory and visual hallucinations, and bizarre behavior. He related having difficulty distinguishing the hallucinations from what was real in his environment. For example, at one point during his intake interview he believed he saw a colorful insect crawling on his arm, and he thought the insect was talking louder than the examiner. His symptoms peaked on the fourth day after carisoprodol cessation. The patient required brief treatment with olanzapine and tapering doses of lorazepam while the symptoms gradually but completely resolved.

Another case of carisoprodol withdrawal syndrome appeared in the literature the following year (Rohatgi, Rissmiller, and Gorman, 2005). A 46-year-old male taking carisoprodol 350 mg three times daily had been abusing the prescription opiates oxycodone and hydrocodone. When his physician refused to continue prescribing narcotics, the patient began taking ten to twelve carisoprodol tablets (3,500-4,200 mg) per day, obtaining the drug from three different internet sites by supplying a written history. Significantly, he denied any opiate withdrawal symptoms while taking the carisoprodol. After decreasing the dosage to seven tablets daily himself, the patient was admitted to a treatment program for detoxification. During tapering of the medication he experienced cardiac palpitations, diaphoresis, chills, stomach cramps, nausea, insomnia, myalgia, tremors, diarrhea, anxiety, psychomotor agitation, and feelings of depersonalization. He continued to have mild symptoms for over about two weeks after complete cessation.

In 2007, Reeves, Hammer, and Pendarvis described in detail two additional case reports involving carisoprodol withdrawal syndrome. The first case was that of a 36-year-old female who was hospitalized because she was apparently experiencing auditory and visual hallucinations. She was actively responding to internal stimuli. The patient had no history of mental illness. Auditory hallucinations included voices of several individuals. She also heard music that she described as "good". Visual hallucinations included animals and people who appeared quite real to her. One was of an annoying individual with whom she argued. She told staff this person was a cousin she did not like. She felt that her dreams continued after awakening and were real. Her hallucinations were so intense she had difficulty distinguishing them from her actual surroundings. It was determined that onset of these symptoms had occurred after cessation of consumption of large doses of carisoprodol. She reported she had been taking approximately 25 carisoprodol tablets daily for several months. Three days prior to admission she had abruptly stopped taking the drug because she could no longer obtain it. The next day she became anxious and jittery and on the day after that she became tremulous. That evening she began hallucinating. The night prior to admission she slept less than one hour. She was hospitalized and given lorazepam and respiridone on an as needed basis to control her symptoms which gradually resolved over the next three days. The patient denied any other alcohol or drug abuse except for occasional use of oxycodone. Urine drug screen was negative at the time of admission. After resolution of this episode she did not resume carisoprodol use and she had no recurrence of psychotic symptoms.

The second case was a description of a 21-year-old female who had been taking approximately 20 carisoprodol tablets per day for over three months. She had been using no other drugs. After being confronted by her family and friends she decided to stop taking carisoprodol "cold turkey". About 24 hours later she developed anxiety, tremulousness, muscle twitching, and insomnia. Between 36 and 48 hours after carisoprodol cessation she began having visual hallucinations consisting of insects and what she referred to as "flying things". She became paranoid about Police who she felt were watching her and about other authority figures. She began taking the carisoprodol again and the symptoms rapidly resolved. About a month later she entered a treatment program and underwent detoxification with lorazepam beginning with 6 mg daily on the first day, with the dosage decreasing by approximately 20% on each subsequent day. On the second through the fourth days she had similar but less intense complaints. After completing detoxification she had no further symptoms of this type.

Proposed Mechanism for Carisoprodol Withdrawal Symptoms

The most likely mechanism to explain withdrawal symptoms concomitant with cessation of intake of large doses of carisoprodol has been proposed to be withdrawal from accumulation of the active metabolite, meprobamate (Reeves, Hammer, and Pendarvis, 2007). Symptoms described in case reports of carisoprodol withdrawal closely resemble those seen in previous reports of meprobamate withdrawal. Meprobamate was widely prescribed for anxiety (under the name Miltown) in the 1950s and 1960s. Abuse was not uncommon, and a withdrawal syndrome was recognized to frequently occur with cessation of intake of the drug. Symptoms of meprobamate withdrawal involved various degrees of anxiety, insomnia, tremors, muscle twitching, anorexia, vomiting, and ataxia. Hallucinations and symptoms resembling delirium tremens were also reported to occur in several patients, and in some cases seizures occurred (Haizlip and Ewing, 1958; Bulla, Ewing, and Buffaloe, 1959). Meprobamate is prescribed much less frequently in current times, but a case describing meprobamate withdrawal in an 80-year-old woman who had taken the drug for 40 years appeared recently appeared in the literature (Shehab et al, 2005).

Many of the symptoms seen during withdrawal from meprobamate are similar to those noted in patients with carisoprodol withdrawal syndrome. Thus, withdrawal from accumulations of meprobamate may be the most likely mechanism for the production of withdrawal symptoms during carisoprodol withdrawal. However, it should be noted that this has not been proven by research methods and other mechanisms may be responsible. The role of the metabolites hydoxymeprobamate and hydroxycarisoprodol in the production of the clinical effects of carisoprodol, or in withdrawal symptoms following carisoprodol cessation, are not well understood.

Clinical Implications

One might think that clinicians would be cautious prescribing a drug that is metabolized to a controlled substance that has a recognized risk of abuse. Most practitioners appear to be aware that meprobamate is a controlled substance with well documented abuse potential. However, a significant proportion are not aware that carisoprodol is metabolized to meprobamate. Many therefore are not alert to the abuse potential of carisoprodol (Reeves et al, 1999).

Some patients who abuse carisoprodol may be cognizant of this fact and attempt to take advantage of the drug's noncontrolled status at the Federal level to obtain it. It is easily conceivable that some clinicians might feel more comfortable prescribing carisoprodol rather than a controlled substance such as a benzodiazepine. Chop (1993) noted that some patients have been "quite aggressive" and manipulative in their attempts to procure carisoprodol, and described one patient actually demanding in an agitated manner, "It's not even controlled, so why won't you give it to me, Doc?" Thus increased awareness of the abuse potential of carisoprodol in the medical community is very much needed.

Controlled Substances Issues

The mounting evidence that carisoprodol has abuse potential and a withdrawal syndrome has not gone unnoticed. Carisoprodol has been classified as a Schedule IV controlled substance in several states, including Alabama, Arizona, Florida, Hawaii, Georgia, Kentucky, Massachusetts, New Mexico, and Oklahoma (Davis and Alexander, 1998; Arizona State Board of Pharmacy, 2003; Florida State Senate, 2003b; Weathermon, 1999). Guidelines for physicans prescribing controlled substances in Kentucky make the recommendation that carisoprodol "should be prescribed with the same caution as opioids and other controlled substances" (Kentucky Board of Medical Licensure, 1996). Certain other states are also apparently considering classifying carisoprodol as a controlled substance. However no such action has been taken at the Federal level. During a telephone interview about carisoprodol by the FDA in 2002, one of the authors (RRR) was told that carisoprodol had not been classified as a controlled substance because of the lack of evidence of withdrawal symptoms.

Classification of carisoprodol as a controlled substance in several states but not at the Federal level represents a curious inconsistency in drug enforcement policy between state and Federal administrations. Carisoprodol is metabolized to a controlled substance with known abuse potential, has clear evidence of abuse potential itself, and has been assigned a Schedule IV controlled substance status in several states. Statistics indicate increasing incidence of abuse, particularly in the southern US. When the case reports cited above are considered as a whole, it could be concluded that carisoprodol has by this time demonstrated convincing evidence of a withdrawal syndrome with abrupt cessation from intake of large amounts of the drug. These facts have lead several clinicians to conclude that it is time for carisoprodol to become a controlled substance at the Federal level (Reeves and Burke, 2007). However, regardless of its controlled substance classification, clinicians should recognize that carisoprodol may have abuse potential, and that a withdrawal syndrome may occur with abrupt cessation of intake the drug, particularly if it is being taken in large dosages.

References

Arizona State Board of Pharmacy (2003). Carisoprodol scheduled as a controlled substance effective September 19, 2003. *Arizona State Board of Pharmacy Newsletter*, October, 2003. Available at www.azpharmacy.gov/pdfs/1003AZNWSLTR.pdf. Accessed April 20, 2008.

Bramness JG, Skurtveit S, Morland J (2004). Impairment due to intake of carisoprodol. *Drug Alcohol Depend* 74:311-318.

Bulla JD, Ewing JA, Bufaloe WJ (1959). Further controlled studies of meprobamate. *Am. Pract. Dig. Treat* 10:1961-1964.

Chop WM Jr (1993). Should carisprodol be a controlled substance (letter)? *Arch Fam. Med.* 2:911.

Davis GG, Alexander CB (1998). A review of carisoprodol deaths in Jefferson County, Alabama. *South Med J* 91:726-730.

Davis K (2004). The Soma pipeline. Drug Free Az news and events, May 13, 2004. Available at www.drugfreeaz.com/news/articles_soma.html. Accessed April 19, 2008.

Del Castilo J, Nelson TE, Jr (1960). The mode of action of carisoprodol. *Ann. NY Acad. Sci.* 86:108-142.

Department of Health and Human Services (2002). Emergency department trends from the Drug Abuse Warning Network, Final Estimates 1994- 2001. Available at www.oas.samhsa.gov/DAWN/final2k1EDtrends/text/EDtrend2001v6.pdf. Accessed April 19, 2008.

Department of Health and Human Services (2006). Drug Abuse Warning Network, 2005: National estimates of drug-related emergency department visits. Available at dawninfo.samhsa.gov/files/DAWN2k5ED.htm. Accessed April 19, 2008.

Elder NC (1991). Abuse of skeletal muscle relaxants. *Am. Fam. Physician* 44:1223-1226.

Florida State Legislature (2002a). Senate staff analysis and economic impact statement for Florida Senate Bill 612. Available at www.leg.state.fl/data/session/2002Senate/bills /analysis/pdf/2002s0612.cj.pdf. Accessed April 19, 2008.

Florida State Legislature (2002b). Florida House Bill 351, passed as Senate Bill 612, effective July 5, 2002. Available at www.leg.state.fl.us/data/session/2002/House /bills/analysis/pdfh0351z.cpcs.pdf. Accessed April 20, 2008.

Haizlip TM, Ewing JA (1958). Meprobamate habituation. *New Eng J Med* 258:1181-1186.

Kentucky Board of Medical Licensure (1996). Kentucky Board of Medical Licensure Guidelines for Prescribing Controlled Substances. Available at www.medsch.wisc.edu /painpolicy/domestic/states/KY/kymbguide96.htm. Accessed April 20, 2008.

Littrell RA, Hayes LR, Stillner V (1993). Carisoprodol (Soma): A new and cautious perspective on an old agent. *South Med. J.* 1993: 86:753-756.

Littrell RA, Sage T, Miller W (1993). Meprobamate dependence secondary to carisoprodol (Soma) use. *Am. J. Drug Alcohol. Abuse* 19:133-134.

Logan BK, Case GA, Gordon AM (2000). Carisoprodol, meprobamate, and driving impairment. *J. Forensic Sci.* 45:619-623.

Luehr JG, Meyerle KA, Larson EW (1990). Mail-order (veterinary) drug dependence. *JAMA* 263:657.

Medical Economics Company (2005). *Physician's Desk Reference*, 59th Ed. Montvale, NJ: Medical Economics Company, pg 1976.

Meyer MC, Straughn A (1977). Meprobamate. *J. Am. Pharm. Assoc.* 17:173-175.

Morse RM, Chua L (1978). Carisoprodol dependence: A case report. *Am. J. Drug Alcohol. Abuse* 5:527-530.

Office of Applied Studies of the Substance Abuse and Mental Health Services (2006). National survey on drug use and health (NSDUH). Available at www.oas.samhsa.gov/nsduh.htm. Accessed April 19, 2008.

Reeves RR, Pinkofsky HB, Carter OS (1997). Carisoprodol: A drug of continuing abuse. *J. Am. Osteopathic Assoc* 97:723-724.

Reeves RR, Carter OS, Pinkofsky HB, et al (1999). Carisoprodol (Soma): Abuse potential and physician unawareness. *J. Addictive Diseases* 18:51-56.

Reeves RR. Carter OS, Pinkofsky HB (1999). Use of carisoprodol by substance abusers to modify the effects of illicit drugs. *South Med. J.* 92:441.

Reeves RR, Liberto V (2001). Abuse of combinations of carisoprodol and tramadol. *South Med J* 94:512-514.

Reeves RR, Parker JD (2003). Somatic dysfunction during carisoprodol withdrawal syndrome. *J. Am. Osteopathic Assoc* 103:75-80.

Reeves RR, Beddingfield JJ, Mack JE (2004). Carisoprodol withdrawal syndrome. *Pharmacotherapy* 24:1804-1806.

Reeves RR, Hammer JS, Pendarvis RO (2007). Is the frequency of cariosprodol withdrawal syndrome increasing? *Pharmacotherapy* 27:1462-1466.

Reeves RR, Burke RS (2007). Is it time for cariosprodol to become a controlled substance at the Federal level? *South Med. J.* 101:127-128.

Roache JD, Griffith RR (1987). Lorazepam and meprobamate dose effects in humans: Behavioral effects and abuse liability. *J. Pharmacol Exp. Ther.* 243:978-988.

Rohatgi G, Rissmiller DJ, Gorman JM (2005). Treatment of carisoprodol dependence: A case report. *J. Psychiatric Pract.* 11:347-352.

Rust GS, Hatch R, Gums JG (1993). Carisoprodol as a drug of abuse. *Arch. Fam. Med.* 429-432.

Shehab AMA, Khanbhai A, Gupta AK, Ferner ER (2005). Meprobamate withdrawal after forty years of drug treatment. *J. Applied Research* 5:193-195.

Sikdar S, Basu D, Malhotra AK, et al (1993). Carisoprodol abuse: A report from India. *Acta Psychiatr. Scand.* 88:302-303.

Ukens C (1992). Carisoprodol abuse on rise, warns Mississippi board. *Drug Topics* January 20, 1992;19.

Weathermon RM (1999). Controlled substances diversion. *U.S. Pharmacist* December, 1999. Available at www.uspharmacist.com/oldformat.asp?url=newlook/files/feat/dec99controlled.cfmandpub_id=456. Accessed April 20, 2008.

Wyller TB, Korsmo G, Gadeholt G (1991). Dependence on carisoprodol (Somadril)? A prospective study among prisoners (in Norweigen). *Tidsskrifft Den Norske Laegeforening* 111:193-195.

In: Substance Withdrawal Syndrome
Editors: J. P. Rees and O. B. Woodhouse

ISBN 978-1-60692-951-3
© 2009 Nova Science Publishers, Inc.

Chapter V

Is Aspirin Withdrawal Detrimental for Patients with or at Risk for Coronary Artery Disease? A Meta-Analysis[*]

Giuseppe G. L. Biondi-Zoccai[1†], Marzia Lotrionte[2],
Pierfrancesco Agostoni[3], Antonio Abbate[4], Massimiliano
Fusaro[1], Giuseppe M. Sangiorgi[5] and Imad Sheiban[1]
[1]Division of Cardiology, University of Turin, Turin, Italy;
[2]Institute of Cardiology, Catholic University, Rome, Italy;
[3]Department of Cardiology, University Medical Center, Utrecht, The Netherlands;
[4]VCU Pauley Heart Center, Department of Medicine,
Virginia Commonwealth University, Richmond, VA;USA
[5]Division of Cardiology, University of Modena, Modena, Italy

Abstract

The protective role of aspirin in the management of patients with or at risk of coronary artery disease has been established for several years. The clinical appropriateness of aspirin therapy depends however on the risk-benefit balance between its potential adverse effects, namely bleeding, and its benefits. Indeed, it is not uncommon for patients to discontinue aspirin according to physician advice or unsupervised, eg before an invasive procedure.

The hazards inherent to aspirin discontinuation in such patients are however incompletely defined. We thus undertook a systematic review and meta-analysis of clinical studies reporting on the impact of aspirin withdrawal in subjects with established coronary artery disease or at moderate-to-high risk for coronary events.

---

[*] A version of this chapter was also published as a chapter in *New Research on Aspririn and Health*, edited by Charles L. Millwood, published by Nova Science Publishers, Inc. It was submitted for appropriate modifications in an effort to encourage wider dissemination of research.
[†] Correspondence concerning this article should be addressed to Dr. Giuseppe Biondi Zoccai, Via Aurelia 5, Ospedaletti (IM) Italy. Tel.: +39-3408626829. Fax: +39-0184502244. Email: gbiondizoccai@gmail.com.

We searched PubMed for pertinent studies, without language restrictions. Study designs, patient characteristics, and outcomes were formally abstracted. Pooled estimates were computed according to random effects methods, when appropriate.

From the 612 studies screened for selection, we finally included in the analysis 6 studies, enrolling a total of 50279 patients. One study involved 31750 patients on secondary prevention for coronary artery disease, 2 studies enrolled 2594 subjects admitted for acute coronary syndromes, 2 studies were focused on 13706 patients undergoing coronary artery bypass grafting, and an additional study involved 2229 patients who had underwent percutaneous coronary revascularization with intracoronary drug-eluting stent implantation. Overall, aspirin withdrawal was associated with a 3-fold higher risk of major adverse cardiac events (3.14 [95% confidence interval 1.75-5.61], P=0.0001). This risk was magnified in patients with intracoronary stents, as such discontinuation of antiplatelet treatment was associated with an even higher risk of adverse events (89.78 [29.90-269.60]).

This systematic overview suggests that aspirin withdrawal has ominous prognostic implication in subjects with or at moderate-to-high risk for coronary artery disease. Such information should be borne in mind when advising patients under such treatment, and aspirin discontinuation should be advocated only when the risk of bleeding or other adverse effects clearly overwhelms that of cardiovascular atherothrombotic events.

Keywords: aspirin, coronary artery disease, discontinuation, meta-analysis, systematic review.

Introduction

Epidemiology of Coronary Artery Disease

Coronary artery disease is among the leading causes of morbidity and mortality worldwide, and its impact is likely to increase even further in the next decades. Indeed, according to recent estimates from the American Heart Association, the current prevalence in the sole United States of coronary disease among those age 18 or older is 5.9%, with the incidence of a first major cardiovascular event rising from 7/1000 to 68/1000 in men at ages 35-44 vs ages 85-94. (Thom, 2006) Furthermore, while cardiovascular disease is the leading cause of death in developed countries, among all such deaths coronary heart disease is the most common culprit.

Primary, secondary and tertiary prevention strategies are pivotal to limit the present and future burden of coronary artery disease. Antithrombotic therapy has been established as a mainstay in the management of subjects at risk for coronary artery disease, as well as for patients with previous coronary events. (Antithrombotic Trialists' Collaboration, 2002) Specifically, antithrombotics can be distinguished in anticoagulants, such as heparin, bivalirudin, or warfarin, and antiplatelet agents, such as ticlopidine, clopidogrel, or aspirin, ie acetylsalicylic acid. (Andreotti, 2006) Indeed, aspirin is the most extensively studied and employed antiplatelet agent used for coronary artery disease prevention and treatment, given its favorable risk-benefit and cost-effectiveness profiles. (Antithrombotic Trialists'

Collaboration, 2002; Andreotti, 2006; Patrono, 2005; Gaspoz, 2002) While other beneficial antiplatelet agents, including dipyridamole, (Antithrombotic Trialists' Collaboration, 2002) ticlopidine, clopidogrel, (Biondi-Zoccai, 2004 (A)) and intravenous glycoprotein IIb/IIIa inhibitors, (Boersma, 2002) have important applications, eg in patients undergoing percutaneous coronary intervention, aspirin is likely to remain for several years the most commonly used antithrombotic agent worldwide. (Tran, 2004).

Risk-benefit balance of aspirin

The relative safety of aspirin has been established in a variety of settings and conditions. (Tran, 2004; Patrono, 2005) In fact, while tolerable to most patients, the impact of adverse effects associated with a long-term aspirin regimen is not negligible, especially given the large number of subjects under aspirin treatment worldwide. While cases of aspirin allergy are known to occur with a low yet predictable rate, (Gollapudi, 2004) most adverse effects of aspirin can nonetheless be expected due to its pharmadynamic properties. In particular, a detailed appraisal of the adverse effects of aspirin is available from a recent randomized trial allocating 19,934 women to 100 mg of aspirin on alternate days for 10 years. (Ridker, 2005) In this study, the 10-year risk was 4.6% for total gastrointestinal bleeding ($p<0.001$ vs placebo), 0.6% for gastrointestinal bleeding requiring transfusion ($p=0.02$), 2.7% for peptic ulcer ($p<0.001$), 15.2% for hematuria ($p=0.02$), 53.0% for easy bruising ($p<0.001$), 19.1% for epistaxis ($p<0.001$), 59.5% for any report of gastric upset ($p=0.59$), and 0.3% for intracranial bleeding ($p=0.31$). (Ridker, 2005) Similar findings were previously reported in males. (Ridker 1997)

More recent data support a superior risk-benefit balance with lower doses of aspirin, ie those ranging around 75-100 mg per day. Evidence in support of this statement comes largely from a recent systematic review, (Antithrombotic Trialists' Collaboration, 2002) and from a randomized clinical trial conducted in patients with acute coronary syndromes. (Peters, 2006)

While secondary prevention of coronary events with aspirin is considered mandatory unless specific contraindications are present, debate continues on the appropriateness, safety and effectiveness of aspirin in primary prevention. (Berger, 2006; Patrono, 2005; Manes, 2005; Nelson, 2005; Ridker, 2005) Nonetheless, in subjects at high risk of coronary events and with a low risk of cerebral hemorrhage (eg diabetics with adequate blood pressure control), aspirin appears to have a favorable clinical profile. (Gaede, 2003; Patrono, 2005; Berger, 2006)

Potential hazards of aspirin withdrawal in patients with or at risk for coronary artery disease

Aspirin discontinuation can occur either under physician supervision or unsupervised. The latter may be due to prescription errors, lack of compliance, intolerance to adverse effects, or, when occurring under physician guidance, before invasive procedures or in case of unspecialized care. (Eagle, 2004) Indeed, spontaneous and unsupervised aspirin discontinuation after 1 year may occur in up to 18% of patients with established coronary artery disease, with older age, female gender, lower educational level, and unmarried status as predictors of withdrawal. (Kulkarni, 2006)

Aspirin withdrawal has been to date incompletely appraised. While potential hazards can be obviously found in interrupting aspirin in subjects who have a clear indication to such therapy, discontinuing this agent might be of value in selected settings if performed for a limited period and under strict supervision. There is however a lack of studies explicitly and thoroughly appraising the subject of aspirin withdrawal in patients with or at risk for coronary artery disease.

Rationale and Aim of the Present Study

Systematic reviews may provide a thorough and sound appraisal of available evidence, by means of sound search strategies, explicit selection criteria, and formal data abstraction. (Randolph, 2002; Higgins, 2003; Biondi-Zoccai, 2004 (B)) Moreover, provided that clinically and statistically homogenous studies are at hand, meta-analytic pooling of individual study findings may be performed, achieving greater statistical power for effect size estimates. (Lau, 1998) Even in the setting of heterogeneous evidence, meta-regression analyses can explore interactions between treatment and patient characteristics, thus providing important hypothesis-generating data. (Lau, 1998)

Given the uncertainty on the hazards of aspirin withdrawal in patients with or at risk for coronary artery disease, we thus undertook a systematic review and meta-analysis of pertinent published studies. This work was conducted according to current guidelines and established standards. (Stroup, 2000; Biondi-Zoccai, 2004 (C))

Methods

Search Strategy

Electronic database searches were conducted for pertinent articles published in BioMedCentral (http://www.biomedcentral.com), Google Scholar (http://scholar.google.com), and PubMed (http://www.pubmed.gov). The detailed PubMed search strategy was designed according to established methods, (Wilczynski, 2004) and is available with the other search strategies in the Appendix. Pertinent previous qualitative and systematic reviews were also checked for additional studies. (Burger, 2005) Finally, forward and backward snowballing was employed. No language restriction was enforced.

Study Selection

Retrieved citations were first screened at the title and/or abstract level. If potentially pertinent, they were then appraised as complete reports according to the following explicit selection criteria.

Inclusion criteria were: a) human studies, b) reporting on the quantitative appraisal of the cardiovascular risk of aspirin withdrawal, and c) in patients at risk for or with established coronary artery disease.

Exclusion criteria were: a) non-human setting, b) duplicate reporting (in which case the manuscript reporting the largest sample or the longest follow-up was selected), c) inability to compute risk estimates due to case report or series design.

Data Abstraction

The following data were formally abstracted: authors, journal, years of conduct and publication, study design, sample size, patient characteristics, index diagnosis, prevention stage (primary vs secondary), coronary lesion characteristics (if available), raw numbers and risks for death, myocardial infarction, stroke, major adverse cardiovascular events (as defined and reported by each investigator) and major bleeding.

Internal Validity and Quality Appraisal

The quality of included studies was appraised according to established methods. (Higgins, 2005) Specifically, we separately estimated the risk of selection, performance, detection and attrition bias, and abstracted additional design features.

Data Analysis and Synthesis

Continuous variables are reported as mean (standard deviation) or median (range). Categorical variables are expressed as n/N (%). Statistical pooling was performed according to a random effect model with generic inverse variance weighting, computing risk estimates (expressed according to the individual report as odds ratios, relative risks, or hazard ratios, with 95% confidence intervals) by means of the RevMan 4.2 freeware, an ad hoc statistical package developed and maintained by The Cochrane Collaboration.

Hypothesis testing was set at the two-tailed 0.05 level. Instead, a two-tailed 0.10 p value at chi-square test was considered as cutoff for statistical heterogeneity, (Higgins, 2005) while I^2 values of 25%, 50%, and 75% were considered to represent, respectively, mild, moderate and extensive statistical inconsistency. (Higgins, 2003)

Results

The reviewing process is summarized in Figure 1. Database searches initially retrieved 612 citations, from which 581 hits were excluded at the title or abstract level. After thorough assessment according to the selection criteria, we further excluded 25 citations.

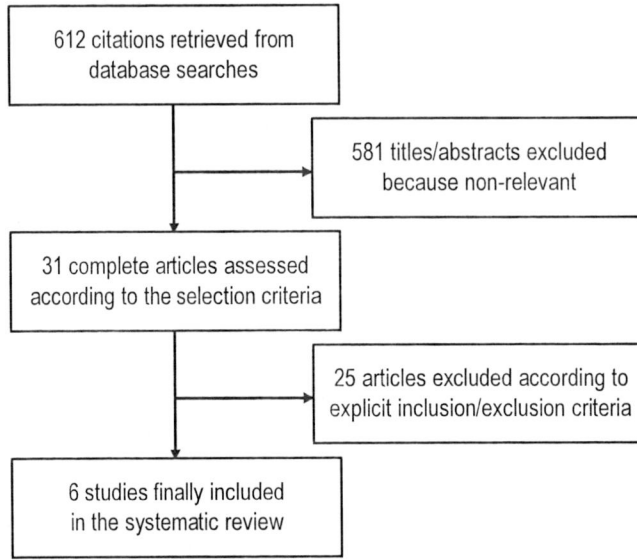

Figure 1. Flow diagram of the reviewing process.

Specific reasons for exclusion were: healthy volunteer setting, (Sonksen, 1999) lack of cardiovascular clinical outcomes, (Lawrence, 1994; Billingsley, 1997; Assia, 1998; Zanetti, 2001; Hui, 2002; Bouvy, 2003; Hamann, 2003; Eagle, 2004; Sud, 2005; Kulkarni, 2006; Newby, 2003; Harker, 1999), lack of a control group, (Madan, 2005) inability or lack of risk estimates due to study design. (Matsuzaki, 1999; Mitchell, 1999; Collet, 2000; Kaluza, 2000; Bachman, 2002; Kovich, 2003; Albaladejo, 2004; McFadden, 2004; Delpierre, 2005; Ong, 2005) Another study was excluded because reporting aspirin substitution with ticlopidine instead of strict aspirin discontinuation. (Pascual Figal, 2000)

We finally included in the analysis 6 studies (Table 1). (Dacey, 2000; Mangano, 2002; Collet, 2004; Ferrari, 2005; Iakovou, 2005; Newby, 2006).

Characteristics of Included Studies

In a prospective study of 1358 patients admitted for acute myocardial infarction and followed for 1 month, Collet and colleagues (2004) demonstrated that subjects who had recently discontinued aspirin were at a significantly higher risk for 1-month death or myocardial infarction, and bleeding, even at multivariable analysis. Infarction occurred 11.9 ± 0.8 days after aspirin withdrawal, and this was in 64% cases primarily a physician decision for scheduled surgery.

Ferrari et al (2005) provided similar data among 1236 patients admitted for acute coronary syndromes. Specifically, aspirin withdrawal was associated with 4.1% of all coronary events, 13.3% of recurrences, and there was a significant association between aspirin discontinuation and presentation with ST-elevation acute coronary syndrome. Intriguingly, the delay between aspirin withdrawal and the acute coronary event was 10.0±1.9 days (range 4 to 17), thus similar to that reported by Collet and colleagues.

Table 1. Characteristics of included studies

Study	Years	Principal investigator	Location	Patients	Setting
Collet (2004)	1999-2002	G Montalescot	France	1358	Patients admitted for acute coronary syndromes
Dacey (2000)	1987-1991	L Dacey	USA	8641	Patients undergoing coronary artery bypass grafting*
Ferrari (2005)	1999-2002	E Ferrari	France	1236	Patients admitted for acute coronary syndromes
Iakovou (2005)	2002-2004	A Colombo	Germany, Italy	2229	Patients treated with drug-eluting coronary stents
Mangano (2002)	1997-2000	DT Mangano	USA	5065	Patients undergoing coronary artery bypass grafting*
Newby (2006)	1995-2002	LK Newby	USA	31750	Secondary prevention after diagnosis of coronary artery disease

*Only combined estimates for subjects continuing aspirin vs those not on aspirin were provided.

Newby et al (2006) reported on the long-term outcomes of patients with consistent use of aspirin after an established diagnosis of coronary artery disease. They found a major protective effect of adherence to aspirin on all-cause mortality (hazard ratio=0.58 [0.54-0.62] over a follow-up of 7 years. Indeed, while not strictly focusing on the hazards of aspirin withdrawal, this study nicely confirm the long-term benefits associated with aspirin use and the risks inherent with aspirin discontinuation.

Iakovou and co-authors (2005) showed that, among 2229 patients undergoing percutaneous coronary intervention with successful drug-eluting stent implantation, antiplatelet therapy discontinuation was strikingly associated with the risk of death, non-fatal myocardial infarction, or stent thrombosis. Indeed, discontinuation of aspirin and/or thienopyridines occurred in 17 patients, leading to a major adverse event in 5 (29%).

Dacey et al (2000) reported on a case-control study performed in 8641 patients undergoing coronary artery bypass grafting. Aspirin use in the week preceding surgery was associated with a decrease in the risk of in-hospital all-cause death, without any major change in the rate of re-exploration for hemorrhage, amount of chest tube drainage, or blood transfusion. Mangano et al (2002) further confirmed and expanded these findings by showing that aspirin treatment resumed as early as 48 hours after coronary artery bypass surgery lead to significant reductions in in-hospital adverse events, including all-cause death, myocardial infarction, stroke, renal failure, mesenteric ischemia, without any major detrimental effect on wound healing.

Characteristics of Excluded Studies

Features of the principal excluded studies are presented in Table 2. Specifically, Collet and co-investigators (2000) provided preliminary and non-quantitative data on the potential hazards of aspirin withdrawal in a retrospective analysis of 475 patients admitted for acute myocardial infarction. Aspirin discontinuation had been occurred in 11 patients of them, and was followed by the thrombotic event after 9.4±3.2 days.

Table 2. Characteristics of main excluded studies

Study	Years	Principal investigator	Patients	Notes and reasons for exclusion
Albaladejo (2004)	1998-2002	P Albaladejo	181	Retrospective analysis on patients admitted for acute lower limb ischemia, without any estimate of the risk of aspirin discontinuation
Collet (2000)	1992-1996	JP Collet	475	Retrospective analysis on patients admitted for acute myocardial infarction, without any estimate of the risk of aspirin discontinuation
Kaluza (2000)	1996-1998	AE Raizner	40	Case series reporting on adverse clinical events after noncardiac surgery in patients treated with coronary stents
McFadden (2004)	2003-2004	PW Serruys	4*	Case series reporting on late drug-eluting coronary stent thrombosis
Ong (2005)	2002-2003	PW Serruys	2006*	Cohort study reporting on 7 cases of late drug-eluting stent thrombosis (3 due to aspirin and thienopyridine withdrawal), without any estimate of the risk of aspirin discontinuation
Pascual Figal (2000)	1994-2000	M Valdés Chàvarri	226	Cohort study reporting on ticlopidine withdrawal without any case of aspirin discontinuation

*For 2 cases duplicate publication is likely.

Kaluza et al (2000) presented data on catastrophic events of noncardiac surgery soon after coronary stenting. Specifically, they reported on 40 consecutive patients meeting such selection criteria, among whom there were 7 acute myocardial infarctions, 11 major bleeding episodes and 8 deaths. All deaths and infarctions, as well as most bleeding episodes, occurred in patients subjected to surgery fewer than 14 days after stenting.

While detailed information on the risk estimates of aspirin withdrawal are not available, the authors clarify that of 8 deceased patients, 1 had no discontinuation of either antiplatelet drug, 2 patients had ticlopidine withdrawn and aspirin continued, and six patients had both drugs stopped 0 to 2 days before going to surgery. In the remaining 32 patients, most had both antiplatelet drugs discontinued 0 to 1 day before and restarted 0 to 1 day after surgery.

The paper by Ong et al, (2005) reported on the incidence and features of late drug-eluting stent thrombosis in patients undergoing percutaneous coronary intervention. While the authors suggested that complete antiplatelet therapy discontinuation (aspirin and thienopyridines) was associated with stent thrombosis in 43% of cases, they did not report risk estimates for aspirin withdrawal, and the study could not thus be included in our meta-analysis.

Albaladejo and colleagues (2004) presented data on the presenting features of 181 patients admitted for acute lower limb ischemia. They found that aspirin discontinuation was associated with such event in 11 patients, with a median time from withdrawal to admission of 23 days (range 7-60). In most cases aspirin had been stopped for a surgical procedure, in the absence of any substitution therapy. Despite these intriguing findings, no formal estimate of risk was undertaken.

Meta-Analysis

Clinical impact of aspirin withdrawal and quality appraisal in included studies is available in Tables 3-4. Generic inverse variance weighting enabled statistical pooling according to a random effect model, providing pooled effect estimates for subgroups and the overall population (Figure 2).

Table 3. Clinical impact of aspirin withdrawal in included studies

Study	Primary end-point	Follow-up	Effect size	Adjustment	Other outcomes
Collet (2004)	All-cause mortality	1 month	Odds ratio=2.05 (1.08-3.89)	Unclear extent, based on univariate analysis	Bleeding
Dacey (2000)	All-cause mortality	In-hospital	Odds ratio=1.82 (1.02-3.23)	Based on univariate analysis and epidemiologic approach	Bleeding
Ferrari (2005)	ST-segment-elevation acute myocardial infarction	NA	Relative risk=2.13 (1.42-3.22)	None performed	NA

Table 3 (Continued)

Study	Primary end-point	Follow-up	Effect size	Adjustment	Other outcomes
Iakovou (2005)	Sudden cardiac death, postprocedural myocardial infarction not clearly attributable to another coronary lesion, or stent thrombosis	9 months	Odds ratio=89.7 8 (29.90-269.60)*	Extensive, but with stepwise selection	NA
Mangano (2002)	All-cause mortality	In-hospital	Odds ratio=2.44 (1.61-3.70)	Extensive, but with stepwise selection	Myocardial infarction, stroke, renal failure, wound healing
Newby (2006)	All-cause mortality	7 years	Hazard ratio=1.72 (1.54-2.38)†	Extensive, but with stepwise selection	NA

*Risk estimates refer to discontinuation of either aspirin or thienopyridines, or both; †originally reported for aspirin continuation (hazard ratio=0.58 [0.42-0.65]); NA=not applicable or available.

Table 4. Quality appraisal of included studies

Study	Design	Multicenter	Selection bias	Performance bias	Detection bias	Attrition bias
Collet (2004)	Prospective cohort	No	A	B	D	A
Dacey (2000)	Prospective cohort	Yes	A	B	D	A
Ferrari (2005)	Prospective cohort	No	A	B	B	A
Iakovou (2005)	Prospective cohort	Yes	A	B	D	A
Mangano (2002)	Prospective cohort	Yes	A	B	D	A
Newby (2006)	Prospective cohort	No	A	B	D	B

*The internal validity of included trials was appraised judging the risk for selection, performance, attrition, and adjudication biases, and expressed as low risk of bias (A), moderate risk of bias (B), high risk of bias (C), or incomplete reporting leading to inability to ascertain the underlying risk of bias (D).

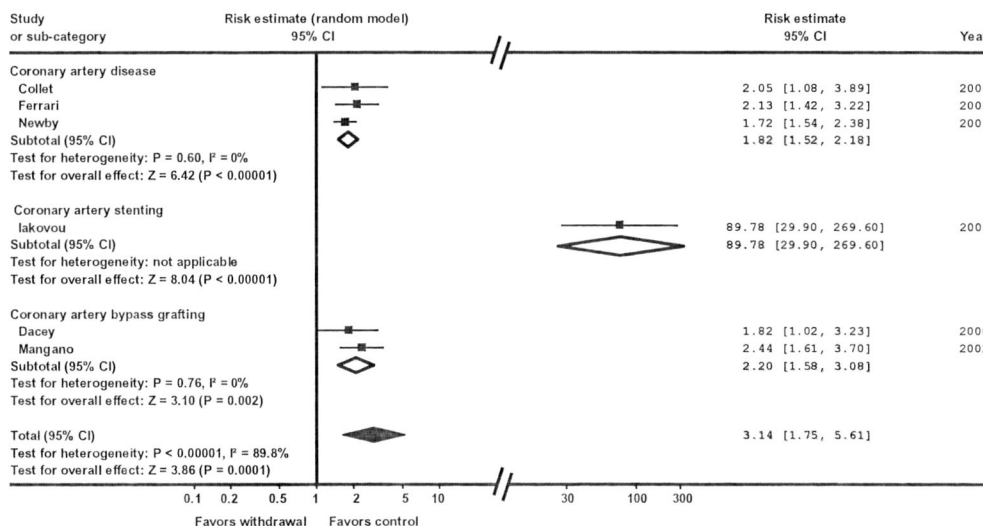

Figure 2. Forest plot of the risk of adverse thrombotic events in patients discontinuing aspirin. The analysis is stratified according to the clinical setting and follow-up duration. There is a statistically significant association between aspirin discontinuation and adverse clinical outcomes overall, and in each subgroup. While every subgroup appears clinically and statistically homogeneous, the risk of antiplatelet discontinuation appear far greater after percutaneous coronary intervention with drug-eluting stent implantation (as reported by Iakovou et al, 2005) than in any other study group. CI=confidence interval.

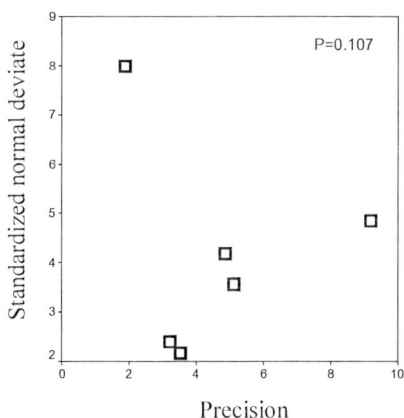

Figure 3. Graphic plot of the Egger test for small study bias, showing no evidence of such publication bias among the studies included in this meta-analysis.

Specifically, in the subgroup of 3 studies enrolling patients with acute coronary syndromes or on secondary prevention for coronary artery disease, the risk of adverse events after aspirin withdrawal was increased 2-fold (1.82 [1.52-2.18], P for effect<0.00001, P for heterogeneity=0.60, I^2=0%). Similarly, combining the 2 studies focusing on cardiac surgery showed the significant detrimental impact of aspirin discontinuation on the risk of adverse events (2.20 [1.58-3.08], P for effect=0.002, P for heterogeneity=0.76, I^2=0%). Pooling all these groups yielded a highly significant association between aspirin withdrawal and adverse events (3.14 [1.75-5.61], P for effect=0.0001, P for heterogeneity<0.00001, I^2=89.8%). While such meta-analysis may be considered robust as performed according to a random effect approach, the presence and extent of statistical heterogeneity limits its conclusiveness and leaves it mainly in the hypothesis-generating realm.

Additional Analyses

A major issue is the time between aspirin discontinuation and subsequent adverse events. While this work was not designed to address this topic (already extensively covered by Berger et al (2005)), pooling available data showed that on average 10.66 (95% confidence interval 10.25-11.07) days elapsed between drug withdrawal and thrombotic events. These results appear in line with the half-life of platelets, and suggest that in case of mandatory aspirin discontinuation for highly invasive interventions in patients at high risk of bleeding, the drug should be resumed well before that 8-10 days have elapsed.

Testing for publication bias yielded non-significant results (P=0.107, Figure 3), suggesting that among included reports the likelihood of such small study bias was not high. Nonetheless, the limited number of studies, and the consequent low statistical power for the Egger test, should be borne in mind.

Sensitivity analyses further confirmed the overall results of our work, as selecting one of the subgroups only, or excluding one study at a time, did not determine major changes in direction or magnitude of statistical findings.

Discussion

Findings of the present systematic review on the hazards of aspirin withdrawal in patients with or at risk for coronary artery disease are several-fold: 1) despite a wealth of data on the favorable risk-benefit balance of initiating aspirin treatment in these subjects, there are still relatively few observational studies focusing on aspirin discontinuation, and no pertinent controlled randomized trial; 2) the few available studies addressing the issue of aspirin withdrawal individually clearly demonstrate the relevant hazards inherent in interrupting aspirin treatment in patients in primary or secondary prevention; 3) meta-analysis combining the available studies further demonstrates the significant increase in the risk of adverse events after an average of 10 days of discontinuing aspirin, across a broad spectrum of patients with or at risk for coronary artery disease.

Current Clinical and Research Context

As clearly reported in the Results section of this work, current data focusing on aspirin discontinuation are still limited and of observational nature. No large randomized trial has been conducted to soundly appraise and define the most appropriate management strategy for patients. Thus, evidence-based recommendations cannot be proposed. Nonetheless, some reports are available suggesting the safety of continuing low-dose aspirin in patients undergoing minor (eg oral) surgery. (Madan, 2005) Moreover, French investigators generated guidelines for the perioperative management of antiplatelet agents. (Samama, 2002) In their consusus statement, they remind that aspirin and non-steroidal anti-inflammatory drugs increase intra- and postoperative bleeding moderately, but not transfusion requirements, and that the common practice of withdrawing antiplatelet agents is now challenged because of the increased incidence of thrombotic events in patients in whom treatment was interrupted. Thus, they recommended that aspirin should not be withdrawn for most vascular procedures and in several additional settings. When a definite increase in intraoperative bleeding is feared, or when surgical hemostasis is difficult, aspirin could be replaced by shorter acting non-steroidal anti-inflammatory drugs, given for a 10-day period and interrupted the day before surgery, and postoperatively antiplatelet treatment should be resumed immediately after surgery (first 6 hours). (Samama, 2002).

Burger et al (2005) have recently reported on a sound and comprehensive systematic review focusing on cardiovascular risks after aspirin perioperative withdrawal versus bleeding risks with its continuation. They found that aspirin withdrawal precedes up to 10.2% of acute cardiovascular syndromes, with time intervals between discontinuation and acute cerebral events of 14.3±11.3 days, 8.5± 3.6 days for acute coronary syndromes, and 25.8±18.1 days for acute peripheral arterial syndromes (P < 0.02 versus acute coronary syndromes). On aspirin-related bleeding risks, 41 studies were retrieved, reporting on 49 590 patients (14 981 on aspirin). Baseline frequency of bleeding complications varied between 0 (skin lesion excision, cataract surgery) and 75% (transrectal prostate biopsy). Whilst aspirin increased the rate of bleeding complications by 1.5, it did not lead to a higher level of the severity of bleeding complications (exception: intracranial surgery, and possibly transurethral prostatectomy). They then concluded that only if low-dose aspirin may cause bleeding risks with increased mortality or sequels comparable with the observed cardiovascular risks after aspirin withdrawal, it should be discontinued prior to an intended operation or procedure.

Pathophysiologically, it is likely that rebound elevations in platelet thromboxane synthesis are among the most important mechanisms underlying the increased thrombotic risk associated with aspirin discontinuation, as shown by Vial et al (1991). However, experimental in vitro and in vivo studies appraising this issues are still limited, and this field appears as a promising avenue for further research.

Contributions of the Present Study

This systematic review, while not overcoming the limitations of the individual studies hereby appraised and pooled, further confirms the major detrimental impact of aspirin withdrawal across a large spectrum of subjects at risk for de novo or recurrent cardiovascular events. Indeed, the similar risk faced by patients with acute coronary artery disease and those undergoing coronary artery bypass grafting clearly demonstrates that the beneficial effects of aspirin continuation are not restricted to a specific patient subset. Moreover, the momentous increase in risk faced by those treated with coronary drug-eluting stents can be easily explained by the highly thrombotic milieu generated by percutaneous coronary intervention with drug-eluting stent implantation, and its consequent dependence on high intensity antiplatelet regimens for several months. (Biondi-Zoccai, 2006)

Another notable finding of this work is the homogeneity in intervals reported from the several included studies from aspirin discontinuation to thrombotic events. Indeed, the typical average interval of 10 days appears coherent with pathophysiologic data on platelet half-life, and has relevant management implications, as in any case of mandatory physician-supervised aspirin withdrawal, the drug should be reinstituted well before these 10 days have elapsed.

Finally, the most relevant result of this scientific endeavor will probably be fulfilled only in the future, if it will be able to guide in the design and conduct of clinically-relevant and adequately powered randomized clinical trials capable of establishing the most appropriate treatment approach in patients scheduled for temporary aspirin discontinuation.

Proposal for Management of Patients on Aspirin Undergoing Invasive Procedures

While common clinical sense should guide most decisions concerning the risk-benefit balance of continuing/discontinuing aspirin in patients undergoing invasive procedures, we find that a synthetic flow-chart may be potentially useful (Figure 4). In our proposal, aspirin could be continued without major concerns in all patients at low risk of bleeding, as well as those at higher risk of bleeding undergoing minor noncardiac surgery (eg, skin surgery) or coronary artery bypass grafting.

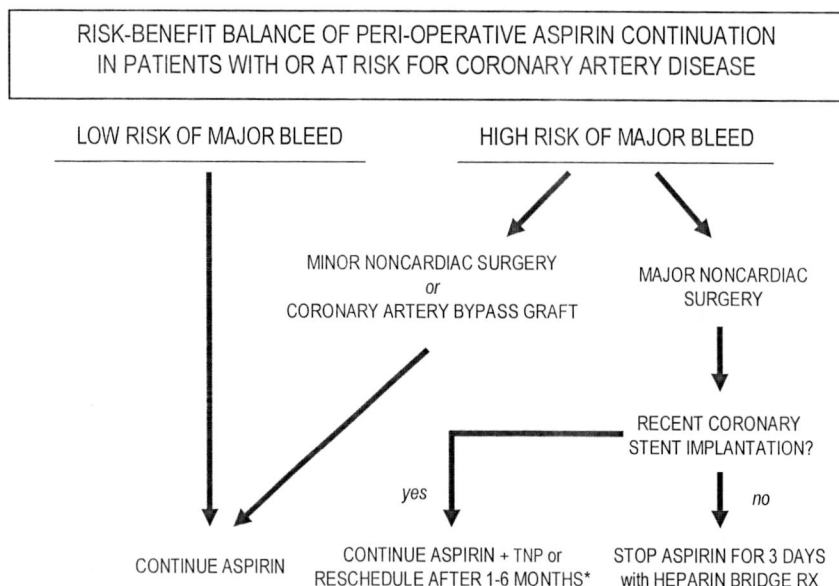

Figure 4. Proposal for management of aspirin treatment in patients with or at risk for coronary artery disease undergoing invasive procedures with variable bleeding and thrombotic risks. *the duration of combined antiplatelet therapy with aspirin and thienopyridines (TNP), ie clopidogrel or ticlopidine, after coronary stent implantation depends on the specific type of stent implanted, and goes from 4 weeks for bare-metal stents to more than 6 months for drug-eluting stents.

For patients scheduled for major cardiac noncardiac surgery, we generally advise aspirin discontinuation 3 days before the intervention, with re-institution no later that 3 days afterwards, and using a parenteral anticoagulant drug such as unfractioned or low-molecular-weight heparin as bridging antithrombotic treatment. However, patients treated with coronary stents should be managed more carefully, especially if only a few weeks have elapsed since the percutaneous coronary intervention with stent implantation. (Kaluza, 2000) Thus, we suggest to continue aspirin and thienopyridines if surgery cannot be postponed until stent endothelialization is completed (at least 4 weeks for bare-metal stents, at least 3 months for sirolimus-eluting stents, and at least 6 months for paclitaxel-eluting stents). Afterwards, short-lived aspirin discontinuation with heparin bridging therapy can be safely envisaged.

Limitations of the Present Study

Drawbacks of this work are those typical of systematic reviews and meta-analyses of clinical studies, (Biondi-Zoccai, 2003) but are not limited to those. Indeed, pooling of observational studies is considered by several investigators as hypothesis-generating only, and should thus be viewed with caution. (Stroup, 2000) Moreover, we should bear in mind that the included studies largely differed in clinical setting, end-point definition, and duration of follow-up, among the others. Thus, this meta-analysis, while providing intriguing findings, should be considered in light of the other available evidence and placed correctly in the hierarchy of evidence among other observational and non-experimental studies.

Conclusion

This systematic overview suggests that aspirin withdrawal has ominous prognostic implication in subjects with or at moderate-to-high risk for coronary artery disease. These findings should be taken into account in the management of patients under such treatment, and aspirin discontinuation should be advocated only when the risk of bleeding or other adverse effects clearly overwhelms that of cardiovascular atherothrombotic events.

Acknowledgements

This study is part of a senior training project of the Center for Overview, Meta-analysis, and Evidence-based medicine Training (COMET), based in Abano Terme, Italy (http://it.geocities.com/comet_milano/Home.htm).

Appendix

PubMed was searched according to the strategy modified from Wilczynski and Haynes, (2004) and incorporating wild cards (identified by *): ((aspirin) AND (therapy OR treatment

OR regimen) AND (discontinue* OR interrupt* OR withdraw* OR stop*)) AND (incidence[MeSH:noexp] OR mortality[MeSH Terms] OR follow up studies[MeSH:noexp] OR prognos*[Text Word] OR predict*[Text Word] OR course*[Text Word])

BioMedCentral and Google Scholar were instead searched with the following strategy: ((aspirin) AND (therapy OR treatment OR regimen) AND (discontinu* OR interrupt* OR withdraw* OR stop*)) AND (incidence OR mortality OR follow* OR prognos* OR predict* OR course*)

References

Albaladejo P, Geeraerts T, Francis F, Castier Y, Leseche G, Marty J. Aspirin withdrawal and acute lower limb ischemia. *Anesth. Analg.* 2004;99(2):440–3.

Andreotti F, Testa L, Biondi-Zoccai GG, Crea F. Aspirin plus warfarin compared to aspirin alone after acute coronary syndromes: an updated and comprehensive meta-analysis of 25,307 patients. *Eur. Heart J.* 2006;27(5):519-26.

Antithrombotic Trialists' Collaboration. Collaborative meta-analysis of randomised trials of antiplatelet therapy for prevention of death, myocardial infarction, and stroke in high risk patients. *BMJ.* 2002;324(7329):71-86.

Assia EI, Raskin T, Kaiserman I, Rotenstreich Y, Segev F. Effect of aspirin intake on bleeding during cataract surgery. *J Cataract Refract Surg.* 1998;24(9):1243-6.

Bachman DS. Discontinuing chronic aspirin therapy: another risk factor for stroke? *Ann Neurol* 2002;51(1):137–8.

Berger JS, Roncaglioni MC, Avanzini F, Pangrazzi I, Tognoni G, Brown DL. Aspirin for the primary prevention of cardiovascular events in women and men: a sex-specific meta-analysis of randomized controlled trials. *JAMA.* 2006;295(3):306-13.

Billingsley EM, Maloney ME. Intraoperative and postoperative bleeding problems in patients taking warfarin, aspirin, and nonsteroidal antiinflammatory agents. A prospective study. *Dermatol Surg.* 1997;23(5):381-3.

Biondi-Zoccai GG, Agostoni P, Sangiorgi GM, Airoldi F, Cosgrave J, Chieffo A, Barbagallo R, Tamburino C, Vittori G, Falchetti E, Margheri M, Briguori C, Remigi E, Iakovou I, Colombo A, for the Real-world Eluting-stent Comparative Italian retrosPective Evaluation Study Investigators. Incidence, predictors, and outcomes of coronary dissections left untreated after drug-eluting stent implantation. *Eur. Heart J.* 2006;27(5):540-6.

Biondi-Zoccai GGL, Agostoni P, Abbate A. Parallel hierarchy of scientific studies in cardiovascular medicine. *Ital. Heart J.* 2003;4(11):819-20. (B)

Biondi-Zoccai GGL, Agostoni P, Testa L, Abbate A, Parisi Q, Burzotta F, Trani C, Mongiardo R, Vassanelli C, Biasucci LM. Increased mortality after coronary stenting in patients treated with clopidogrel without loading dose. Evidence from a meta-analysis. *Minerva Cardioangiol.* 2004;52(3):195-208. (A)

Biondi-Zoccai GGL, Testa L, Agostoni P. A practical algorithm for systematic reviews in cardiovascular medicine. *Ital Heart J.* 2004;5(6):486-7. (C)

Boersma E, Harrington RA, Moliterno DJ, White H, Theroux P, Van de Werf F, de Torbal A, Armstrong PW, Wallentin LC, Wilcox RG, Simes J, Califf RM, Topol EJ, Simoons ML. Platelet glycoprotein IIb/IIIa inhibitors in acute coronary syndromes: a meta-analysis of all major randomised clinical trials. *Lancet*. 2002;359(9302):189-98.

Bouvy ML, Heerdink ER, Leufkens HG, Hoes AW. Patterns of pharmacotherapy in patients hospitalised for congestive heart failure. *Eur J Heart Fail*. 2003;5(2):195-200.

Burger W, Chemnitius JM, Kneissl GD, Rucker G. Low-dose aspirin for secondary cardiovascular prevention - cardiovascular risks after its perioperative withdrawal versus bleeding risks with its continuation - review and meta-analysis. *J Intern Med*. 2005;257(5):399-414.

Collet JP, Himbet F, Steg PG. Myocardial infarction after aspirin cessation in stable coronary artery disease patients. *Int. J. Cardiol*. 2000;76(2-3):257-8.

Collet JP, Montalescot G, Blanchet B, Tanguy ML, Golmard JL, Choussat R, Beygui F, Payot L, Vignolles N, Metzger JP, Thomas D. Impact of prior use or recent withdrawal of oral antiplatelet agents on acute coronary syndromes. *Circulation*. 2004;110(16):2361-7.

Dacey LJ, Munoz JJ, Johnson ER, Leavitt BJ, Maloney CT, Morton JR, Olmstead EM, Birkmeyer JD, O'Connor GT, for the Northern New England Cardiovascular Disease Study Group. Effect of preoperative aspirin use on mortality in coronary artery bypass grafting patients. *Ann. Thorac. Surg*. 2000;70(6):1986-90.

Delpierre S, Vantelon C, Samandel S, Lacaille S, Legrain S. Fatal coronary stent thrombosis after withdrawal of aspirin treatment before performing a colonoscopy. *Rev. Med. Interne*. 2005;26(8):675-7.

Eagle KA, Kline-Rogers E, Goodman SG, Gurfinkel EP, Avezum A, Flather MD, Granger CB, Erickson S, White K, Steg PG. Adherence to evidence-based therapies after discharge for acute coronary syndromes: an ongoing prospective, observational study. *Am. J. Med*. 2004;117(2):73-81.

Ferrari E, Benhamou M, Cerboni P, Baudouy M. Coronary syndromes following aspirin withdrawal. *Chest* 2003;124(Abstract supplement October):148S.

Ferrari E, Benhamou M, Cerboni P, Marcel B. Coronary syndromes following aspirin withdrawal: a special risk for late stent thrombosis. *J. Am. Coll Cardiol*. 2005;45(3):456-9.

Gaede P, Vedel P, Larsen N, Jensen GV, Parving HH, Pedersen O. Multifactorial intervention and cardiovascular disease in patients with type 2 diabetes. *N. Engl. J. Med*. 2003;348(5):383-93.

Gaspoz JM, Coxson PG, Goldman PA, Williams LW, Kuntz KM, Hunink MG, Goldman L. Cost effectiveness of aspirin, clopidogrel, or both for secondary prevention of coronary heart disease. *N. Engl. J. Med*. 2002;346(23):1800-6.

Gollapudi RR, Teirstein PS, Stevenson DD, Simon RA. Aspirin sensitivity: implications for patients with coronary artery disease. *JAMA*. 2004;292(24):3017-23.

Hamann GF, Weimar C, Glahn J, Busse O, Diener HC. Adherence to secondary stroke prevention strategies--results from the German Stroke Data Bank. *Cerebrovasc Dis*. 2003;15(4):282-8.

Harker LA, Boissel JP, Pilgrim AJ, Gent M, for the CAPRIE Steering Committee and Investigators. Comparative safety and tolerability of clopidogrel and aspirin: results from CAPRIE. Clopidogrel versus aspirin in patients at risk of ischaemic events. *Drug Saf.* 1999;21(4):325-35.

Higgins JPT, Green S, McDowell N. The Cochrane handbook for systematic reviews of interventions 4.2.5 [updated May 2005]. Available at: http://www.cochrane.org/ resources/handbook/hbook.htm (accessed 4 March 2006).

Higgins JPT, Thompson SG, Deeks JJ, Altman DG. Measuring inconsistency in meta-analyses. *BMJ.* 2003;327(7414):557-560.

Hui CK, Lai KC, Yuen MF, Wong WM, Lam SK, Lai CL. Does withholding aspirin for one week reduce the risk of post-sphincterotomy bleeding? *Aliment Pharmacol Ther.* 2002;16(5):929-36.

Iakovou I, Schmidt T, Bonizzoni E, Ge L, Sangiorgi GM, Stankovic G, Airoldi F, Chieffo A, Montorfano M, Carlino M, Michev I, Corvaja N, Briguori C, Gerckens U, Grube E, Colombo A. Incidence, predictors, and outcome of thrombosis after successful implantation of drug-eluting stents. *JAMA.* 2005;293(17):2126-30.

Kaluza GL, Joseph J, Lee JR, Raizner ME, Raizner AE. Catastrophic outcomes of noncardiac surgery soon after coronary stenting. *J. Am. Coll Cardiol.* 2000;35(5):1288-94.

Kovich O, Otley CC. Thrombotic complications related to discontinuation of warfarin and aspirin therapy perioperatively for cutaneous operation. *J. Am. Acad. Dermatol.* 2003;48(2):233–7.

Kulkarni SP, Alexander KP, Lytle B, Heiss G, Peterson ED. Long-term adherence with cardiovascular drug regimens. *Am. Heart J.* 2006;151(1):185-91.

Lau J, Ioannidis JP, Schmid CH. Summing up evidence: one answer is not always enough. *Lancet.* 1998;351(9096):123-7.

Lawrence C, Sakuntabhai A, Tiling-Grosse S. Effect of aspirin and nonsteroidal antiinflammatory drug therapy on bleeding complications in dermatologic surgical patients. *J. Am. Acad. Dermatol.* 1994;31(6):988-92.

Madan GA, Madan SG, Madan G, Madan AD. Minor oral surgery without stopping daily low-dose aspirin therapy: a study of 51 patients. *J. Oral Maxillofac. Surg.* 2005;63(9):1262-5.

Manes C, Giacci L, Sciartilli A, D'Alleva A, De Caterina R. Aspirin overprescription in primary cardiovascular prevention. *Thromb Res.* 2005 Nov 28; doi:10.1016/j.thromres.2005.09.013.

Mangano DT, for the Multicenter Study of Perioperative Ischemia Research Group. Aspirin and mortality from coronary bypass surgery. *N. Engl. J. Med.* 2002;347(17):1309-17.

Matsuzaki K, Matsui K, Haraguchi N, Nagano I, Okabe H, Asou T. Ischemic heart attacks following cessation of aspirin before coronary artery bypass surgery: a report of two cases. *Ann. Thorac. Cardiovasc Surg* 1999;5(2):121–2.

McFadden EP, Stabile E, Regar E, Cheneau E, Ong AT, Kinnaird T, Suddath WO, Weissman NJ, Torguson R, Kent KM, Pichard AD, Satler LF, Waksman R, Serruys PW. Late thrombosis in drug-eluting coronary stents after discontinuation of antiplatelet therapy. *Lancet.* 2004;364(9444):1519-21.

Mitchell SM, Sethia KK. Hazards of aspirin withdrawal before transurethral prostatectomy. *BJU Int.* 1999;84(4):530.

Nelson MR, Liew D, Bertram M, Vos T. Epidemiological modelling of routine use of low dose aspirin for the primary prevention of coronary heart disease and stroke in those aged > or =70. *BMJ.* 2005;330(7503):1306.

Newby LK, Bhapkar MV, White HD, Moliterno DJ, LaPointe NM, Kandzari DE, Verheugt FW, Kramer JM, Armstrong PW, Califf RM, for the SYMPHONY and 2nd SYMPHONY investigators. Aspirin use post-acute coronary syndromes: intolerance, bleeding and discontinuation. *J. Thromb. Thrombolysis.* 2003;16(3):119-28.

Newby LK, LaPointe NM, Chen AY, Kramer JM, Hammill BG, DeLong ER, Muhlbaier LH, Califf RM. Long-term adherence to evidence-based secondary prevention therapies in coronary artery disease. *Circulation.* 2006;113(2):203-12.

Ong AT, McFadden EP, Regar E, de Jaegere PP, van Domburg RT, Serruys PW. Late angiographic stent thrombosis (LAST) events with drug-eluting stents. *J. Am. Coll Cardiol.* 2005;45(12):2088-92.

Pascual Figal DA, Valdes Chavarri M, Ruiperez JA, Cortes R, Lopez Palop R, Pico Aracil F, Garcia Alberola A. Subacute thrombosis with antiplatelet treatment in a non-selected population of intracoronary stents: incidence and predictors. *Rev. Esp. Cardiol.* 2000;53(6):791-6.

Patrono C, Garcia Rodriguez LA, Landolfi R, Baigent C. Low-dose aspirin for the prevention of atherothrombosis. *N. Engl. J. Med.* 2005;353(22):2373-83.

Peters RJ, Mehta SR, Fox KA, Zhao F, Lewis BS, Kopecky SL, Diaz R, Commerford PJ, Valentin V, Yusuf S, for the Clopidogrel in Unstable angina to prevent Recurrent Events (CURE) Trial Investigators. Effects of aspirin dose when used alone or in combination with clopidogrel in patients with acute coronary syndromes: observations from the Clopidogrel in Unstable angina to prevent Recurrent Events (CURE) study. *Circulation.* 2003;108(14):1682-7.

Randolph A, Bucher H, Richardson WS, Wells G, Tugwell P, Guyatt G. Prognosis. In: Guyatt G, Rennie D, editors. Users' guides to the medical literature. A manual for evidence-based clinical practice. *Chicago: American Medical Association Press.* 2002:141-154.

Ridker PM, Cook NR, Lee IM, Gordon D, Gaziano JM, Manson JE, Hennekens CH, Buring JE. A randomized trial of low-dose aspirin in the primary prevention of cardiovascular disease in women. *N. Engl. J. Med.* 2005;352(13):1293-304.

Ridker PM, Cushman M, Stampfer MJ, Tracy RP, Hennekens CH. Inflammation, aspirin, and the risk of cardiovascular disease in apparently healthy men. *N. Engl. J. Med.* 1997;336(14):973-9.

Samama CM, Bastien O, Forestier F, Denninger MH, Isetta C, Juliard JM, Lasne D, Leys D, Mismetti P; French Society of Anesthesiology and Intensive Care. Antiplatelet agents in the perioperative period: expert recommendations of the French Society of Anesthesiology and Intensive Care (SFAR) 2001—Summary statement. *Can. J. Anaesth.* 2002;49(6):S26-35.

Sonksen JR, Kong KL, Holder R. Magnitude and time course of impaired primary haemostasis after stopping chronic low and medium dose aspirin in healthy volunteers. *Br. J. Anaesth.* 1999;82(3):360-5.

Stroup DF, Berlin JA, Morton SC, Olkin I, Williamson GD, Rennie D, Moher D, Becker BJ, Sipe TA, Thacker SB. Meta-analysis of observational studies in epidemiology: a proposal for reporting. Meta-analysis Of Observational Studies in Epidemiology (MOOSE) group. *JAMA.* 2000;283(15):2008-12.

Sud A, Kline-Rogers EM, Eagle KA, Fang J, Armstrong DF, Rangarajan K, Otten RF, Stafkey-Mailey DR, Taylor SD, Erickson SR. Adherence to medications by patients after acute coronary syndromes. *Ann. Pharmacother.* 2005;39(11):1792-7.

Thom T, Haase N, Rosamond W, Howard VJ, Rumsfeld J, Manolio T, Zheng ZJ, Flegal K, O'Donnell C, Kittner S, Lloyd-Jones D, Goff DC Jr, Hong Y, Adams R, Friday G, Furie K, Gorelick P, Kissela B, Marler J, Meigs J, Roger V, Sidney S, Sorlie P, Steinberger J, Wasserthiel-Smoller S, Wilson M, Wolf P. Heart Disease and Stroke Statistics—2006 Update: A Report From the American Heart Association Statistics Committee and Stroke Statistics Subcommittee. *Circulation* 2006;113(6):e85-151.

Tran H, Anand SS. Oral antiplatelet therapy in cerebrovascular disease, coronary artery disease, and peripheral arterial disease. *JAMA.* 2004;292(15):1867-74.

Vial JH, McLeod LJ, Roberts MS. Rebound elevation in urinary thromboxane B2 and 6-keto-PFF1 alpha exacerbation after aspirin withdrawal. *Adv Prostaglandin Thromboxane Leukot Res.* 1991;21A:157–160.

Wilczynski NL, Haynes RB, for the Hedges Team. Developing optimal search strategies for detecting clinically sound prognostic studies in MEDLINE: an analytic survey. *BMC Med.* 2004;2:23.

Zanetti G, Kartalas-Goumas I, Montanari E, Federici AB, Trinchieri A, Rovera F, Pisani E. Extracorporeal shockwave lithotripsy in patients treated with antithrombotic agents. *J. Endourol.* 2001;15(3):237-41.

In: Substance Withdrawal Syndrome
Editors: J. P. Rees and O. B. Woodhouse

ISBN 978-1-60692-951-3
© 2009 Nova Science Publishers, Inc.

Chapter VI

Changes Observed in Circulatory and Alimentary Systems in Alcohol Dependent Patients during the Withdrawal Period[*]

Maria Kłopocka, Jacek Budzyński,
Grzegorz Pulkowski and Marcin Ziółkowski[1]
Department of Gastroenterology, Vascular Diseases and Internal Medicine,
Nicolaus Copernicus University, CM Bydgoszcz, Poland
[1]Department of Psychiatry Nursing, Nicolaus Copernicus University,
CM Bydgoszcz, Poland

Abstract

This chapter includes up-to-date information concerning the most important changes in morphological and functional status of cardiovascular system and gastrointestinal tract, observed in alcohol dependent patients after alcohol withdrawal. The results of our own studies on this subject are also presented and discussed.

Alcohol abuse is associated with well-known psychosomatic health and social problems. It leads to multi-organ, especially cardiovascular system, alimentary tract, liver, pancreas and immunologic system dysfunction. Therefore withdrawal and anti-relapse therapy should be undoubtedly undertaken in every case. Nevertheless our knowledge on alcohol withdrawal consequences is still insufficient. Within abstinence period, especially during the first month, not only psychiatric, but also systemic and metabolic (mainly endocrine, haemostatic and immunologic) changes occur. As a result of such changes, some differences in circulatory system function, exercise capacity and autonomic nervous system activity can be observed. Some of them may be even life-threatening, leading to sudden cardiac death or acute cardiovascular events.

[*] A version of this chapter was also published as a chapter in *Trends in Alcohol Abuse and Alcoholism Research*, edited by Rin Yoshida, published by Nova Science Publishers, Inc. It was submitted for appropriate modifications in an effort to encourage wider dissemination of research.

The most expressed alterations in cardiovascular diseases risk factors values occur within first four weeks after alcohol misuse period, although, as it was proved in our studies, they can be also noted after six months of observation. In such long abstinence period pro-atherogenic metabolic changes expressed by the decrease of HDL and increase of LDL- cholesterol plasma concentration occurred. These unfavorable changes were less expressed in patients treated with naltrexone, what probably should be taken into consideration, when anti-relapse pharmacotherapy is planned. Other factors important in atherosclerosis progression and acute coronary syndromes pathogenesis are platelets activation and plasma blood coagulation and fibrinolysis system function. In our studies some indirect markers of platelets activation were determined in the early abstinence period. The highest level of fibrinogen, thrombomodulin, antithrombin, markers of trombinogenesis activation in vivo (thrombin- antithrombin, TAT complexes), tissue type plasminogen activator antigen (t-PA:Ag), antigen of plasminogen activator inhibitor type 1 (PAI-1:Ag), markers of fibrinolysis activation in vivo, such as D-dimers, plasmin- alpha2- antiplasmin (PAP) complexes were recorded shortly after alcohol drinking cessation. Mentioned changes were strongly expressed in patients with determinable TNF-alpha plasma level. Abstinence keeping improved effort capacity and positively modulated autonomic nervous system activity via vagal nerve influence on heart rate variability.

Similarly, in alcohol withdrawal period can be observed some morphological and functional changes in alimentary tract, although they are less expressed and mostly beneficial as a result of cytotoxic action cessation. The most important clinical manifestations of alcohol abuse are mucosal lesions in the upper part of the gastrointestinal tract, motility disorders, pancreatitis and liver function impairment. In our studies some changes in examined parameters values, which occurred within the withdrawal period were estimated by endoscopic examinations, esophageal and gastric pH-metry, esophageal manometry, abdominal ultrasonography and blood samples biochemical analysis. Favorable effect of alcohol withdrawal on liver function tests values was affected by pituitary-thyroid and pituitary- gonadal axes hormones level, cytokine TNF-alpha serum level, nutrition status, Helicobacter pylori infection presence and gastric acidity value.

The results of our analysis also indicated, that some of studied haematological and biochemical parameters, such as mean platelets volume and nitric oxide metabolites plasma level may be taken into consideration as new, potentially valuable markers of alcohol abuse as well as drinking relapse predictors.

Conclusion: Alcohol withdrawal and early abstinence is a dynamic period with potentially harmful health consequences, especially in cardiovascular system. In some cases appropriate treatment, also pharmacologic, should probably be recommended. The results of latest papers on the alcohol withdrawal benefit and harmful effects suggest the necessity of scrupulous multicentre studies to estimate the real clinical importance of occurring changes and cost- benefits analysis of selected interventions.

Introduction

Alcoholism, exactly alcohol dependence, heavy alcohol abuse and withdrawal syndrome cause and promote a plethora of diseases and injuries. The financial and social health care costs of harmful alcohol consumption consequences are enormous. It was estimated, that about 20 million Americans, no mention their families and community, suffer from alcohol abuse dependence. This leads to annual losses of more than 80 billion dollars and 100 000 lives in the United States [1], but the same, probably underestimated problem is of prime concern to all modern societies. Approximately 21% of all the intensive care unit admissions are directly alcohol related [2], and 20-40% of all persons admitted to general hospitals have alcohol-related health problems [3]. Similar group of often undiagnosed alcoholics visit general practitioners, being treated for the consequences of their drinking, especially in the elderly, when the number of alcohol-related health problems are similar to those of other origin. Even moderate doses of alcohol have cognitive and psychomotor effects that lead to increased risk of injury while driving, operating machinery, in sports and recreational activities [4]. For many chronic diseases the risk of disease increases with increasing average daily alcohol consumption. The best documented example when the disease risk is clearly affected by the amount and the pattern of alcohol consumption is the risk for cardiovascular disease (CVD), especially coronary heart disease (CHD). Meta- analysis show, that this relationship is represented by a J-shaped curve. It means, that compared with abstinence, low-to-moderate consumption of alcohol is associated with lower risk for CHD incidence and mortality, the lowest risk being found at 20 grams per day [5]. For higher levels of alcohol consumption, with average amount of more than 70 grams per day this risk becomes greater, than for abstainers [6]. In addition to its effect on CHD, excessive alcohol consumption, especially even irregular heavy drinking is connected with other negative cardiovascular effects, as stroke, more often hemorrhagic, arterial hypertension, cardiomyopathy and sudden cardiac death [7]. Many studies have reported relationships between alcohol misuse and different types of cancer. A recent meta-analysis showed the association between drinking on average 25 grams of alcohol per day and significantly elevated risk for the following cancer sites: oral cavity, pharynx and larynx, female breast, esophagus, stomach, colon, rectum and the liver [8]. Alcohol use is also related to other chronic health consequences, as neuropsychiatric disturbances and digestive diseases. Its casual role in alcoholic liver disease, chronic pancreatitis, some gastrointestinal symptoms and nutritional deficiencies is well established [9].Ethanol is a hydrophilic and lipophilic substance, so it may effect nearly every organ. Many relationships exist, both detrimental and beneficial between alcohol consumption and disease. The relationship between average volume of consumption and all-cause mortality in males and females older than 45 is J-shaped. In younger population, a linear relationship prevails, what means that light-to-moderate drinking has no protective effect [10, 11, 12, 13, 14]. Stronger links has alcohol use to morbidity, disability and quality of life, as evidenced by recent studies [11].

Consuming alcohol initially produces the acute effects, e.g. sedation and incoordination. Regular, long-term heavy alcohol drinking induces some adaptation processes to restore the neurochemical balance. As a result, the effects of a given doses of alcohol are diminished, what is known as tolerance. If alcohol consumption is decreased or completely removed the adaptation is still exposed, unbalancing the brain's chemistry in the opposite direction. This results in symptoms, that are opposite to alcohol's initial effects, as agitation and seizures, which are the main components of withdrawal syndrome. These disturbances continue until the adaptation is removed from the brain, or until alcohol is consumed again [16]. There are still controversies regarding the risk, outcome, complications and clinical management of withdrawal syndrome. Individual risk for experience withdrawal symptoms is difficult to estimate, results from patient's pattern of drinking, genetic influences, the presence of coexisting illnesses and mentioned above neurochemical mechanisms. Despite the variability and severity of symptoms the diagnostic criteria for alcohol withdrawal are well defined [17]. It can be recognized, when two or more of the following signs and symptoms develop within hours to a few days after cessation of or reduction in alcohol use, that has been heavy or prolonged: autonomic hyperactivity (sweating, arrhythmia), hand tremor, insomnia, transient visual, tactile, auditory hallucinations or illusions, grand mal seizures, psychomotor agitation, anxiety, nausea or vomiting. The symptoms cause clinically significant distress or impairment in social, occupational, or other important areas of functioning, are not attributable to a general medical condition or another mental disorder. Some complications of acute alcohol withdrawal are life- threaten. The mortality rate among patients exhibiting delirium tremens, which is characterized by hallucinations, mental confusion and disorientation is 5 to 25 percent. As many as 15 percent of alcoholics with depressive symptoms are at risk for death by suicide. Repeated acute alcohol withdrawal states can increase the severity of certain symptoms and complications [18]. Some syndromes, which usually occur during alcohol withdrawal, as Wernicke's and Korsakoff's syndromes are the nervous systems disorders caused by thiamine deficiency, but alcoholics account for most cases. Wernicke's syndrome is characterized by severe cognitive impairment, delirium, ataxia and paralysis of certain eye muscles [19]. Korsakoff's syndrome includes severe amnesia for past events along with impaired ability to commit current experience to memory. Some clinical evidence exists, that a part of symptoms may persist for a longer time, and even some new may develop later, after acute withdrawal period. The significance of this protracted withdrawal syndrome is perhaps underestimated [20]. Protracted withdrawal syndrome manifestations associated with acute withdrawal, but persist beyond typical time course include: sleep disturbances, anxiety and depressive symptoms, tremor, increased blood pressure, pulse, breathing rate, body temperature and tremor. Other symptoms, which appear to oppose symptoms of acute withdrawal could reflect the brain's slow recovery from the reversible nerve cell damage common in alcoholism. These symptoms include decreased energy, lassitude and decreased overall metabolism. Protracted withdrawal syndrome seems to be very important, because may predispose abstinent alcoholics to relapse in an attempt to alleviate the symptoms [20]. In this time other, often not well estimated changes in many organs and systems structure and function take place.

Besides of favorable abstinence effects, some other unfortunately may be harmful. The best known are these connected with cardiovascular events risk, like proatherogenic metabolic changes (decrease in HDL cholesterol level and increase in LDL cholesterol concentration), platelet aggregability and plasma thrombotic activity increase.

Elucidate the processes, which take place in withdrawal period, their significance, clinical benefits and risk, possible connections between biochemical parameters and symptoms, as well as influence of available treatment may be very important to elaborate the best cost-effective long-term treatment strategy for every alcohol dependent patient, especially that mentioned harmful effects of early abstinence period may lead to potentially life threaten cardiovascular events.

The aim of this chapter is the short up- to- date rewiev and presentation of our own studies concerning beneficial and harmfull effects of alcohol withdrawal on some,especially cardiovascular and alimentary, systems function in alcohol dependent pateins.

Consequences of Alcohol Abuse and Withdrawal in the Gastrointestinal Tract

Main Points of Authors' Studies Results

- The features of esophageal inflammation, both in macroscopic and in microscopic examination, were frequent in alcohol dependent patients and lasted also in the withdrawal period
- Gastritis, most often not intense, was diagnosed in nearly all of patients in the distal part of the stomach and in half of them in gastric corpus shortly after alcohol drinking cessation. Some trends towards to improvement in microscopic appearance were noticed after four weeks of controlled abstinence
- The prevalence of Helicobacter pylori infection seemed to be greater in alcoholics, than in overall Polish population
- Esophageal and gastric 24-hours pH-metry parameters values were similar in the first examination performed no later, than two weeks after alcohol drinking cessation and in the second one, performed four weeks later, in the time of controlled abstinence
- The results of esophageal 24-hours pH-metry indicated on the impairment in esophageal chemical clearance in chronic alcoholics
- In patients with coexistence of depression and/or alexythimia, in comparison to patients without such disorders occurred features of more intensive esophageal exposition to gastric content, as well as esophageal motility disturbances
- About half of alcoholics had determinable plasma concentration of TNF-alpha cytokine measured after alcohol drinking cessation, and in this group biochemical features of liver injury were more expressed, as well as Helicobacter pylori gastric mucosa colonization and gastric lumen alkalization.
- Esophageal motility patern in alcoholics is characterized mainly by the higher value of contractions amplitude

Introduction

Acute, as well as chronic alcohol abuse produces well-known gastrointestinal symptoms, leads to structural and functional changes in the gastrointestinal tract and is the main causative factor of liver and pancreas injury.

Alcoholic patients show high prevalence of gastrointestinal signs and symptoms such as heartburn, chest and abdominal pain or discomfort, nausea, vomiting, gastrointestinal bleeding, flatulence and diarrhea [26, 27].Intensity of these symptoms usually decreases in the abstinence period, however some of them still exist even in the long-time of withdrawal period. In many cases manifestations could not be attributed to apparent alcohol-derived organic diseases what indicates that some other factors, such as systemic action of ethanol, disturbances in the brain-gut axis and changes in hormonal and neurotransmitters balance may be important [27 28].

Alcoholic liver disease (ALD), and especially its most severe form, cirrhosis accounts for the majority of all medical death among alcoholics. The spectrum of ALD ranges from asymptomatic hepatomegaly and tranasient abnormal liver function tests to hepatocellular failure from alcoholic hepatitis or cirrhosis. ALD is divided into three major types: alcoholic fatty liver, alcoholic hepatitis and cirrhosis. Clinical diagnosis of these stages is difficult, because they may overlap in any combination and a number of less common variants may also occur. It remains still unsolved, which of the risk factors are most important to cause serious liver injury. No more than 35% of heavy drinkers develop alcoholic hepatitis and only in 20% liver cirrhosis is diagnosed. Identification and next modification of such powerful factors seems to be a great challenge, because some of them are probably also important in the pathogenesis of some other alcohol-related harmful processes, such as inflammation, cardiovascular and metabolic disturbances. Ethanol, after ingestion is rapidly absorbed from the gastrointestinal tract. It's at first metabolised by the gastric mucosa   alcohol dehydrogenases in the stomach, however the total ethanol oxidizing capacity of the stomach is rather low, so alcohol is mainly metabolized to acetaldehyde in the liver. Liver hepatocytes contain three pathways for ethanol metabolism. The most important depends on alcohol dehydrogenase (ADH) activity in the cytosol, the second is mediated by cytochrome P450IIE1 (CYP2E1) in the endoplastic reticulum and the third by catalase, located in peroxisomes. Acetaldehyde is next oxidized by aldehyde dehydrogenase (ALDH) to acetate, Both ADH and ALDH mediate reactions in which free reduced nicotinamide adenine dinucleotide (NADH) are generated, what in excess contributes to formation of reactive O2 species. Such reactions lead to oxidative stress cascade initiation, oxidation and peroxidation of DNA, proteins and lipids. Increased levels of cytosolic and mitochondrial NADH stimulate fatty acid synthesis and inhibit their oxydation what, among other things, result in accelerated synthesis of triglycerides. These substances are next secreted by the liver as very-low-density-lipoprotein (VLDL), what is the most important reason of observed hyperlipidemia. Accumulation of free fatty acids and triglycerides in the hepatocytes is conducive to fatty liver formation. This usually benign condition may however turn into fibrosis or cirrhosis, even without alcoholic hepatitis as an intermediate stage. Evidence exists, that fatty liver cells are much more sensitive to bacterial lipopolysaccharide (LPS) action, what is probably important in the pathogenesis of ALD[25]. These endotoxins derived from the cell wall of gram-negative bacteria transfering from the gastrointestinal tract can stimulate monocytes, macrophages and some other, e.g. endothelial cells to produce alcoholic hepatitis or cirrhosis.

Elevated plasma endotoxin concentration is observed in alcoholics, independently of the degree of liver disease severity [30, 31]. binding protein (LBP), an acute phase reactan, facilitates LPS binding to humoral factors or CD14 (receptor located on monocytes and macrophages) and its soluble form, sCD14, what enables endothelial cells activation[32 On the other hand LBP transfers LPS to plasma lipoproteins, LDL and particularly HDL, what results in neutralization of LPS activity. The key role in interaction process between HDL and LBP plays apolipoprotein (Apo) A1 [33, 34].

This short introduction realizes how many relationships exist between gastrointestinal tract structure and function integrity and the liver status, balance between inflammation processes and host defence, plasma lipoproteins concentrations with respect to the cardiovascular consequences of alcohol abuse, but also regulation mechanisms important in directed against the effect of LPS.

In our studies we have estimate some of above mentioned factors in alcohol-dependent patients in the early withdrawal period.

The Upper Digestive Tract Morphological and Functional Status

The upper digestive tract morphological and functional status in alcohol-dependent patients was estimated no later than two weeks after alcohol abuse. Examinations were repeated after four weeks of controlled abstinence. The other aim of the study was to identify potentially important clinical and biochemical factors which might influence the gastrointestinal tract status and developing within the abstinence period changes. The presence as well as the intensity of esophageal and gastric inflammation features was estimated during the upper digestive tract endoscopy and in microscopic examination. Esophageal and gastric 24-hour pH-metry as well as 24-hour esophageal manometry was performed.

Esophageal Lesions

Esophageal lesions were found in more than 30% of patients. According to four-stages Los Angeles [35] classification less advanced inflammation occurred more frequently. In the control endoscopy similar percentage of esophageal inflammation features was observed, however improvement was found in more advanced stages. In microscopic examination esophagitis was diagnosed in more than 60% of patients and this value didn't change significantly in the second estimation [36].This observation seems to be important, because even in the absence of clinical symptoms, consequences of undiagnosed and untreated esophagitis, as ulceration, stenosis, hemorrhage and carcinogenesis are harmful. In the largest prospective study of gastroesophageal reflux disease (GERD) patients, regular alcohol use was one of the independent predictors of erosive GERD [37] but there is no available data concerning changes in esophageal inflammation during withdrawal period.

Gastritis Features

Macroscopic features of gastritis, most often not intense, were found in 39% of patients in gastric corpus and nearly in all (98%) in the antral part of the stomach in the initial examination. The results were similar in the repeated after four weeks endoscopy. In microscopic examination gastritis was confirmed in gastric corpus and antrum respectively in 62 and 94% of patients. The inflammation degree was generally not intense, in more advanced cases improvement was observed in the controlled estimation, however the total percentage of patients with antral gastritis was the same (94%) and with corpus gastritis lower (47%) but without statistical significance. Excessive acute alcohol consumption may breed massive bleeding from esophageal-gastric junction lesions which can arise after repeated retching and vomiting (Mallory-Weiss syndrome), as well as induce gastric mucosal hemorrhagic lesions. Though opinions concerning short-time and rapidly reversible consequences of alcohol abuse on gastric mucosa integrity and permeability are rather unanimous, nevertheless the authors vary on the subject concerning chronic alcohol misuse and withdrawal influence on gastric morphology. Gastric lesions observed after alcohol administration in endoscopic study were alcohol- dose dependent, and were less extensive with alcohol beverages, like wine and beer than with pure alcohol solutions [38]. It means, that some substances in alcohol beverages exert a protective effect on gastric mucosa, similar as they influence gastric secretion. Prolonged alcohol exposure disturbs the microcirculation, gastric mucosal barrier and increases the mucosa permeability, as well as leads to progressive structural mucosa injury [39]. Bienia et all [40] observed, that the progression of inflammatory process is related to the duration of addiction. Atrophic gastritis and lower values of hydrochloric acid secretion were connected with addiction period of at least 10 years. Though most of the authors have found a higher incidence of chronic gastritis in alcoholics [41, 42], nevertheless others shake the opinion of causal alcohol role in gastric inflammation process [43,44]. Uppal [43] in his study observed the improvement in macroscopic appearance after 3 to 4 weeks of abstinence, but histologic findings were essentially unchanged. Eradication of Helicobacter pylori (H. pylori), which prevalence was high in the studied group led to resolution of gastritis and was strongly correlated with reduction of dyspeptic symptoms. Authors suggested that H. pylori, rather than alcohol, causes chronic gastritis in alcoholics. In our study however, some histologic improvement was observed after 4 weeks of abstinence, although other factors, like H. pylori colonization didn't change at all. The high incidence of gastritis seen in alcoholics indicates, that they may be particularly prone to colonization with this microorganism, but studies on this subject have yielded inconsistent results. In our study H. pylori infection was detected in histologic examination and urease gel test in 76% of patients. Our data in this regard is similar to reported by Hydzik [45], who in the group of 66 alcohol dependent persons confirmed H. pylori infection in 80% of patients. The prevalence of H. pylori seems to be greater in alcoholics, then in overall Polish population (about 50%) [46], but these studies had limited power due to small sample size. The infection is acquired in childhood in most cases and is strongly influenced by socioeconomics conditions and childhood poverty, what explains, even partially its high incidence in our patients, who were derived mostly from straitened life circumstances. The prevalence of H. pylori infection differs and changes according to the part of the world and socioeconomic indicators. In the recently published studies it has been estimated at about 42% in the Czech Republic [47], 63% in Brazil [48] and about 30% in Sweden [45]. In the study by Hauge et al. [45] no differences were seen according to tissue pathology which showed chronic gastritis and H. pylori infection in about 30% of alcoholics and in controls as well. Brenner et all. and Murray et all.[50, 51]observed the inverse relationship between alcohol consumption and active H. pylori infection. This relation was stronger for wine and indicated the protective effect of moderate (approximately 7 units a week) wine consumption against H. pylori infection. The heavy drinkers however, like in our study, used to drink strong alcohols in great amounts, so effect on gastric acid output and intensity of inflammation may differ on such conditions. Alcoholic beverages, especially wine, display strong antimicrobial activity [52], and probably facilitate eradication of the microorganism. Dose and beverage type specific effects on the gastric mucosa and other layers of gastric wall, on the stomach emptying process and on acid secretion may also influence H. pylori, as well as other microorganisms acquisition or elimination from this part of gastrointestinal tract. Hauge [49] in spite of rather low H. pylori colonization in alcoholics, found significantly more bacteria, mainly gram-positive aerobic cocci in the gastric and duodenal biopsies of alcoholics than in those of the controls. This increased frequency of bacterial overgrowth may contribute to the common gastrointestinal symptoms as diarrhea, nausea, abdominal pain or discomfort. Some other consequences may also arise from bacterial overgrowth, the most important seems to be endotoxemia, which plays a great role in pathogenesis of liver injury, atherosclerosis processes, pulmonary hypertension, hyperdynamic circulation, endocrine glands dysfunction and even carcinogenesis observed in alcohol dependent persons [53, 54, 55].

Gastric and Esophageal 24-hours pH-metry. Esophageal 24-hours Manometry

One of our studies aim was to evaluate esophageal and gastric acidity and esophageal motor activity in alcohol dependent patients within the withdrawal period. The decrease in pH value may cause esophageal and gastric injury, provoke reflux and dyspeptic symptoms so common in alcohol abusers. On the other hand alkalization of gastric lumen facilitates bacterial overgrowth with mentioned above consequences. Effect of ethanol on gastric acid output depends on concentration and the kind of alcohol beverages. Lower concentrations of pure ethanol (up to 5% v/v) have a small stimulatory effect on gastric acid output, whereas higher concentrations (up to 40% v/v) have no effect or even inhibit acid secretion [56]. Alcoholic beverages produced by fermentation like wine and beer contain succinic acid and maleic acid, substances which are responsible for the maximal acid secretion, as well as the release of gastrin. Beverages with high alcohol concentration that are produced by distillation do not stimulate acid output and the release of gastrin [57]. Alcohol dependent persons are therefore prone to have normal, decreased or increased gastric acid output. Most of our patients used to drink strong alcohol beverages in great amounts what predisposes to lower secretion of hydrochloric acid and progression of the inflammatory process in the stomach. 24-hours esophageal and gastric pH-metry and esophageal 24-hours manometry were performed no later, then two weeks after alcohol abuse period. This time interval was probably to long for careful analysis concerning the early abstinence period, but it was difficult to perform such examination, which requires very good patient's collaboration (with two sensors positioned in esophagus for 24 hours, after nasal and esophageal intubation) in persons often suffering from sever withdrawal symptoms. The second examination was conducted after four weeks of controlled abstinence. The same procedures were carried on in the control group of patients without alcohol dependence. No differences in gastric pH-metry parameters between alcohol dependent patients and control group were found in both examinations. After four weeks of abstinence in alcohol dependent patients was observed a decrease in percentage of total monitoring time with gastric pH range 3-4, no other significant changes were noticed [58]. Importance of this finding is uncertain, however changes in pH ranges below 3 and above 4 may have some clinical outcome. Firstly, intragastric pH values above 3-4 were found to be appropriate for management of gastric and esophageal lesions and gastroesophageal symptoms control, but on the other hand lower gastric acidity facilitates bacterial overgrowth in the upper gastrointestinal tract with subsequent endotoxemia, cytokines generation and multiorgan consequences [54, 55, 59].

When esophageal pH-metry parameters in alcoholics were analyzed, no significant differences between the results of the first and controlled examination were found [60]. It suggested, that alcohol effect on antireflux barrier disappeared soon after alcohol drinking cessation or maintained longer, than one month. In comparison with the control group, alcohol dependent patients in our study had significantly lower values of acid gastroesophageal reflux, as well as lower values of esophageal exposure to content with pH above 7. However, regular alcohol use is one of the independent predictors of erosive GERD [37], and our observation is consistent with this conclusion, moreover we have demonstrated, that esophageal lesions persisted also in a withdrawal period [58]. This discrepancy is not easy to explain. Acute ethanol consumption leads to a transient decrease in the lower esophageal sphincter (LES) pressure and inhibits the primary peristalsis of the distal esophagus body. These functional changes result in an impaired esophageal clearance and increased gastroesophageal reflux [18,61]. Chronic alcohol consumption causes different disturbances in esophageal motor function. The most typical are secondary motility disorders in the middle third and distal esophagus with prolonged contractions of a high amplitude, simultaneous and double-peaked contractions. The influence on the LES pressure is opposite to that of acute alcohol consumption [18, 62, 63, 64]. This may explain our finding of higher amplitude of esophageal contractions in alcoholics, mainly in the group with depression and/or alexithymia who drank more alcohol [65]. Chronic alcohol consumption, besides of mentioned above effect on gastric acid output, delayed gastric emptying [6, 67], what facilitates bacterial overgrowth and may intensify gastric content reflux to the esophagus. In chronic alcoholics moreover, impairment in chemical esophageal clearance takes place, what seems to be important in interpretation of our finding. It concerns mainly the lower flow rate of saliva, with diminished amounts of bicarbonates, total protein, amylase and epidermal growth factor, all of them important in esophageal chemical defense [68]. It should be noticed that esophageal lesions may also result from direct cytotoxic effect of ethanol, as well as its more toxic metabolite, acetaldehyde. This substance originates already in the stomach as the result of ethanol metabolism by alcohol dehydrogenases occurring in gastric mucosa, as well as in bacteria, also H. pylori, present in gastric lumen. In the context of no essential changes in gastric pH-metry values [58] in alcoholics and in control group we suggest, that the results of significantly lower values of esophageal pH-metry parameters both of acid and alkaline reflux may result mainly from an impaired esophageal chemical defense.

Interesting results concerning esophageal motility appeared, when other factors, as psychosomatic disorders were taken into consideration. Among our patient's population was a group suffering from atypical chest pain. Psychosomatic disorders, like depression and alexithymia are common in addictive disorders, post traumatic stress disorders, as well as in patients with chest pain and normal coronary arteries in angiographic examination [69]. Psychosomatic factors also play a pathophysiological role in the pathogenesis of digestive tract diseases (hypersensitive esophagus, dyspepsia, endoscopically negative GERD, gastric and duodenal ulcer, irritable bowel disease) [70, 71, 72]. Hypothesis advanced to explain the pathophysiological role of such factors involves central disturbances in catecholamine discharge in the locus caeruleus and its multiple projection to various regions of the brain, including the entire cerebral cortex [69]. The influence of emotional disorders on gastrointestinal symptoms can be also explained by changes in serotonergic neurotransmission in the central nervous system and the digestive tract [73]. Modification of some receptors function is probably of importance as well, e. g:

– cholecystokinin (CCK) receptors, involved in the mediation of pain impulses in the gastrointestinal tract and nociception in the central nervous system
– opioid receptors which mediate pain perception in the brain, spinal cord and peripheral nervous system
– muscarinic M3-receptors, substance P, neurokinin A and B receptors important in motor adaptation and pain transmission in inflammation processes
– gabba receptors involved in nociception and cannabinoid receptors important in the control of acetylocholine release in the gut [28].

All of these mediators and receptors may influence autonomic nervous system activity and gut motility. as well as increase visceral sensitivity (decreasing the pain threshold) often occurring in functional disorders.

We have compared the results of upper digestive tract examinations in alcoholics with or without depression and/or alexithymia diagnosed with atypical chest pain[65]. To make our appreciation scrupulous and reliable we also estimated autonomic nervous system activity by heart rate variability analysis [24, 25, 74] and measured the level of plasma nitric oxide metabolites, the nonadrenergic noncholinergic inhibitory neurotransmitter [75], which together with excitatory cholinergic innervations and vasoactive intestinal polypeptide (VIP) regulate normal esophageal motility and mucosal circulation [76]. Diagnostic procedures were undertaken in 52 alcohol dependent male patients. Depression and/or alexithymia were diagnosed in 37 subjects (71%), 26 of them (50%) had both disorders simultaneously, so in final analysis patients with at least one of the two disorders were classified to one group. Alcoholics with depression and/or alexithymia, in comparison to patients with scores in normal range according to the BDI and TAS scales, were slimmer and had stronger expression of some environmental factors potentially harmful for digestive tract mucosa, as smoking and alcohol drinking intensity. The frequency of gastrointestinal symptoms and their relation to esophageal pH and motility were similar in both groups, as well as appearance of esophageal, gastric and duodenal mucosa, with the exception of H. pylori gastric mucosa colonization, which was borderline less intensive in patients with depression and/or alexithymia. In this patients group greater, but within the physiological range, esophageal mucosa acid exposition was found (significantly longer duration of the longest acid reflux, greater percentage of total monitoring time with esophageal pH below 4), in spite of similar gastric acidity. Moreover esophageal motility was also more effective (higher contractions amplitude and longer mean contraction duration) in this group. Additionally group of patients with psychosomatic disturbances, who furthermore drank more, and are probably more susceptible to alcohol drinking relapse, higher percentage of hypertensive contractions in the distal esophagus was observed. In the light of above mentioned results it seems, that the reason of greater esophageal exposition to gastric content in this patients group may be more frequent transient lower esophageal sphincter relaxations and/or less effective chemical clearance, due to saliva secretion, in part dependent on acid-induced esophago-salivary reflex [77, 78]; however the influence of other factors, such as heavy smoking and diet cannot be excluded. We found no significant differences in heart rate variability (HRV) analysis parameter values and nitric oxide metabolite plasma concentration between patient groups, so the observed differences seem to be caused by psychosomatic and environmental factors. Esophageal motility changes may also result from some other, not well determined substances, whose secretion is related to brain-gut axis function, for example galanin [79], corticotropin-releasing factor (CRF) [80] or other enterohormones (VIP, secretin, cholecystokinin, gastrin) [81].

Tumor Necrosis Factor Alpha (TNF-alpha) Concentration in the Aspect of Liver Injury Pathogenesis

As was discussed in the previous parts of this chapter, bacterial overgrowth [53] and greater permeability of the upper gastrointestinal tract observed in alcoholics [43, 59] are the main reasons of endotoxemia, which plays a great role in pathogenesis of numerous alcohol-related complications with, the perhaps most harmful, liver injury [57, 58, 59, 34, 35]. An important stage in this process is stimulation of pro-inflammatory cytokines synthesis (mainly tumor necrosis factor alpha- TNF-alpha) and the decrease of anti-inflammatory cytokines synthesis.

In our research we've compared the values of liver tests and TNF –alfa plasma concentration looking for some relationships and changes occurring within the withdrawal period [82]. However, we didn't analyze liver biopsies to determine the liver status, because of lack of clinical indications to perform this invasive procedure. The features of liver failure were one of the exclusion criteria in assumption to exclude potential confounding factors, which could have an influence on parameters, we have planned to estimate. Obtained results were for sure dependent on such selection and the results perhaps would differ with another premises.

Another limitation in the complete analyze is, that we didn't determine TNF-alpha level in the control group, so the estimation of the isolated alcohol misuse effect on TNF-alpha level was impossible. Our observations were therefore limited to determine the effect of alcohol dependence duration and severity (using Short Alcohol Dependence Data and Michigan Alcohol Screening Test) and the interrelations between analyzed factors.

About half of alcoholics had determinable plasma concentration of TNF-alpha no later, then two weeks after alcohol drinking cessation, and in this group higher alanine aminotransferase- ALT and gamma-glutamyltransferase-GGT, biochemical markers of liver injury and alcohol abuse were observed. All of these parameters values decreased after four weeks of controlled abstinence. This suggested, that alcohol abuse and withdrawal may influence TNF-alpha production and that relationships existed between this cytokine level and liver function tests values after alcohol drinking cessation.

It is known, that cytokine synthesis is related to many factors, both genetic, as individual and environmental. To estimate, which features diversified the patients group and determined

TNF-alpha level, the multiple regression analysis was performed. TNF-alpha level was positively related to alcohol dependence duration and severity indicators, liver injury biochemical markers (ALT plasma activity), intensity of Helicobacter pylori gastric mucosa colonization and duration of monitoring time with gastric pH above 3. The last two factors seemed to be the most interesting, and the possible importance of gastric mucosa alkalization in bacterial overgrowth, endotoxin production and liver injury was discussed in this chapter. In this place we only want to note, that Helicobacter pylori gastric infection may probably also stimulate TNF-alpha secretion, what was already reported [83]. This interesting subject needs of course careful estimation, moreover some reasonable premises appear to continue investigations on gastric and intestinal bacterial contamination and therapy with immunomodulators on the course of alcoholic liver disease and other alcohol-related organ disturbances.

Cardiovascular Effect of Alcohol Withdrawal

Main Points of Author's Reasearch Results

- Changes in cardiovascular system function, as well as in important biochemical and hemostatic parameters values after alcohol withdrawal are very complicated, interrelated and inconstant. This dynamic process can be observed for at least six months long period. It may clinically manifest as: acute coronary syndrome, cardiac arrhythmia, especially atrial fibrillation, stroke, congestive heart failure exacerbation. These life-threating events can be ilustrated by the left arm of J-shaped (or U-shaped) curve showing the relationship between alcohol use and cardiovascular as well as total mortality.

- Within six month long abstinence period proatherogenic changes in plasma lipids level proceed. They are expressed by decrease in HDL_2 and HDL_3 cholesterol, as well as apolipoprotein A-I and A-II levels and increase of LDL cholesterol plasma concentration

- Within first month of alcohol withdrawal period blood platelets activity increased. It is clinically expressed as augmentation of platelets aggregability and increase of mean platelets volume (MPV), indirect marker of platelets turn-over and alcohol abuse.

- Alcohol withdrawal is the reason of permanent intravascular activation of thrombin generation, with secondary activation of fibrinolysis system and these processes last for at least 6 months after alcohol misuse period. This is probably a consequence of platelets activation, changes in haemostatic factors blood levels, as well as functional and morphological endothelial injury. The last one is expressed by the increase in endothelial derived hemostatic factors plasma level and decrease of vasorelaxant factors (nitric oxide).

- About half of alcoholics had increased plasma concentration of cytokine, TNF-alpha after alcohol misuse period, and they had simultaneously more intense

proatherogenic changes in lipid and haemostatic atherosclerosis risk factors level within six-month long abstinence period.
- Four weeks long abstinence period was sufficient enough to improve the vagal nerve influence on heart rhythm and physical competence in alcoholics
- In normotensive alcohol dependent males, alcohol abstinence had a favorable effect on the proper response of blood pressure values to physical exercise. Clinical importance of this factor in cardiovascular risk estimation is considered to be similar as reduction in resting hypertension.

Introduction

Cardiovascular disease still are the main cause of deaths in the development countries in spite of an favorable effects of the prophylactic actions, such as physical activity, low-lipid diet, anti-tobacco, and slim silhouette promotion, and progress in diagnostics and therapy of hypertension, hyperlipidemia and diabetes. The powerful, but on the other hand hazardous method to protect heart and vessels seems to be among other things moderate and regular alcohol drinking [5, 6, 7, 11, 12]. Such supposition results from epidemiological studies, which show the negative relationship between the prevalence of coronary artery disease (CAD) and quantity of alcohol consumption [12]. These relationships are presented as J-shaped curve, what means, that moderate alcohol drinkers have lower cardiovascular risk that abstainers and heavy drinkers. On the other hand well known social, somatic and psychiatric complications of alcohol abuse are enormous and similar to cardiovascular disease they increase total morbidity, mortality and consume finance of medical care [1, 2, 3, 4]. These data motivate application in each case the most effective anti-alcohol relapse therapy. However, in the context of above mentioned relationships between quantity of alcohol consumption and atherosclerotic complications this therapy may increase cardiovascular event risk, because persons, who take up anti-relapse therapy, should maintain a complete alcohol abstinence resigning from favorable effects of moderate alcohol drinking.

By this reason it's obviously very important to be aware of kind and intensity of metabolic, functional and morphological changes, which occur in cardiovascular system after alcohol withdrawal, mainly to prevent connected with them harmful and even life-threating complications.

Plasma Lipids

Cardiovascular disease, especially coronary artery disease (CAD) is the leading cause of death in the developed countries. Increased plasma cholesterol level, especially LDL cholesterol are the main cardiovascular risk factors, which role was overwhelmingly confirmed in many epidemiological investigations [84, 85], whereas fasting plasma lipids, especially increased LDL-cholesterol concentration are considered to be an important pathogenetic factor involved in atherosclerosic processes and the risk factor of CAD events. Moreover, more and more evidence has insisted on the low HDL-cholesterol concentration and increased triglycerides level as factors contributing to cardiovascular event occurrence. These three fractions abnormalities are often termed as "lipid triad" or "atherogenic lipoprotein phenotype" [86]. Randomized clinical trails have provided strong evidence that decreasing plasma cholesterol with statins reduces the risk of cardiovascular events, particularly in high-risk patients, irrespective of baseline cholesterol levels, both in primary and secondary prevention [87, 88, 89]. The improvement was confirmed not only in cardiovascular (even up-to 42%), but also in general (even up-to 30%) mortality following 4-10 years of lipid-lowering therapy [84, 89]. It is generally accepted, that the decrease in total cholesterol (TC) concentration by 1% may decrease cardiovascular event risk by 2-3%. Similar effect produces an increase of HDL cholesterol level by 1mg/dl. On the basis of these data, plasma lipids concentration is the main target of prophylactic and therapeutic procedures, and no increase of suicides prevalence after lipid lowering therapy was observed, how it was postulated by advocates when the casual role of hypocholesterolemia in pathogenesis of psychiatric disorders, depression, suicides and neoplastic disorders was suggested [90]. Lack of relationships between low plasma lipids level and risk of suicidal attempts in patients with alcohol dependence confirmed also Deisenhammer et al. [91].

The epidemiological evidence showed J-shaped (or U-shaped) relationships between quantity of alcohol drinking and CAD events prevalence [5, 6, 12, 13, 14, 92, 93]. Analysis made by Langer et al. [94] revealed, that more than half of cardioprotective effects of moderate alcohol drinking depends on its influence on lipids metabolism. It has been evidenced, that alcohol intake caused the increase in HDL cholesterol and trigliceryles concentration, as well as decrease in total and LDL cholesterol level [92]. Evidence exists, that these alteriation may be also influenced by gene polymorphism, especially concerning alcohol dehydrogenese type 3 activity [12] and drinking pattern [95]. These effects, beside the direct effect on lipoprotein, resulted from altered activities of plasma proteins and enzymes involved in lipoprotein metabolism: cholesteryl ester transfer protein (CETP), phospholipid transfer protein (PTP), lecithin:cholesterol acyltransferase (LCAT), lipoprotein lipase (LL), hepatic lipase (HL), paraoxonase-1 and phospholipases. Alcohol intake also leads to modification of lipoprotein particles: low sialic acid content in apolipoprotein components of lipoprotein particles (e.g., HDL apo E and apo J) and acetaldehyde modification of apolipoproteins. In addition, "abnormal" lipids, as phosphatidylethanol, fatty acid ethyl esters formed in the presence of ethanol connect with normal lipoproteins in plasma [93]. These qualitatively alcohol-related changes in lipoproteins are recognized as factors contributing to proatherogenic effects of heavy ethanol drinking. It is supposed, that the lipid-effect of alcohol withdrawal results from the opposite reactions than mentioned above, alcohol- related. This hypothesis was also confirmed by the results of our investigations [96, 97], in which fractions of plasma lipids levels, including lipoprotein(a)-Lp(a), were determined, both fast, and five hours after fatty meal (0,5g butter per one kilo of body mass with two 50g slices of rye bread). The premises for determination of postprandial plasma lipids level in alcoholics were the results of work by Nikilla et al [98], who pointed the triglycerides level five hours after lipid meal as the better cardiovascular risk predictor than HDL cholesterol concentration. Similar clinical importance of this parameter suggested also Slyper et al. [99] and Gotto et al. [100]. This evidence has afforded, that magnitude of postprandial lipemia has been identified as independent risk factor for the development of

CAD [101, 102]. It seems obvious, because vessels for majority of day-time are exposed not for fasting, but for postprandial lipemia. It is known, that postprandial lipemia is determined by many factors, affecting lipids absorption, synthesis and clearance [103, 104]. Among them, the most important seems to be: lipids content in the meals, absorption, lipoprotein lipase activity, and polymorphisms within the genes for apolipoprotein AI, apolipoprotein E, apolipoprotein B, apolipoprotein CI, apolipoprotein CIII, apolipoprotein AIV, apolipoprotein AV, lipoprotein lipase (LLP), hepatic lipase (HL), fatty acid-binding protein-2, the fatty acid transport proteins, microsomal triglyceride transfer protein and scavenger receptor class B type I [105]. Alcohol drinking may potentially affect all, besides of genetic, above mentioned factors, via decrease in appetite, induce liver (decrease in bile acids secretion), pancreas (lipase source) and intestine (microvilli are the place of chylomicrons formation) injury, alteration of LLP activity [106]. Reference data suggest, that the final outcome leads to postprandial hiperlipemia in heavy drinkers [107], what, besides qualitative changes in lipoproteins profile, may additionally explain proatherogenic effect of alcohol abuse. However, recently recognized effect of gene polymorphism, which correlates with coronary artery disease prevalence, implies the individual influence of alcohol abuse and withdrawal on the postprandial triglycerides concentration [12, 105]. This subject will be touched in the further part of this chapter.

After alcohol misuse period alcohol dependent male patients had similar to the control group mean plasma lipids levels, however, after four weeks of abstinence, the significant decrease of Lp(a) and fasting HDL concentration as well as the increase of fasting LDL concentration and the values of plasma lipids proatherogenic indexes (TC/HDL, TC-HDL/HDL, LDL/HDL, Lp(a)/HDL) were noticed [97]. Moreover, in this withdrawal period, significantly augmented the percentage of patients with TC-HDL/HDL ratio value above 4 (from 20% to 40%), what was indicative of the cardiovascular event risk increase. In the following abstinence period, especially after the first control estimation, the level of studied lipids in alcohol dependent patients showed the tendency towards returning to similar values, as were observed at the study beginning. In spite of this, after six months, in comparison with the initial estimations, alcoholics still had significantly lower fasting (by 13%) and postprandial (by 16%) mean HDL values. The mean TC level increased within this period in average by 6% and LDL by 18%. Postprandial levels of studied plasma lipids, except of HDL, didn't differ significantly in the sixth month long observation period. In patients, who failed to maintain abstinence for the whole observation period, in comparison to abstinent alcoholics, we found higher fasting and postprandial HDL levels, as well as the tendency to lower values of LDL level, LDL/HDL ratio, Lp(a) concentration and Lp(a)/HDL ratio. These observations corroborated with results obtained by the other authors [12, 13, 92]. Interesting where also the results of individual analysis which showed, that among our patients was a group with proatherogenic changes in plasma lipids and the other, where observed changes had even anti-atherogenic profile. These differences resulted probably from mentioned genetic polymorphism [12, 105], affecting both fasting and postprandial plasma lipids concentration after alcohol drinking cessation, as well as during following weeks of withdrawal period. The hyperlipemic (proatherogenic) effect of first four-weeks of alcohol withdrawal was related to at least several factors: the kind of pharmacotherapy [naltrexone], liver status (greater gamma- glutamyltransferase (GGT) activity), pituitary-thyroid axis status

(TSH plasma concentration), alcohol dependence severity, quantity of alcohol consumption in the time preceding anti-relapse therapy [97].

In our randomized, placebo controlled investigation concerning the effect of pharmacotherapy with naltrexone, carbamazepine, and lithium carbonate on abstinence keeping in alcohol dependent male patients, we have observed, that after 16 weeks of the study, in subjects treated with naltrexone, TC and TG concentrations were lower than before such therapy was undertaken [96]. Moreover, this patients group had lower TC, LDL cholesterol and TG level than groups randomized to taking carbamazepine, lithium carbonate or placebo in the same observation period. In subjects randomized to receiving carbamazepine, a significant increase of TC concentration after 16 weeks of pharmacotherapy was found [87, 108]. Because the results of meta-analysis of many clinical trials showed that coronary artery disease risk decreased directly in proportion to the percentage of decrease in TC and LDL levels [87, 108] and time duration of TC level reduction [109], it might be supposed, that observed in our naltrexone-treated subjects decrease of TC concentration by 10% may decrease their CAD event risk by 18%. The work by Law et al. [109] also showed, that decrease in TC concentration by 23 mg/dl, similarly as in our naltrexone-group, led to a decrease in coronary events risk by 7% during the first 2 years and by 25% when the lipid-lowering therapy period was longer than 5 years. Additionally, anti- atherogenic, favorable effect of naltrexone, applied during abstinence period in heavy drinkers, had also implied the reduction of fasting TG concentration by 30%. So far no similar results were reported.

The revealed hypolipemic effect of naltrexone (reduction of concentration of TC by 10% and TG by 30%) was weaker, than usually obtained when typical lipid-lowering drugs are used, but was comparable to the diet effect [110, 111]. The mechanisms of serum cholesterol-lowering pharmacotherapy resulted from the influence on cholesterol synthesis (statins), cholesterol absorption (ezetimibe) or bile acid synthesis (resins). Naltrexone effect, on the other hand, can be explained by blockade of opioids receptors, which are probably involved in stress induced hyperlipidemia [112]. In our study, we have also revealed the effect of carbamazepine, increasing plasma lipids concentration. It may be explained by recently discussed potentially proatherogenic action of anti-epileptic drugs proceeded via at least three metabolic ways: altered metabolism of homocysteine, influence on lipids and lipoproteins as well as uric acid levels[113].

We have also noticed, that patients with greater plasma GGT and aminotransferases activities after alcohol withdrawal had simultaneously higher plasma concentrations of studied lipids. In the multi- factorial analysis, we have showed, that GGT was the independent factor determining plasma lipids level at the beginning of the abstinence and within following weeks of withdrawal period. These results were consisted with the results of recent studies by Valle et al. [114], Meisinger et al. [115], Ruttmann et al. [116], which have found, that elevated serum GGT activity may predict cardiovascular complications [114, 115, 116, 117]. Formerly, Hartung et al. [118] showed, that changes in GGT and the other liver enzymes values in alcoholics resulted from the changes in activities of the microsomal enzymes and metabolic pathways involved in lipids metabolism. This observation has been supported by revealed in our study strong linear correlation between HDL cholesterol concentration and GGT activity.

In our study we didn't perform a genetic determination (for example GABRA2 or ADH type 3 gene), but the role of this factors was estimated indirectly in personal history: possessing of alcohol dependent relatives and age of alcohol dependence onset (type of Cloninger typological differentiation). We found, that hyperlipemic reaction on alcohol withdrawal was more frequently present in patients without first degree relatives addicted to alcohol. There was supposed, that heavy alcohol consumption altered the effect of apoE polymorphism on apoB levels, via a defect in sialylation of apoE, formation of acetaldehyde adducts on apoB, or both of them [119]. Whereas, in available papers we didn't find any conclusion concerning the relationships between genetic predisposition to alcohol dependence and the kind of lipid profile changes after alcohol withdrawal.

Well documented is also the importance of the kind of alcoholic beverages drunk on plasma lipids. It seems, that this factor may also contribute to the differences observed in plasma lipids concentration after alcohol withdrawal. Well known is the reported promising cardioprotective effect of red wine intake (so called "french paradox") [92, 120, 121, 122, 123], and only some authors didn't confirm it [124]. However, there is still no data explaining the reasons of observed differences in lipids profile changes occurring in individual persons after alcohol misuse period.

The pituitary- thyroid axis plays, among other factors, a well documented role in plasma lipids profile. In our study (data not published) patients with higher plasma level of thyreothropin (relative hypothyroidism) had as well greater plasma lipids values during abstinence period. Similar influence displayed also the greater than average quantity of alcohol consumed during 90-days before including into the investigation. It suggested, that well known from epidemiological studies proatherogenic effect of heavy drinking was prolonged and observed even in the abstinence period.

In the context of still up- to- date inflammatory atherosclerosis definition and, for example, the results of JUPITER study [87], very interesting seems to be the hypothesis of the possibly pathogenetic role of inflammatory cytokines effect on the observed differences in the cardiovascular risk factors values after alcohol withdrawal. We revealed, that the changes in plasma lipids level during six-months long abstinence period were related to the presence of detectable amounts of tumor necrosis factor – alpha (TNF-alpha) after alcohol drinking cessation. Patients, in whom this cytokine was determinable, had also higher plasma lipids concentration in the sixth month of the study than the group without detectable TNF-alpha level. There were previously reported striking positive correlations between TNF-alpha and plasma triglycerides, VLDL triglycerides and VLDL cholesterol concentrations in patients with coronary artery disease [125]. These observation suggested also, that immune response to alcohol drinking (TNF-alpha) was diversified and, similar as for example GGT activity, may predict the response to alcohol drinking cessation in the context of atherosclerosis progression. This is confirmed by Kloner et al. [12], who cited also the work by Maraldi et al., in which mild alcohol drinking was related to the decrease in all-cause mortality, and benefits were more marked among patients with high baseline IL-6 level.

Above mentioned relationships, which were observed in our study and than revealed in uni-variate analysis were next confirmed in multi-factorial analysis. We found, that the level of respective plasma lipids fractions at the beginning of the study and after four weeks of controlled abstinence was independently related to patients age, severity of alcohol dependence (Short Alcohol Dependence Data score, delirium tremens in personal history), TSH concentration and liver function tests (INR, albumin, GGT, bilirubin, transaminases). The references data have also underlined the role of drinking pattern in pathogenesis of cardiovascular complications related to alcohol drinking [126, 127]. The results of some investigations pointed out, that only regular and moderate drinking displayed a favorable effect on cardiovascular system and plasma lipids, but so called binge drinking exerts harmful influence, expressed mainly by hyperlipemic and haemorragic consequences as well as pro-coagulative changes during hangover. In our investigation we didn't undertake such analysis, because all of alcoholics from the studied group were heavy drinkers for a long time.

In conclusion, alcoholics demonstrated varied, individual pattern of changes in plasma lipids concentration after cessation of heavy alcohol drinking. In about 80% of them after four weeks of abstinence the decrease of HDL cholesterol and increase of LDL cholesterol level were found, but in the rest of them the LDL concentration lowered, and HDL cholesterol value didn't change or increased. The trend of plasma lipids level changes, which was observed after the first four weeks of abstinence, didn't predict their later values within following 16 and 20 weeks of the withdrawal period. Majority of the initial changes turned over within this time, thus the cholesterol concentration in some subjects returned to the initial value, moreover most evident proatherogenic plasma lipids disturbances maintained in alcoholics with no alcohol dependent relatives in anamnesis. Less important factors responsible for the long-term proatherogenic alcohol withdrawal effect mediated via changes in plasma lipids level appeared to be: TSH concentration, secretive liver function, severity of alcohol dependence, quantity of alcohol consumption and mental consequences of alcoholism presented after alcohol drinking cessation.

Mentioned observations, corresponding with the references data, may imply some clinical significance, most important seems to be the following: (1)increased plasma lipids level is the risk factor of cardiovascular event, (2)there are some clinical factors which may predict lipid- related reaction on alcohol withdrawal, (3)there are some pharmacological and non-pharmacological methods to prevent proatherogenic lipids changes after alcohol heavy drinking cessation, (4)plasma lipids profile may be a marker of alcohol abstinence keeping or alcohol abuse. Firstly, after six months of abstinence period, in comparison to the initial values, alcoholics in average had significantly lower fasting (by 13%) and postprandial (by 16%) mean HDL values. The mean TC level increased within this period in average by 6% and LDL by 18%. In the context of reference data these plasma lipid changes may be responsible for about forty percentage increase of CAD event risk in our alcoholics treated against alcohol drinking relapse. This suggests necessity to investigate the usefulness of some interventions preventing these disturbances. Secondly, in alcoholics, who were in the greatest risk of lipid-mediated proatherogenic consequences after alcohol misuse perid were found: determinable (>0,05pg/ml) level of TNF-alpha, abnormal GGT activity and the lack of alcohol dependent first degree relatives in personal history. Thirdly, identification of predictors indicating on possible unfavorable plasma lipids changes suggested the possibility of applying some intervention methods, which could prevent such disturbances. Among already known methods of plasma lipids decrease, some seems to be useful. There are appropriate diet, physical activity, body mass normalization and control of the other cardiovascular risk factors, such as smoking, blood pressure, glucose concentration. There is a doubt about the recommendation of lipids-lowering drugs, such as statins or fibrates, because of their potential hepatotoxic adverse effects, but this problem should be analyzed in the context of studies results, which established safety of these drugs in spite of liver function tests abnormalities [128]. We have discussed above the hypolipemic effect of naltrexone use, so this therapeutic agent may be as yet the best choice, regarding both lipids lowering and anti-relapse effects [96, 129]. On the basis of references data and our observations, suggesting more proatherogenic changes in patients with determinable level of TNF –alpha after alcohol withdrawal, this cytokine seems to be promising therapeutic target. There were found lipid-lowering, anti-inflammatory [130, 131] and hepatoprotective properties of probiotics [132], which usefulness in these patients group should be further investigated. Fourthly, there are many biochemical markers of alcohol abuse, such as GGT, AST, ALT activities, transferrin isoforms with a reduced number of sialic acids (asialo-, monosialo-, and disialotransferrin) called carbohydrate-deficient transferrins (CDTs). It seems, that similar importance and significance may be attributed to following parameters: plasma concentration of total cholesterol, HDL cholesterol, LDL cholesterol and LDL to HDL level ratio [133].

Platelets

Platelets play an important role in haemostasis, atherosclerosis progression and acute coronary syndromes pathogenesis. Their importance in this processes is pointed out from pathophysiological premises, as well as from interventional investigations which showed the effect of about 25-50% decrease in cardiovascular event risk as a result of anti-platelets drugs use (aspirin, ticlopidine, clopidogrel, abciximab, integreline, eptifibatide, tirofiban) [134] and lack of this effect in patients with resistance to such therapy [135]. Discussed above favorable, anti- atherogenic effect of moderate alcohol drinking, was also supposed to be proceeded via anti-platelet action of ethanol and non-alcoholic components of beverages, mainly flavonoids [92]. That platelets-mediated mechanism of favorable moderate alcohol drinking was confirmed in many epidemiological studies [92]. Whereas, only several investigations corroborated the changes in platelets count and activity after alcohol misuse period as well. During alcohol abuse period and after drinking cessation thrombocytopenia was described, what used to be explained by injury of bone marrow and liver (secondary hypersplenism), foliate deficiency, and direct ethanol effect on the platelets structure, function and metabolism [136]. In following time of abstinence, in patients without clinically crucial alcohol related organ complications, platelets count predominantly increased and between fifth and twenty first day of abstinence reached even 2-19 times greater value than soon after alcohol drinking cessation. Subsequently, platelets count decreased to normal values. In our observation, two weeks after alcohol misuse period, alcoholics, in comparison to the control group, had greater platelets count and greater platelets adhesion index. After the next four weeks of controlled abstinence in alcoholics, who successfully continued the withdrawal, significant increase of mean platelets volume (MPV) and aggregation to collagen was found, whereas in subjects, who failed to remain abstinent for the whole six-month long observation period, again the significant decrease of MPV value had occurred. Yazici et al. [137] reported the decrease in MPV value after 20 weeks of life style modification (among other things, limited alcohol consumption) in prehypertensive patients. These observations may have some clinical implications, for at least three reasons:

Firstly, in several recent studies was documented the significance of MPV determination as a predictor of coronary events [138]. The pathophysiological background confirming such observations resulted from this, that large platelets contain more dense granules, their metabolism and enzymatic function is more active than the smaller ones. They have also greater thrombotic potential, partially related to the increased expression of procoagulatory surface proteins, such as P-selectin and glycoprotein IIIa. In the context of these data, our results evidenced the increased risk of cardiovascular events in alcoholics after alcohol drinking cessation, lasting for at least four weeks. These results corresponded to the mentioned left arm of J-shaped curve, expressing the relationships between coronary artery disease prevalence and quantity of alcohol intake [139]. The effect of alcohol drinking and withdrawal on platelets function was reviewed by Renaud and Ruf [140] and Goldberg and al. [92]. They summarized many investigations and concluded, that already 10-20 minutes after alcohol intake decrease, in the platelets was observed aggregation to ADP and epinephrine and aggregation to collagen. In moderate and regular drinkers this inhibitory effect was lasting for several hours. Whereas, by contrast, in binge drinkers or in alcoholics after alcohol withdrawal, response to aggregation, especially that induced by thrombin, is markedly increased. To this rebound phenomenon was attributed the supposed explanation of ischemic strokes or sudden death more frequent occurrence after episodes of drunkenness. The platelet rebound effect of alcohol drinking was not observed with moderate red wine consumption in men, most probably due to polyphenols, especially resveratrol and quercetin, an antiaggregability effect on human platelets [140, 141, 142]. The protection afforded by wine has been recently duplicated in rats fed with alcohol solutions with grape tannins added, and was recognized to be associated with a decrease in the level of conjugated dienes in the first step of lipid peroxidation. In our study we didn't find any relationships between platelets count or activity expression and plasma lipids, as well as parameters of pro- antioxidative systemic balance, although their occurrence was suggested in some reports [142].

Secondly, changes induced by alcohol drinking in platelets function may also cause hemorrhagic complications, clinically expressed most often as hemorrhagic stroke. Disturbances of platelets hemostasis should also be taken into consideration in alcohol users after motor vehicle crashes, other accidents and surgery, who are in risk of potentially dangerous injury and major bleeding. It should be also underlined, that immobilization after surgery procedures is on the other hand associated with increased risk of thrombo-embolic complications as a result of mentioned rebound effect, which concerns not only platelets haemostasis, but also plasma and vascular haemostatic factors.

Finally, the third clinical implication concerns the MPV value, which changes in relation to varying alcohol consumption and therefore should be better estimated as a potential new alcohol abuse marker (similarly, as discussed in another part of this chapter usability of some plasma lipids determination). We found only the work of Coccini et al [143] in this subject. They suggested temporal pattern of platelet derived B-type monoamine oxidase B (MAO-B) activity to be an useful marker for the diagnostic assessment of alcoholism and early abstinence, regardless of gender and smoking status. This enzyme activity was the lowest after drinking cessation, increased after 8 days of withdrawal, and remained stable thereafter.

Plasma Blood Coagulation System

Plasma coagulation pathway, similar as platelets function plays an important role in hemostatic processes, which regulate maintenance of blood in liquid state inside of vascular system. The relationships between plasma coagulation system and cardiovascular event risk was previously well documented. It is known, that the main cause of thrombus formation are disturbances of balance between activators and inhibitors both of coagulation and fibrinolysis systems. The main factors responsible for arterial thrombosis are platelets activation as well as increased levels of fibrinogen, von Willebrand (vWf) and VII factors. To the new hemostatic markers of increased cardiovascular events risk belong: high levels of protein C metabolism factors (thrombomodulin- TM, protein C, protein S, Leiden V factor), platelet receptors GPIIb/IIIa, plasminogen activator inhibitor type 1 (PAI-1), and lipoprotein(a) [144]. Disturbances in their levels may lead to thrombotic and hemorrhagic complications, which are often present in alcoholics, both during misuse and abstinence periods.

In our study we found, that alcoholics after alcohol drinking cessation had in average four times higher plasma concentration of thrombin- antithrombin complexes (TAT-complexes; marker of thrombin generation in vivo) than the upper level of normal range and than were obtained in control group. The level of D-dimers, another marker of coagulation, but also fibrinolysis activation in vivo, was in normal range at the study start. After four weeks of abstinence period significant decrease of D-dimers, fibrinogen and antithrombin levels were observed. Abstinent patients, after 6 months, compared with the initial values, had significantly lower antithrombin activity, thrombomodulin, fibrinogen and D-dimers levels as well as longer prothrombin time, expressed as INR value. Whereas, in the final estimation after 6 months, in patients who failed to remain abstinent for the whole observation period, in comparison to abstinent alcoholics, we found, similarly as it was observed for MPV value, once more the decrease of INR value and increase of TAT complexes concentration. We didn't find any significant effect of the kind of alcohol beverages (beer, wine, vodka, or "non-beverage" alcohol defined as liquids containing alcohol but not aimed for consumption, such as glass-washing or defroster liquids), as well as the liver function tests, body mass and smoking on changes in studied haemostatic parameters during six months long abstinence period. Our results were not always consisted with the results of other authors, although not many studies concerned alcoholics after alcohol drinking cessation. Trotti et al. [145] found, that the levels of coagulation activation markers, such as TAT-complexes, prothrombin fragment F1+2, D-dimers, were higher in chronic alcohol abusers than in moderate drinkers. On the other hand, McConnell's et. al. [146] study showed, that consumption of a single, daily alcoholic beverage for 6 weeks did not change significantly the levels of such haemostatic parameters as vWf, prothrombin fragment F1+2, TAT complexes. Van Golde et al. [147] found also, that the consumption of large amounts of wine does not influence the coagulation parameters levels, such as aPTT, TAT complexes, factors VII and VIII, and von Willebrand factor. The main point of our observations, as well as the other authors results is, that in alcoholics after alcohol withdrawal, the intra-vascular, persistent, slight increase of thrombin generation takes place. This plasma coagulation activation might be probably due to endothelial cell dysfunction or cytokine acting, as well as changes in plasma coagulation factors in alcoholics during abstinence period [92]. Many epidemiological investigations presented negative relation between quantity of alcohol consumption and fibrinogen concentration [148, 149] as well as antithrombin activity [149, 150]. In our study alcohol withdrawal showed procoagulative changes in plasma coagulation factors, expressed by the increase of fibrinogen and antithrombin concentration, and shortening of the prothrombin time, what corroborated with the results of previously made investigations [151, 152]. The global interpretation of this results suggests that some, not well identified factors, acting after alcohol withdrawal have stimulated both chronic thrombin generation in vivo and the increase of coagulation factors and inhibitors synthesis and/or secretion. It may be, that the increase of coagulation factors and their inhibitors levels resulted from chronic compensative processes secondary to their increased consumption and atherosclerosis progression [148, 150]. Independently on this mechanism, in the vicious circle mechanism, increased fibrinogen concentration and shorter prothrombin time may facilitate thrombotic processes acceleration, what was suggested in the studies indicating on TAT-complexes [153], fibrinogen [152, 154], antithrombin [155], shorter prothrombin time [156] as the potent predictors of cardiovascular events. It should be brushed up, that thrombin, fibrinogen and fibrin are the well known platelets activators. This implies, that increased thrombin generation after alcohol withdrawal may lead not only to forming red-clot, but also white-clot, composed with platelets. Increased consumption of blood platelets after alcohol misuse period was also suggested on the ground of the mean platelets volume increase, observed after four weeks of abstinence period.

Besides of the mentioned changes in plasma coagulation factors, very important for global cardiovascular event risk estimation in alcoholics after misuse period is for sure endothelial dysfunction, which is thought to play a pivotal role in the development, progression, and clinical complications of atherosclerosis. Several recent studies have addressed the clinical implications of endothelial dysfunction for cardiovascular events, atherosclerosis, restenosis, and heart failure [157]. In our investigation we estimated the levels of such endothelium function markers as: antigen von Willebrant factor (vWf:Ag), soluble thrombomodulin (sTM), tissue type plasminogen activator antigen (t-PA:Ag), and plasminogen activator inhibitor antigen type1 (PAI-1:Ag). We determined also the levels of nitric oxide metabolites, but it will be discussed in the further part of the chapter. Within six-months long abstinence, the significant decrease in soluble TM, t-PA:Ag and PAI-1:Ag plasma concentration was found, but vWf level didn't change in this period. Whereas, in alcoholics, who failed to remain abstinent for half of a year, the repeated increase of t-PA:Ag and PAI-1:Ag was found. The thrombomodulin is an anticoagulant expressed during endothelial activation and damage. It acts as a receptor which binds thrombin, next activates protein C, which inactivates factors Va, VIIIa and PAI-1. Von Willebrant factor (vWf) under high shear arterial blood flow binds the platelet receptor glycoprotein (GP) Ib-alpha, leading to platelet adhesion, activation and thrombosis. Tissue type plasminogen activator (t-PA) is a factor released from endothelium, which is responsible for intravascular thrombus dissolution via plasmin activation, and PAI-1 inhibits its action. Increased levels of TM soluble form, vWf, PAI-1:Ag and t-PA:Ag are associated with the sever coronary artery disease, stroke or peripheral occlusive arterial disease and such increase is not noticed in healthy or asymptomatic subjects [158, 159, 160]. Observed in our study, increased plasma level of endothelial function markers after alcohol withdrawal and following decrease of their values after six-months long abstinence period, indicates on the presence of endothelial injury or dysfunction after alcohol drinking cessation. This observation is in agreement with the results of some other investigations, and explains above described, presented in our alcoholic patients activation of thrombin generation in vivo. Mukamal et al. [161] have shown, that light-to-moderate alcohol consumption was associated with lower levels of fibrinogen, plasma viscosity, von Willebrand factor, and factor VII. This association was most pronounced in consumers of no more, than 3 drinks weekly, but in subjects, who drank heavier, impaired fibrinolytic potential, reflected by higher levels of plasminogen activator inhibitor antigen-1 (PAI-1:ag) and t-PA:Ag was found. These relationships were also consistent with J-shaped curve expressing relationships between the quantity of alcohol intake and coronary artery disease prevalence, what suggests an impotant role of endothelium and fibrinolysis in cardioprotective effect of moderate alcohol drinking and harmful influence of alcohol abuse [12, 147, 162, 163].

In conclusion, presented results have shown procoagulative effect of alcohol withdrawal and in consequence the increase of cardiovascular event risk, especially within first month after alcohol misuse period [164]. The last supposition, mainly on the basis of theoretical premises, needs confirmation, although is consistent with mentioned J-shaped curve expressing relationships between CAD events prevalence and quantity of alcohol drinking. Lastly, it should be underlined, that thrombotic complications in alcoholics may concern not only coronary, cerebral and peripheral arteries and veins, but also abdominal vessels [165]. It seems to be important because of the frequent occurrence in this patients group traumas, acute and chronic pancreatitis, liver diseases with secondary thrombophilia and blood congestion in portal circulation, immobilization and dehydratation (after vomiting) and sometimes, neoplasmatic diseases [166]. Taking these disturbances into diagnostic consideration in alcoholics seems to be very important, because of at least three factors. Firstly, symptoms related to intestinal ischaemia are very similar to the symptomatology of other diseases, more often occurring in general population, and in alcoholics as well. The obvious examples may be: gastritis, peptic ulcer, and pancreatitis. In each from these diseases abdominal pain occurs and changes in intestinal movement are presented. Such symptoms mimic and mask those connected with abdominal vessels thrombosis, what may result in high mortality. Secondly, all of mentioned pathologic processes, especially when described platelets, plasma coagulation and fibrinolysis system disturbances coexist, may predispose to thrombotic complications, in abdominal vessels as well. In clinical diagnosis such overlapping of diseases is not easy to recognize. Thirdly, the consumption of coagulation factors in thrombotic processes may mask changes in hemostasis system, depending on alcohol drinking and withdrawal, if personal history concerning alcohol drinking would not be obtained.

Mentioned procoagulative effect of alcohol withdrawal stands in opposition to the known increased risk of haemorrhagic complications during alcohol misuse period [92, 167]. The reason of such situation results from liver injury, coagulation factors acetylation or consumption in the processes of disseminated intravascular coagulation [168]. Both of these effects, pro- (after drinking cessation) and anti-coagulative (during alcohol abuse) expressed with different force, what depends on alcohol drinking-related period, should be taken into consideration in patients after accidents and surgery, because of potential thrombotic and bleeding complications. Moreover, our result suggests the necessity to carry out interventional studies, especially in patients with anti- alcohol relapse therapy, in order to estimate the effectiveness of not pharmacological methods (simultaneous smoking cessation, diet modification, exercise, body mass control), anticoagulants, and/or anti-platelets drugs in cardiovascular events prevention after alcohol drinking cessation.

Plasma Blood Fibrinolysis System

Plasma fibrinolysis activation depends on plasminogen conversion into plasmin. This process may be an effect of endogenic activators, derived from intrinsic pathway (kallikrein) and extrinsic pathway (tissue type plasminogen activator- t-PA, urokinase type plasminogen activator- u-PA) as well as egzogenic plasminogen activators, mostly applied as a drugs (streptokinase, alteplase, urokinase). Active plasmin dissolves fibrinogen and fibrin deposits. Its excessive activity is restricted by receptor mechanisms and plasmin inhibitors (alpha2-antiplasmin, alpha2- macroglobulin), plasminogen activators inhibitors (plasminogen activator inhibitor type 1, or type 2- PAI-1, PAI-2), and so called "other inhibitors", which inhibit activity of respective pathways of fibrinolysis system, as C-1-esterase inhibitor (kallikrein inhibitor), protease nexins, thrombospondin, and above mentioned lipoprotein(a)-Lp(a) [97].

Fibrinolysis system plays a well documented role in pathogenesis of atherosclerosis, acute coronary syndromes, and haemorrhagic complications. Imbalance between blood coagulation and fibrinolysis, or between fibrinolysis inhibitors and activators may be clinically manifested as cardiovascular thrombotic events or haemorrhage. Increased levels of t-PA and PAI-1 antigens (respectively, t-PA:Ag, and PAI-1:Ag), and D-dimers (products of fibrin degradation) are considered as fibrinolytic markers of increased cardiovascular event risk [169].

In vitro, alcohol increased t-PA:Ag and u-PA:Ag transcription and decreased PAI-1 gene expression in endothelial cells culture [162]. In human studies t-PA:Ag, PAI-1:Ag and D-dimers level correlated with quantity of alcohol intake [161,169, 170, 171, 172, 173], although there are some reports, which results denied cardioprotective effect of moderate alcohol drinking proceeded via fibrinolysis activation [147, 174]. In our study alcohol abusers had significantly greater plasma concentration of PAI-1:Ag, D-dimers and plasmin-alpha2- antiplasmin complexes (PAP-complexes) than non-drinkers in the estimation performed.two weeks after alcohol drinking cessation, The last factor, similarly as D-dimers, is recognized as a marker of fibrinolysis activation in vivo, and exactly as a marker of plasminogenesis in vivo. After consecutive four weeks of abstinence, the concentration of fibrinolysis activation in vivo marker decreased significantly, but plasma concentration of t-PA:Ag and PAI-1:Ag didn't change at all. Whereas, in alcoholics, who failed to remain abstinent for half of an year, again was observed the increase of t-PA:Ag, PAI-1:Ag, t:PA:Ag/PAI-1:Ag ratio value, as well as PAP-complexes and D-dimers concentrations. As a result, relapsed patients had significantly greater level of this parameters than abstinent subjects. Generally, these results have shown an increased fibrinolysis activation in vitro during early abstinence period. Values of estimated parameters were greater in alcoholics, who consumed more alcohol, for a longer time, with onset of alcohol dependence in younger age and longer alcohol dependence time. In similar patients group we found simultaneously increased level of thrombinogenesis activation in vivo markers (TAT-complexes), what suggested, that fibrinolysis activation was secondary to increased coagulation, and depended on two pathways, intrinsic (kallikrein- related) and extrinsic (t-PA-related). Greater activity of extrinsic pathway of fibrinolysis, in the context of increased level of PAI-1:Ag, resulted probably from higher value of t-PA:Ag to PAI-1:Ag ratio and possibly from increased protein C plasma activity. Protein C is activated by thrombomodulin, which increased level after alcohol drinking cessation was confirmed in our study as well as by other authors [175]. Active protein C, besides coagulation inhibition, binds also PAI-1 and facilitates t-PA pro-fibrinolytic activity. In the references, there are reports concerning the relationships between alcohol abstinence and fibrinolysis [92, 147], but existing data show, that alcohol withdrawal leads to weakening of fibrinolysis, via pro-oxidative acting, impaired endothelial function, reversed fibrinolysis activation, and decrease of elevated PAI-1 level, observed within alcohol drinking period [12, 172, 176, 177]. The recent investigation showed, that binge drinking, even red wine, may inhibit plasma fibrinolysis in human [178]. These observations are consist with J-shaped relationships between quantity of alcohol drinking and cardiovascular and general mortality [12].

In conclusion, heavy drinkers in the withdrawal period and binge drinkers presented activation of fibrinolysis system, but simultaneously coagulation activation took place, so, as the result, the increased risk of rather thrombotic than haemorrhagic complications occurred. This interpretation is consistent with the above mentioned reports, which results have shown an increased cardiovascular event risk in persons with elevated levels of t-PA:Ag, PAI-1:Ag, and D-dimers [169, 173]. Some papers, published in the recent years, have indicated on the other clinical implications concerning also the results of our work. They came down from known interactions between t-PA and the N-methyl-D-aspartate (NMDA) receptor, which, among other things, is considered to be an important target of acute and chronic effects of ethanol overuse. In this context, t-PA would participate in the mechanisms leading to the development of physical dependence on ethanol and seizures after alcohol drinking cessation [179].

However, as this was already mentioned, plasma fibrinolysis system doesn't act in human body separately, but is connected with the other systems. In the context of its role in atherosclerosis pathogenesis, there should be underlined the relationships between coagulation and fibrinolysis system and some other factors involved in atheroslerosis progression, such as smoking, body mass, blood pressure, plasma lipids and so on [84, 85]. This is in agreement with recommended global cardiovascular risk stratification [180].

Cigarette smoking, one among main and traditional cardiovascular event risk predictors [84, 181], was together with the other three risk factors (diabetes, hyperlipidemia, and hypertension) presented in more than 80% of 122458 patients enrolled in 14 international randomized clinical trials of CHD [85]. It is not only an independent factor, but affects the levels of some others, especially haemostatic factors, as platelets, fibrinogen, t-PA, PAI-1, and so on. There is proved a frequent association between alcohol abuse and addiction to nicotine [170]. This also suggested that many metabolic, potentially unfavorable changes after alcohol withdrawal, might be avoided, if smoking would be simultaneously discontinued [181]. In this way, cardiovascular risk increase via lipids-related changes by about 40%, might be balanced with smoking cessation by 36%.

Moreover, there exist some important relationships between fibrinolysis system and some other factors affecting cardiovascular risk in alcoholics after alcohol withdrawal. The significant role demonstrates its connection with plasma lipids, especially lipoprotein(a)-Lp(a). Lp(a) plays a special role in atherogenesis, mainly: as LDL-lipoprotein, which, after oxidation, may accumulate in foam cells and activate inflammatory processes, also as a false plasminogen, fibrinolysis inhibitor, which competes with t-PA and u-PA for binding to plasminogen, as well as an inductor of PAI-1 synthesis and secretion, and as a factor facilitating binding of plasmin to alpha2-antiplasmin. Moreover, Lp(a) activates also platelets adhesion, aggregation, and vascular smooth myocyte migration and proliferation. As a result of these processes, Lp(a) level above 30 mg/dl is associated with the twofold increase of cardiovascular events risk[182]. In our investigation [97], in opposite to the other reports [183], Lp(a) level was the greatest at the study start, and gradually, but significantly decreased in the following six months of abstinence period. Changes in this lipoprotein concentration were related to the platelets count, the fibrinogen and thrombomodulin concentrations, antithrombin activity, as well as to the t-PA:Ag, PAI-1:Ag, D-dimers and PAP-complexes levels. The lack of negative relationships between Lp(a) concentration and the level of fibrinolysis parameters showed, that the role of Lp(a) as an anti-fibrinolytic agent was not clinically important. On the other hand, we have found correlation between t-PA:Ag and HDL cholesterol concentration (positive) and triglycerides concentration (negative). These observations may suggest the favorable influence of HDL lipoprotein on endothelial function [184] and pro-coagulative triglicerydes properties [185].

Nitric Oxide

Nitric oxide (NO) plays a great role in circulatory, digestive, neural and immunological systems function regulation. It takes part in blood pressure control, inhibits mast cells degranulation, possess antioxidant and antiaggregant properties, regulates vascular tone and inhibits both proliferation of smooth muscle cells and adhesion of leukocytes and platelets. It also controls activity and morphological state of digestive tract, respiratory and urinary systems. In neural system, NO acts as neurotransmitter and regulates many functions, both in its central and in peripheral part. Some reports showed, that NO may be also involved in molecular mechanisms for substances abuse and dependence to opioids, ethanol, and to psychostimulants, as cocaine, marihuana and nicotine, as well as to psychotropic drugs [186]. Moreover, NO participates in the development of rapid tolerance to ethanol and inhibitors of nitric oxide synthase (NOS), modulates withdrawal from opioids, nicotine and ethanol, diminishing many signs of withdrawal syndrome, especially anxiety [187, 188, 189].

In human body, besides neuronal type of NOS (type I, nNOS), as constitutive form of NOS acts also endothelial NOS (type III, eNOS). The disturbances in eNOS activity, as well as endothelial dysfunction leads to decrease in vessel relaxation reserve. The third isoenzyme of NOS is the inductive NOS (type II, iNOS), which isn't normally present in the cells and requires transcriptional activation by cytokines, bacterial cell wall products or other inflammatory stimuli. Alcohol drinking may influence the nitric oxide synthesis, both via changes in constitutive and inductive NOS activities, as well as both after acute and chronic administration [190], but the investigations results are ambiguous and show both suppressive and stimulating alcoholic beverages effect on NO synthesis [172, 191, 192]. Increase of NO synthesis and secretion is consider to be one of the mechanisms responsible for cardioprotective moderate alcohol drinking effect. In our study we have estimated NO metabolites level changes within six-months long abstinence period [193, 194]. At the study beginning, alcoholics had lower NO metabolites plasma level than the control group. Within following weeks, abstinent alcoholics presented significant decrease of mean nitrites concentration, however in subjects who relapsed, increase of NO metabolites level was observed. As a result, significantly higher NO metabolites plasma level was noticed in patients, who relapsed, than in those, who remained abstinent at six-months visit. It was interesting however, that this difference of mean NO metabolites concentration appeared already within first four weeks, when all hospitalized subjects kept abstinence, and the relapse occurred before six-month visit. On this base we supposed, that the increase of NO metabolites level or their decrease by no more than 4,4mcmol/l may be predictive for alcohol drinking relapse during next five months observation, after hospital discharge. This hypothesis was confirmed in logistic regression method. Moreover, in multiple regression analysis was found, that in abstinent alcoholics, besides the positive correlation with quantity of alcohol intake before the study beginning, plasma level of NO metabolites was also related positively with t-PA:Ag/PAI-1:Ag ratio value, GGT plasma activity, and negatively with parameters of alcohol dependence (age of alcohol dependence onset, length of dependence, Michigan Alcoholism Screening Test score, decrease in alcohol tolerance, history of withdrawal epilepsy and family history of alcoholism).

These observations, in majority consisting with the results of the other authors, might suggest some clinical implications. Firstly, the greatest NO metabolites level after alcohol misuse period and their gradually decrease within six-months long abstinence time may suggest that its synthesis was stimulated either by alcohol drinking or by alcohol withdrawal, what confirmed the other studies results [172, 191, 195]. Secondly, the plasma level of NO metabolites in alcoholics might result from stimulation of all three isoforms of NOS. The neural isoform of NOS as a source of nitrites in our patients was supposed indirectly, on the basis of the relationships between NO metabolites level and alcohol dependence severity in psychological score, and on the occurrence of alcohol drinking relapse. Whereas, on the endothelial origin of nitrites, pointed simultaneous rise of some other endothelial function markers plasma concentration, such as t-PA:Ag and PAI-1:Ag. This supposition was also supported by the results of multiple regression analysis, which showed, that t-PA/PAI-1 ratio independently, positively correlated with NO metabolites plasma level. It is known, that NO, prostacyclin and t-PA are mutually released from endothelial cells. Finally, the potential role of inductive NOS as a source of NO in studied alcoholics was suggested by the presence of TNF-alpha, and bacterial endotoxins in their plasma. The increased level of these substances, which may stimulate endothelial cells to NO synthesis and secretion is mostly explained by the decrease in intestinal epithelium integrity and intestinal barrier injury, secondary to cytotoxic effect of ethanol. Thirdly, although in our alcoholics the greatest NO metabolites level was found within first 14 days after alcohol drinking cessation, it was about 35% lower than in non-alcoholics control. This might result from endothelium dysfunction, decreased NOS reaction on stimuli, limitations in availability of NO synthesis substrates (L-arginine), or NO consumption in reactions with free radicals leading to overproduction of peroxynitrites (ONOO). Endothelial dysfunction in alcoholics might be potentially induced by inflammatory factors (cytokines, endotoxins), by oxidized LDL, or by peroxynitrites, formed during NO reaction with free radicals overproduced during ethanol metabolism or smoking [196]. Endothelial dysfunction induced by alcohol misuse may be a potential factor responsible for increased cardiovascular events risk in heavy drinkers, known from epidemiological study results (the right arm of J- shaped curve illustrating the relationships between coronary artery disease prevalence and quantity of alcohol drinking).

Nitric oxide may be involved in pathomechanism of alcohol dependence, withdrawal symptoms and alcohol drinking relapse via central, neural mechanism and via peripheral, vasomotoric effect. Cerebral mechanism of NO acting pointed from its function as neurotransmitter and different activity in respective brain regions [197]. The potential peripheral mechanism leading to mentioned disturbances going on after alcohol drinking cessation might result from the vasomotor effect of NO. The excess of NO may generate vascular dilatation, thus causing rush, tachycardia and sweating, which are the typical withdrawal syndrome symptoms [195]. Aggravation of these symptoms may make abstinence difficult to maintain. From these premises arose the fourth clinical implication of our consideration. The usefulness of nitric oxide metabolites level determination as a predictor of alcohol drinking relapse needs confirmation in further studies. The selection of patients in the greatest risk of alcohol drinking relapse just at the beginning of abstinence period may give the possibility to prolong psychotherapy and/or apply more effective in these cases, but in overall more expensive and doubtful pharmacotherapy. On the other hand, our results, like the other authors reports, have implied NO synthesis blockade as a promising method of alcohol withdrawal syndrome treatment and alcohol drinking relapse prevention [187]. However, in the context of NO role in vascular reserve regulation, such therapeutic methods may provoke the appearance of cardiovascular noxious effects. There is the next, important reason to undertake the complex studies for better estimation of NO role in the pathogenesis both of alcohol withdrawal syndrome and alcohol drinking relapse, in the connection with various, especially cardiovascular complications appearing after alcohol abuse period.

Tumor Necrosis Factor Type Alpha (TNF-alpha)

Since atherosclerosis has been considered as a chronic low-grade inflammatory disease, cytokine and adhesion molecules took an attention of investigators. Although cytokines play an important role in many diseases, their significance in chronic alcohol abuse consequences, especially atherosclerosis, liver disease, acute and chronic pancreatitis, seems to be not overestimate. It is known, that increased levels of inflammatory markers, including C-reactive protein (CRP), tumor necrosis factor- type alpha (TNF-alpha), and interleukin-6 (IL-6), predict the onset of poor health outcomes in these diseases. On the other hand, increased level of this inflammatory markers is considered as a risk factor of atherosclerosis progression, cardiovascular event, and heart failure.

Alcohol exerts a different, dose related effect on cytokine level, acting as immunomodulator. Recent studies showed that moderate alcohol intake is associated with lower levels of some acute-phase markers, including fibrinogen and CRP [12, 198, 199]. Imhof et al. [198] and Albert et al. [199] noted a U-shaped association between alcohol consumption and C-reactive protein (CRP) value, with a less strong association among women. Badia et al. [200] found, that moderate alcohol consumption, especially alcoholic beverages with high polyphenolic concentration, such as red wine, may reduce the adhesion of human monocytes to endothelial cells through the down-regulation of adhesion molecules on the monocyte surface, mainly VLA-4. Our patients, however, were all heavy drinkers. In such subjects alcohol drinking increased cytokine production and secretion, especially TNF-alpha [201]. The vascular effect of TNF-alpha depends on endothelial dysfunction, atherosclerosis plaque destabilization, suppression of re-endothelialization of denuded arteries and inhibition of endothelial cell proliferation, what may contribute to vasoconstriction, vessel occlusion or development of restenosis, if angioplasty was made [162]. There were suppositions, that cytokine source is the liver, stimulated to their synthesis by endotoxins released by intestinal bacterial flora [202]. The increased quantity of this toxins in heavy drinkers may result from increased gastric and intestinal bacterial growth, an effect of gastric acid secretion suppression related to alcohol drinking, slowdown of intestinal peristalsis, decrease in sIgA secretion, as well as cytotoxic ethanol effect, contributive to intestinal barrier injury and its increased permeability. Alcohol heavy drinking may additionally decrease the macrophage response to bacterial lipopolisaccharydes (LPS) and gamma-interferone [203]. On the other hand, TNF-alpha synthesis, stimulated by alcohol drinking, depends on TNF-alpha gene polymorphism [201], what might explain some differences in the results of respective investigations. Some of them showed a stimulating alcohol effect on TNF-alpha synthesis [202], while the others pointed on the different influence [203] or lack of any effect [204, 205]. Whereas, we found that among 47 alcoholics more or less 50 percent had determinable (>0,05pg/ml) TNF-alpha plasma level within two weeks after alcohol abuse [206]. After alcohol withdrawal they had significantly higher TNF-alpha plasma concentration, than the control group of healthy non-drinkers. After six-month observation period TNF-alpha concentration decreased significantly. In multivariate analysis, TNF-alpha plasma concentration at the start of the investigation was positively related to history of delirium tremens, plasma ALT activity, percent of time spent at gastric pH above 3 (in 24-hours gastric pH-metry), intensity of antral Helicobacter pylori gastric mucosa colonization, age of alcohol dependence onset, and negatively to length of alcohol dependence and score in Michigan Alcoholism Screening Test (MAST) questionnaire. Moreover, we showed, that alcoholics, in whom at the beginning of the study determinable TNF-alpha level was found, in comparison to "TNF-negative" subjects, had greater plasma lipids concentration and greater mean platelets volume (MPV) at the study start. After four weeks and six months abstinence period they have presented also greater collagen induced platelets aggregation-ability and lower total antioxidative plasma potential. The last observation was consistent with the work by Brown et al. [207].

In conclusion, we suggested, that in studied alcoholics alcohol abuse had stimulated TNF-alpha synthesis and secretion (the greatest cytokine level at the study start). Plasma occurrence of TNF-alpha within two weeks after alcohol drinking cessation predicted unfavorable changes in atherosclerosis risk factors levels during anti-relapse therapy. In this way, TNF-alpha may act as proatherogenic factor not only by direct mechanism, but also via influence on the traditional (main) atherosclerosis risk factors.

Blood Pressure

Hypertension is one of the main risk factors for atherosclerosis, CAD, stroke, heart failure, left ventricular hypertrophy and peripheral embolism. Heavy alcohol drinking is in turn important factor influencing hypertension prevalence and its refractory to applied pharmacotherapy [12, 208, 209]. On the basis of this premises, alcohol abstinence or alcohol drinking limitation is recommended in prophylaxis and non-pharmacological therapy of hypertension [196, 210]. However, observations exist, that alcohol may display biphasic effects on blood pressure (BP), according to the J-shaped curve [211, 212]. Klatzky et al. [208] have revealed, that also moderate alcohol drinking (one to two drinks per day) may increase prevalence of systemic hypertension, although he has suggested, that such results appeared to be partially due to underreporting of alcohol intake. In our investigation we have studied the long-time effect of alcohol withdrawal on blood pressure, both resting, and maximal achieved during treadmill stress test in 54 alcoholics within six-month long abstinence period. In studied subjects no significant changes in resting blood pressure during observation period were found, but after six months of abstinence significant decrease in maximal, responding to exercise systolic and diastolic, blood pressure was observed. We noticed also higher blood pressure (BP) values in patients, who drank alcohol for more than 51 days during 90 days before the study start, as well as in those of them, who had increased gamma-glutamyl transferase (GGT) plasma activity at the study start. In multiple regression analysis, values of blood pressure, both resting and responding to exercise, at the beginning of the study and after four weeks of abstinence period were determined by quantity of alcohol intake during 90 days before the study start, nitric oxide metabolites plasma level, severity of alcohol dependence, depression score (Beck Depression Inventory), clinical (body mass index-BMI, waist to hip ratio- WHR) and biochemical (glucose, lipids and uric acid plasma concentrations) parameters of metabolic syndrome and values of frequency domain analysis of heart rate variability (HRV), such as high (HF) and low (LF) frequency component of HRV analysis, and LF to HF ratio value (expressing sympathovagal balance).

So, we found only not significant decrease in resting systolic and diastolic blood pressure. While, the significant decrease of systolic BP after alcohol drinking reduction or cessation, have shown Minami et al. [212], Yazici et al. [137] and Kähkönen et al. [210]. The first group found simultaneous augmentation of parasympathetic indices of heart rate variability. In Asian men with hypertension, restriction of alcohol intake reduces daytime BP but not night-time values of 24-hour blood pressure monitoring [213]. Moreover, it was pointed out, that an association between alcohol drinking and higher systolic BP was more pronounced in women than men [214], as well as in heterozygotes and individuals with mutation of ALDH2 gene [215]. It also may be, that no significant decrease in resting BP values after six month of abstinence period in our subjects resulted from lack of physical training, when they were hospitalized. It was documented, that in rats exercise training attenuates the chronic ethanol-induced hypertension via reduction of body weight, clearance of ethanol, and augmentation of the aortic endothelial relaxation response [216].

After alcohol withdrawal and in the following time of abstinence, resting blood pressure was higher in alcoholics with increased GGT activity. As was mentioned above, GGT activity is considered as a cardiovascular event risk factor, associated with increased level of known main risk factors for CAD event. This may explain our observation, especially, that similar results, although in general population, have obtained Sakuta et al. [217]. Increased GGT is the feature of subjects with alcoholic and non-alcoholic steatohepatitis and patients with metabolic syndrome. Hypertension is one of the main components of this syndrome. In our study, in multi- variate analysis we have found the relationships between resting BP value and the other components of metabolic syndrome. These observations were similar, as the results obtained by Yamada et al. [218]. Drinking pattern had no influence on BP values. Alcohol consumption had similar pressing effect in weekend as well as in daily drinkers. This influence occurred throughout a 24 hours period, had a rapid onset/offset in weekend drinkers but was more stable in daily drinkers [213].

Nevertheless, in the opposite to the cited papers, in our normotensive alcoholics within six-months long abstinence period, we have shown a significant decrease not in resting blood pressure, but in maximal BP achieved during treadmill stress test, called pressor response to exercise. In available reports, we didn't find similar observations concerning alcoholics. However, the results of recent work implied, that an exaggerated systolic blood pressure response to exercise was strongly associated with carotid atherosclerosis, independently of established risk factors in healthy men [219]. Moreover, blood pressure response after exercise with a two-step method was associated with an increased risk of hypertension, independently of resting blood pressure [220]. Similar effect showed previously Singh et al. [221] and Miyai et al. [222], as well. In conclusion, decrease in pressure response to exercise in alcoholics after alcohol drinking cessation belongs to such factors, which level in withdrawal period changes in advisable direction. So, alcoholics who decided to anti-relapse therapy, may avoid complications depending on hypertension, sometimes leading to death or severe disability.

Alcohol drinking and withdrawal impact on blood pressure is explained mainly by influence on the autonomic nervous system activity, endothelial dysfunction, increase in body mass [209] and L-type Ca2+ channels action, which modifies vascular reactivity[210]. This hypothesis may be supported by observed simultaneous with BP value decrease in endothelial function markers levels (TM, t-PA:Ag, PAI-1), and increase in parasympathetic influence on heart rhythm regulation.

Heart Rate Variability

Heart rate variability (HRV), expresses the fluctuation of the heart beat to beat differences. In many studies it is considered to be a reliable, noninvasive marker of cardiac autonomic nervous system activity [24, 25, 223, 224]. Moreover, decrease in HRV has been found to predict CHD morbidity and mortality in apparently healthy populations and in patients after an acute coronary event [134]. Relatively few studies have investigated the alcohol drinking and alcohol withdrawal effect on HRV activity. Because of this we have also analyzed the effect of alcohol drinking cessation on values of HRV parameters in 54 alcohol dependent male patients. We tested the hypothesis, that prolongation of alcohol abstinence period may improve the autonomic nervous system balance in alcoholics, what indirectly might show on the decrease of cardiovascular event risk or death. In our alcohol dependent patients examined no later than 2 weeks after alcohol abuse period were found greater: mean daily heart rate, lower values of the mean R-R interval duration (MRR), the standard deviation for all 5 minutes segments of the analysis (SDNN_I) and low frequency component of HRV spectrum (LF) than in control group. The percentage of differences between R-R intervals that are greater than 50ms (pNN50) in our alcoholics were lower than in healthy non-drinkers with borderline statistical significance. In alcohol dependent males after four weeks of alcohol abstinence the significant increase of the standard deviation of all R-R intervals (SDNN) and pNN50 values were observed. The values of standard deviation of the mean R-R intervals for all 5 minutes segments of the analysis (SDNN_I) and LF increased not significantly. Moreover, within this period we have also found the decrease of percentage of alcoholics with HRV parameters below cut-off, prognostic values, what may indicate the diminished risk of sudden cardiac death. After following five months of abstinence there were no more significant changes in values of HRV analysis parameters. Nevertheless, all these changes suggested increase of vagal nerve influence on sinus rhythm variability, what is considered as prognostic factor of good outcome. Previously, there were performed relatively not numerous studies concerning the relationships between alcohol drinking and HRV analysis in the meaning of cardiovascular prognostic value and indicator of autonomic nervous system activity, and even less works have presented changes of these parameters after alcohol withdrawal. In the recent work by Janszky et al. [224], the increase of heart rate variability in women with coronary artery disease, who drunk red wine was found. Authors have not observed any influence of drinking beer, spirits and the total amount of alcohol intake on the HRV parameters, what supported the earlier suggested cardioprotective effect only of red wine [126]. While, the other investigations results showed an unfavorable decrease in values of HRV analysis parameters, especially concerning indexes of vagal nerve activity, both after acute alcohol intake [195, 212, 225, 226, 227], and chronic alcohol abuse [228, 229]. These results are in agreement with ours, obtained in the first examination. Similar interpretation came down from the works on alcohol drinking restriction or alcohol abstinence on values of HRV analysis parameters. In Minami's et al. paper [212], the daytime and nighttime heart rate and value of low (LF) to high frequency (HF) components of frequency domain HRV analysis ratio (LF/HF ratio) were significantly lower as well as pNN50 and HF values were greater after three-weeks long alcohol drinking restriction period than in alcohol users. These results, similar to ours, demonstrated that alcohol abstinence augmented parasympathetic indices of heart rate variability in male drinkers [212, 230]. Nevertheless, the effect of a small alcohol amount intake on hemodynamics and HRV was modified by ALDH2 genotypes in Japanese men, and presented only in heterozygotes and patients with mutation of this allele [215]. Similar effect displayed also a one-week long period of smoking cessation [231].

In conclusion, alcohol abstinence resulted in a favorable effect on cardiac autonomic nervous system activity studied by heart rate variability. This was expressed by the increase of vagal nerve participation in regulation of heart rhythm already after four weeks of abstinence. These results may suggest, that in early abstinence period alcoholics are susceptible to complications related to sympathicotonia, such as aggravation of withdrawal syndrome symptoms, tachycardia, arrhythmia, oxygen wasting effect in myocardium, insulin resistance, hyperlipidemia, hypertension, greater hematocrit value (increase of blood viscosity) and platelets activity. These disturbances may increase sudden cardiac death and atherosclerosis progression risk.

Physical Activity

Decrease in exercise tolerance is a common symptom related by out-patients. It may be an effect of central (systemic) as well as peripheral mechanism. To the central mechanism responsible for decrease in physical activity level belong: heart failure, respiratory insufficiency, anemia, obesity, and the level of motivation (low in patients with depression coexistence, for example in the course of double diagnosis). Whereas, the peripheral mechanisms determining effort capacity are: muscle metabolism efficiency and training, efficient peripheral blood flow, electrolytes balance, autonomic nervous system activity. Thus changes in effort competence may be an effect of many factors overlap. On the other hand, alcohol drinking related problems concern about 30% of individuals visiting out-patients departments. Alcohol is an energy source, psychoactive and vasoactive substance, as well as cytotoxin, and all of these effects may influence effort competence. Because of this, it was suggested, that the decrease in physical activity, not only in declared alcoholics, but also in some out-patients with different health problems may be related to excessive alcohol drinking. On the basis of these premises, using treadmill stress test we have estimated physical efficiency in alcohol dependent male patients during six-months long abstinence period. They didn't have significant abnormalities in blood morphology, echocardiography and respiratory system functional tests (spirometry), whereas, in comparison to control group, they had greater heart rate value at the beginning of stress test. More of them (21%) had significant (>1mm) decrease of ST interval during the test, both at the beginning of the study and after four weeks of abstinence. Already after four weeks, in alcoholics significant prolongation of exercise test duration (effort capacity) was found, and after following five months significant decrease in maximal heart rate achieved during the test was observed. Moreover, alcohol dependent patients, in whom determinable TNF-alpha concentration at the study beginning was found, continued test for a longer time and performed greater load. Additionally, alcoholics with abnormal plasma GGT activity at the study start, had greater value of double product (the product of maximal value of heart rate and systolic blood pressure achieved during stress test, which is considered as a marker of myocardial perfusion), but needed shorter time to maximal ST interval depression. Values of respective treadmill stress test parameters correlated negatively with quantity of alcohol drunk during 90 days before the study beginning, body mass index, plasma LDL cholesterol concentration, fasting glucose concentration and positively with TNF-alpha plasma concentration, values of heart rate variability (HRV) analysis, such as LF, low frequency component of HRV analysis (expresses the influence of sympathetic system on cardiac sinus node) and HF, high frequency component of HRV analysis, expressing vagal nerve effect on heart rhythm regulation.

Summarizing the results of our study, it may be concluded, that alcohol abstinence have improved effort competence in alcoholics. About one to five among them had electrocardiographic signs of "silent myocardial ischaemia". We didn't find any significant changes in systemic mechanisms determining exercise tolerance during six-months long abstinence period, so observed improvement in effort competence may resulted from peripheral mechanisms amelioration. Exercise tolerance in the context of alcohol drinking was investigated by some authors. These works concerned the effect of both occasional and chronic alcoholic beverage drinking. Acute, moderate alcohol drinking increased exercise tolerance [135, 207], but not all of authors confirmed this observation [232]. Chronic alcohol drinking leads to decrease of exercise tolerance [232, 233]. Sulander et al. [235], showed U-shaped relationships between functional ability and quantity of alcohol drinking, what is quite similar as for other alcohol related health consequences.

Alcohol influence on exercise capacity may be explained both via systemic, as peripheral mechanisms. Heart injury related to excessive alcohol drinking clinically appears as congestive cardiomyopathy. There is supposed, that it results from disturbances in intracellular calcium metabolism, membrane canal injury (Ca-ATP-ase, Na/K-ATP-ase), impaired calcium binding in endoplasmatic reticulum, and injury of mitochondria (the place of ATP synthesis). Moreover, chronic alcohol consumption decreases the use of glucose, fatty acids (main energy source of myocardium) and amino acids by skeletal muscles and cardiomyocytes, changes energy supply and impairs the metabolic processes during exercise. Alcohol abuse is connected with the decrease in beta-adrenergic receptors density, facilitates atherosclerosis progression and leads to heart injury by ischemic mechanisms [236]. Some influence on effort competence in alcoholics may have pulmonary hypertension, mostly secondary to portal hypertension, which value increases after alcohol drinking, especially in patients with alcoholic liver disease [237], as well as chronic pulmonary disease resulted from chronic smoking, and recurrent gastric content aspiration into airways. Moreover, via peripheral mechanisms, alcohol drinking may favor "oxygen waste" by simultaneous hypersympathycothonia, which presence was confirmed in our study in HRV analysis, as well [230].

The next observation resulted from our study was the alcohol influence on coronary blood flow, which was suggested indirectly by presence of "silent ischaemia" in 20% of subjects at the study start. Already Herbeden in 1768y described favorable effect of low alcohol dose on angina pectoris course. Whereas mechanism by which ethanol exerts this action remain not fully known, especially that some authors have shown vasoconstrictive effect of alcohol drinking and withdrawal [238, 239]. In available papers, the postulated potential mechanisms of vasorelaxative alcohol drinking impact were increase of NO synthesis and induction of prostacyclin secretion. Moreover, Gazieri et al. [240] in recent work have suggested, that low ethanol concentration may release calcitonin gene-related peptide (CGRP) within coronary arteries via stimulation of transient receptor potential vanilloid 1 (TRPV1) in perivascular sensory nerve terminals, and in this way increase coronary flow and induce arterial dilatation. On the other hand, vasoconstrictive alcohol drinking effect may result from increased sympathetic nervous system activity. This disturbance, throughout "oxide waste" effect induction caused by tachycardia and arrhythmia, insulin resistance, hyperlipidemia, hypertension, hematocrit value and platelets activity may also induce myocardial ischaemia independently to coronary vessels diameter.

Moreover, in our study we have found some differences between alcoholics with determinable (>0.05pg/ml) and undeterminable plasma TNF-alpha as well as between subjects with increased and normal GGT activity. Paradoxically, alcoholics with increased TNF-alpha plasma level presented better treadmill test course, expressed by longer test duration time and greater load overcame during exercise, although theoretically the should have worse exercise performance. However, these results are indirectly consistent with the work by Itoh et al. [241] and Cicoira et al [242]. They showed that noradrenaline and brain natriuretic peptide (BNP, marker of heart failure) rose parallel to the degree of exercise intolerance, while the plasma level of receptors for TNF_alpha (TNFR-I and –II) rose only if exercise intolerance reached severe levels. The second parameter, which affected the treadmill exercise test course in our alcoholics was GGT activity. Subjects with GGT value above laboratory norm had greater maximal ST interval depression during the test, and needed shorter time to achieve it. GGT is the well known marker of alcohol abuse, and one among important liver function test. Recently, it is also considered as a risk factor of cardiovascular complications. Persons with an elevated serum GGT of 40 U/l or above had significantly higher odds ratio for all the coronary risk factors as compared with those with normal GGT, even after adjusting for alcohol consumption, age, body mass index, cigarette smoking and physical activity [243]. It may be, that our subjects with increased GGT activity had more pronounced coronary artery disease, which via ischaemic mechanism decreased their effort competence. Gradual increase of exercise tolerance after alcohol drinking cessation showed favorable effect of abstinence. Physical activity on the other hand produces favorable effects on alcohol withdrawal-related metabolic changes, such as general cardioprotective acting, desirable changes in plasma lipids and the other components of metabolic syndrome, even anti-neoplasmatic acting, so it seems obvious, that it should be recommended as the useful method of training in alcoholics during withdrawal period. This procedure would be for sure the cheapest, efficient and free from adverse effects therapeutic method. There was revealed, that even moderate intensive walking for 60 and 90 min slightly, but insignificantly, reduced postprandial lipemia after two mixed meals with moderate fat content in healthy young men, compared to inactive persons [244].

Glucose Tolerance

Glucose metabolism disturbances, clinically expressed by insulin resistance, glucose intolerance and diabetes mellitus are an important risk factor of multi-organ complications, especially concerning cardiovascular system. Alcohol drinking may predispose to liver steatosis or steatohepatitis, secondary insulin resistance and metabolic syndrome appearance, and lifetime drinking pattern is significantly correlated with the prevalence of the metabolic syndrome [139, 245]. On the other hand, daily alcohol intake of >9.2 and > or =3-9 g was positively associated with adiponectin and insulin sensitivity, independently to existing obesity, and metabolic control [246]. Moderate alcohol drinking in patients with diabetes mellitus exerted a cardioprotective effect [247]. In our study we have estimated, in 54 alcoholics without diabetes mellitus, the effect of alcohol drinking cessation on glucose tolerance using standard glucose tolerance test (GTT). In all subjects the results of fasting glucose concentration within six month long abstinence period were normal, but in ten of them (18%) glucose plasma concentration was abnormal two hours after taking 75g glucose in GTT. After following four weeks and six months of abstinence these disturbances disappeared, therefore none of patients had incorrect results of glucose tolerance. This implied that alcohol abuse exerted unfavorable effect on glucose tolerance and insulin resistance. However, reference data have suggested, that one among benefits of moderate alcohol drinking is improvement in insulin sensitivity and glucose tolerance [248]. In the other, cross- over study in healthy, moderate to heavy male drinkers, a four weeks long reduction in alcohol intake from 7.2 to 0.8 standard drinks per day, didn't influence insulin sensitivity as measured by insulin sensitivity index or homeostasis model assessment (HOMA) score [249]. Independently on these data, our results suggested that in some, probably genetically predisposed subjects, heavy alcohol drinking may induce glucose tolerance disturbances, but four weeks long alcohol abstinence was enough to improve it.

Sex Hormones

Alcohol is metabolized mainly via alcohol dehydrogenase (ADH) pathway. However, this enzyme activity is regulated by endocrine and nutritional factors. Estrogens and thyroid hormone deficiency increased and androgens decreased ADH activity. Growth hormone (GH) secretion pattern may also influence ADH activity: frequent pulse, presented in females, increases ADH activity, rare pulse of GH secretion inhibits it. Similar regulation influence activities of liver cytochromes, CYP2C12 (female) and CYP2C11 (male) as well as liver peroxisome proliferator- activated receptors (PPAR), which are important in lipids metabolism regulation. Many consequences of alcohol drinking, for example liver injury and lipoproteins acetylation, depend in great part on the level of acetaldehyde, intermediate product of ethanol metabolism, therefore changes in ADH activity may be responsible for the individual differences in susceptibility to alcohol abuse dependent organ complication. These interrelationships, called hypothalamo-pituitary gonadal – liver axis [250], are also important in some other aspects. Liver is the organ, in which takes place carrier proteins synthesis, hormone metabolism and plasma clearance, so liver injury may change these processes, what results also in gonads function. Moreover, the role of sex hormones in alcoholics may be considered in the context of anti-atherogenic action of estradiol.

In the purpose to estimate the effect of alcohol abuse on sex-hormones plasma concentration, we have performed the investigation in thirty-seven females and twenty-five males with alcohol dependence, who were abstinent for less than 7 days before the study. We determined biochemical liver function tests values and the levels of sex hormones, such as prolactin, follicle-stimulating hormone (FSH), luteinizing hormone (LH), estradiol, progesterone and testosterone; in females three times during the menstrual cycle and in males at the study beginning. In comparison to male alcoholics, alcohol dependent females, had significantly greater concentration of prolactin, estradiol, and lower level of testosterone in all three determination, whereas greater level of progesterone during ovulation and before menstruation, as well as greater LH level during ovulation, however, these differences resulted mainly from sex. To decrease or even eliminate this effect, in the further analysis we have compared frequency of abnormal hormones values presence in respective subjects groups. Alcohol dependent females had significantly more frequently incorrect values of sex hormones, than male alcoholics, according to set producers range values. Moreover, female alcoholics with abnormal liver function tests values, more frequently than females with correct values, had greater than normal LH and FSH concentrations during ovulation and in luteal phase of menstrual cycle and lower than normal range estradiol concentration during ovulation. Whereas, in male alcoholics presence of abnormal liver function tests didn't affect the frequency of incorrect hormone values. The multi- factorial analysis showed, that alcohol dependent females were more susceptible than males to disturbances in prolactin and estradiol secretion and less to FSH and LH secretion. Whereas, when into model of log-linear analysis gender and liver injury as the independent variables were included, we found, that abnormal biochemical liver function tests values, as the independent factor, have affected only presence of increased (above normal value) prolactin concentration during early alcohol abstinence period. Differences in abnormal hormones values prevalence was independently related only to patients gender.

We have also compared the concentration of sex-hormones in female alcoholics and women, who denied alcohol drinking (control group). This analysis has shown, that alcohol dependent subjects, in comparison to the control group, had lower average LH level and lower value of LH/FSH ratio during ovulation. Moreover, female alcoholics with increased aminotransferases activities (>40U/l), had significantly greater level of FSH during ovulation and before menstruation, higher LH level in follicular phase, lower estradiol level during ovulation. The concentration of prolactin, progesterone and testosterone in each of three phases of menstrual cycle were similar in female alcoholics with and without biochemical markers of liver injury. Significant linear correlations between GGT activity and the levels of LH, FSH, estradiol, and LH/FSH ratio value were found. The number of drinking days during one month before start of the study have correlated with prolactin concentration in all three phases of menstrual cycle, and number of drinks drank in this period correlated with LH/FSH ratio and estradiol level during luteal phase. The majority of our observations corroborated the results obtained by the other authors [251, 252, 253, 254].

Concluding, our observations have suggested, that alcohol abuse, in relationship to quantity of alcohol intake, produced important disturbances in the levels of sex hormones in majority of females, while in males it caused mainly the increase of prolactin level. Moreover we have pointed out, that biochemical markers of liver injury value was the second, besides of gender, independent factor affecting the abnormal increase of prolactin concentration. The clinical importance of these observation was the demonstration of alcohol abuse effect on hypothalamic –pituitary – gonadal axis, which appeared independently to susceptibility to alcohol induced liver injury. On the other hand such results underline the necessity of alcohol problem exclusion in women with menstrual cycle disturbances and infertility.

References

[1] McGinnis, JM; Foege, WH. Actual causes of death in the United States. *JAMA*, 1993, 270, 2207-2212.

[2] Marik, P; Mohedin, B. Alcohol- related admissions to an inner city hospital intensive care unit. *Alcohol Alcoholism*, 1996, 31, 393-396.

[3] Adams, WL; Yuan, Z; Barboriak, JJ; Rimm, AA. Alcohol-related hospitalizations of elderly people: Prevalence and geographic variation in the United States. *JAMA*, 1993, 270, 1222-1225.

[4] Cherpitel, CJ. The epidemiology of alcohol-related trauma. *Alcohol Health Research World,* 1992, 16, 191- 196.

[5] Corrao, G; Rubbiati, L; Bagnardi, V; Zambon, A; Poikolainen, K. Alcohol and coronary heart disease: A meta-analysis. *Addiction*, 2000, 94, 1505-1523.

[6] Rehm, J; Bondy, S; Sempos, CT; Vuong, CV. Alcohol consumption and coronary heart disease, morbidity and mortality. *American Journal of Epidemiology*, 1997, 146, 495-501.

[7] Rehm, J; Sempos, CT; Trevisan, M. Average volume of alcohol consumption, patterns of drinking and risk of coronary heart disease-A review. *Journal of Cardiovascular Risk,* 2003, 10, 15-20.

[8] Bagnardi, V; Blangiardo, M; La Vecchia, C; Corrao G. A meta-analysis of alcohol drinking and cancer risk. *British Journal of Cancer,* 2001, 85, 1700-1705.

[9] Lieber, C. Hepatic and other medical disorders of alcoholism: from pathogenesis to treatment. *Journal of Studies on Alcohol,* 1997, 59, 9-25.

[10] Rehm, J; Gutjahr, E; Gmel, G. Alcohol and all-cause mortality. A pooled analysis. *Contemporary Drug Problems*, 2001, 28, 337-361.

[11] Schuckit MA. Alcohol-use disorders. *Lancet,.* 2009, 373, 492-501.

[12] Kloner, RA; Rezkalla, SH. To drink or not to drink? That is the question. *Circulation,* 2007, 116, 1306-1317.

[13] Hart, CL; Smith, GD. Alcohol consumption and mortality and hospital admissions in men from the Midspan collaborative cohort study. *Addiction,* 2008, 103, 1979-1986.

[14] Klatsky AL. Alcohol and cardiovascular diseases. *Expert Rev Cardiovasc The,*. 2009, 7, 499-506.

[15] Murray, CJL; Lopez, AD. Global mortality, disability, and the contribution of risk factors: Global burden of disease study. *Lancet*, 1997, 349, 1436-1442.

[16] Littleton, J. Neurochemical mechanisms underlying alcohol withdrawal. *Alcohol Health Research World*, 1998, 22, 13- 24.

[17] American Psychiatric Association. Diagnostic and statistical manual of mental disorders. 4th ed., text revision. Washington, D. C.: American Psychiatric Association, 2000, 216.

[18] Trevisan, LA; Boutros, N; Petrakis, IL; Krystal, JH. Complications of alcohol withdrawal. *Alcohol Health Research World*, 1998, 22, 61- 66.

[19] Charness, ME. Brain lesions in alcoholics. *Alcoholism Clinical Experimental Research, 1993,* 17, 2- 11.

[20] Satel, SL; Kosten, TR; Schuckit, MA; Fischman, MW. Should protracted withdrawal from drugs be included in the DSM-IV? *American Journal of Psychiatry*, 1993, 150, 695- 704.

[21] Bauer, LO; Costa, L; Hesselbrock, VM. Effects of alcoholism, anxiety and depression on P300 in women: a pilot study. *Journal of Studies on Alcohol,* 2001, 62, 571-579.

[22] Ziółkowski, M; Gruss, T; Rybakowski, JK. Does alexithymia in male alcoholics constitute a negative factor for maintaining abstinence? *Psychotherapy and Psychosomatix*, 1995, 63, 169-173.

[23] Stendal, Ch. *Practice guide to gastrointestinal function testing.* Oxford: Blackwell Science, 1997.

[24] Toichi, M; Sugiura, T; Murai, T; Sengoku, A. A new method of assessing cardiac autonomic function and its comparison with spectral analysis and coefficient of variation of R-R interval. *Journal of the Autonomic Nervous System,* 1997, 62, 79-84.

[25] Heart rate variability. Standards of measurements physiological interpretation and clinical use. Task Force of The European Society of Cardiology and The North American Society of Pacing and Electrophysiology [editorial]. *European Heart Journal,* 1996, 17, 354-381.

[26] Fields, J; Turk, A; Durkin, M. Increased gastrointestinal symptoms in chronic alcoholics. *American Journal of Gastroenterology*, 1994, 95, 382-386.

[27] Siegmund, S; Spanagel, R; Singer, MV. Role of the brain-gut axis in alcohol-related gastrointestinal diseases- what can we learn from new animal models? *Journal of Physiology and Pharmacology,* 2003, 54 (Suppl 4), 191-207.

[28] Hunt, RH; Tougas, G. Evolving concepts in functional gastrointestinal disorders: promising directions for novel pharmaceutical treatments. *Best Practice and Research in Clinical Gastroenterology,* 2002, 16, 869-83.

[29] Watson, RR; Borgs, P; Witte, M; McCuskey, RS; Lantz, C; Johnson, MI; Mufti, SI; Earnest, DL. Alcohol, immunomodulation and disease. *Alcohol and Alcoholism,* 1994, 29, 131-139.

[30] Schafer, C; Schips, I; Landig, J; Bode, JC; Bode, C. Tumor necrosis factor and interleukin-6 response of peripheral blood monocytes to low concentrations of lipopolysaccharides in patients with alcoholic liver disease. *Zeitschrift fur Gastroenterologie,* 1995, 33, 503-508.

[31] Bode, C; Kugler, V; Bode, JC. Endotoxemia in patients with alcoholic and non-alcoholic cirrhosis and in subjects with no evidence of chronic liver disease following acute alcohol excess. *Journal of Hepatology*, 1987, 4, 8-14.

[32] Hailman, E; Vasselon, T; Kelley, M; Busse, LA; Hut, MC-T; Lichenstein, HS; Detmers, PA; Wright, SD. Stimulation of macrophages and neutrophils by complexes of lipopolysaccharide and soluble CD 14. *Journal of Immunology,* 1996, 156, 4384-4390.

[33] Massamiri, T; Tobias, PS; Curtiss, LK. Structural determinants for the interaction of lipopolysaccharide-binding protein with purified high density lipoproteins: role of apolipoprotein A-1. *Journal of Lipid Research,* 1997, 38, 516-525.

[34] Schumann, RR; Zweigner, J. A novel acute-phase marker: lipopolysaccharide binding protein (LBP). *Clinical Chemistry and Laboratory Medicine,* 1999, 37, 271-274.

[35] Armstrong, D; Bennett, JR; Blum, AL; Dent, J; De Dombal, FT; Galmiche, JP; Lundell, L; Margulies, M; Richter, JE; Spechler, SJ; Tytgat, GN; Wallin, L. The endoscopic assessment of esophagitis: a progress report on observer agreement. *Gastroenterology,* 1996, 111, 85-92.

[36] Kłopocka, M; Budzyński, J; Świątkowski, M; Ziółkowski, M. The influence of four-weeks abstinence on macro- and microscopic appearance of the upper gastrointestinal tract mucosa and on esophageal and gastric pH-metry in alcohol-dependent male patients. *Alkoholizm i Narkomania,* 2003, 16, 87-99.

[37] Labenz, J; Jaspersen, D; Kulig, M; Leodolter, A; Lind, T; Meyer-Sabellek, W; Stolte, M; Vieth, M; Willich, S; Malfertheiner, P. Risk factors for erosive esophagitis: a multivariate analysis based on the ProGERD study initiative. *American Journal of Gastroenterology,* 2004, 99, 1652-1656.

[38] Knoll, MR; Kolbel, CB; Teyssen, S; Singer, MV. Action of pure ethanol and some alcoholic beverages on the gastric mucosa in healthy humans: A descriptive endoscopic study. *Endoscopy,* 1997, 29, 1-9.

[39] Bode, C; Bode, JC. Effect of alcohol consumption on the gut. *Best Practice and Research in Clinical Gastroenterology,* 2003, 17, 575-592.

[40] Bienia, A; Sodolski, W; Luchowska, E. The effect of chronic alcohol abuse on gastric and duodenal mucosa. *Annales of University Mariae Curie Sklodowska,* 2002, 57, 570-582.

[41] Figlie, NB; Benedito-Silva, AA; Monteiro, MG; Souza-Formigani, ML. Biological markers of alcohol consumption in nondrinkers, drinkers and alcohol-dependent Brazilian patients. *Alcohol Clinical Experimental Research,* 2002, 26, 1062-1069.

[42] Potet, F; Florent, C; Benhamou, E; Cabrieres, F; Bommelaer, G; Hostein, J; Bigard, MA; Bruley De Varannes, S; Colombel, JF; Rampal, P. Chronic gastritis: prevalence in the French population. CIRIG. *Gastroenterology and Clinical Biology,* 1993, 17, 103-108.

[43] Uppal, R; Lateef, SK; Korsten, MA; Paronetto, F; Lieber, ChS. Chronic alcoholic gastritis. Roles of alcohol and Helicobacter pylori. *Archives of Internal Medicine,* 1991, 151, 760-764.

[44] Borch, K; Jonsson, KA; Petrsson, F; Redeen, S; Mardh, S; Franzen, LE. Prevalence of gastroduodenitis and Helicobacter pylori infection in a general population sample: relations to symptomatology and life-style. *Digestive Diseases and Science,* 2000, 45, 1322-1329.

[45] Hydzik, P; Kosowski, B. Macroscopic and microscopic picture of the gastric mucosa in ethanol dependent persons. *Przegląd Lekarski,* 2001, 58, 306-314.

[46] Muszynski, J; Biernacka, D; Sieminska, J; Stepka, M; Zalewski, L; Ehrmann, A; Gornicka, B. Changes in gastric mucosa and Helicobacter pylori infection in young health volunteers. *Polski Merkuriusz Lekarski,* 1996, 1, 169-173.

[47] Bures, J; Kopacova, M; Koupil, I; Vorisek, V; Rejchrt, S; Beranek, M; Seifert, B; Pozler, O; Zivny, P; Douda, T; Kolesarova, M; Pinter, M; Palicka, V; Holcik, J; European Society for Primary Care Gastroenterology. Epidemiology of Helicobacter pylori infection in the Czech Republic. *Helicobacter,* 2006, 11, 56-65.

[48] Santos, IS; Boccio, J; Santos, AS; Valle, NC; Halal, CS; Bachilli, MC; Lopes, RD. Prevalence of Helicobacter pylori infection and associated factors among adults in Southern Brazil: a population-based cross-sectional study. *BMC Public Health,* 2005, 10, 118.

[49] Hauge, T; Persson, J; Danielsson, D. Mucosal bacterial growth in the upper gastrointestinal tract in alcoholics (heavy drinkers). *Digestion,* 1997, 58, 591-595.

[50] Brenner, H; Rothenbacher, D; Bode, G; Adler, G. Inverse graded relation between alcohol consumption and active infection with Helicobacter pylori. *American Journal of Epidemiology*, 1999, 149, 571-576.

[51] Murray, LJ; Lane, AJ; Harvey, IM; Donovan, JL; Nair, P; Harvey, RF. Inverse relationship between alcohol consumption and active Helicobacter pylori infection: the Bristol Helicobacter project. *American Journal of Gastroenterology,* 2002, 97, 2750-2755.

[52] Weisse, ME; Eberly, B; Person, DA. Wine as a digestive aid: comparative antimicrobial effects of bismuth salicylate and red and white wine. *BMJ,* 1995, 311, 1657-1660.

[53] Lin, RS; Lee, FY; Lee, SD; Tsai, YT; Lin, HCh; Lu, RH; Hsu, WCh; Huang, ChC; Wang, SS; Lo, KJ. Endotoxemia in patients with chronic liver diseases: relationships to severity of liver diseases, presence of esophageal varices, and hyperdynamic circulation. *Journal of Hepatology,* 1995, 22, 165-172.

[54] Napolitano, LN; Koruda, MJ; Zimmerman, K; McCowan, K; Chang, J; Meyer, AA. Chronic ethanol intake and burn injury: evidence for synergistic alteration in gut and immune integrity. *Journal Trauma,* 1995, 38, 198-207.

[55] Bujanda, L. The effects of alcohol consumption upon the gastrointestinal tract. *American Journal of Gastroenterology,* 2000, 95, 3374-3382.

[56] Chari, ST; Teyssen, S; Singer, MV. Alcohol and gastric acid secretion in humans. *Gut,* 1993, 34, 843-847.

[57] Teyssen, S; Gonzales-Calero, G; Schimiczek, M; Singer, MV. Maleic acid and succinic acid in fermented alcoholic beverages are the stimulants of gastric acid secretion. *Journal of Clinical Investigation,* 1999, 103, 707-713.

[58] Kłopocka, M; Budzyński, J; Świątkowski, M; Ziółkowski, M. Changes in gastric pH during a four week period of abstinence in alcohol dependent male patients. *Alkoholizm i Narkomania,* 2000, 13, 503-511.

[59] Bercik, P; Verd, EF; Armstrong, D; Cederberg, C; Idstrom, JP; Stolte, M; Blum, A. Apparent increase in acid output during omeprazole after cure of H. pylori infection. *Gastroenterology,* 1997, 112, A70.

[60] Kłopocka, M; Budzyński, J; Pulkowski, G; Ziółkowski, M; Świątkowski, M. The results of esophageal pH-metry in alcohol dependent male patients after alcohol withdrawal. *Valetudinaria,* 2005, 10 (Suppl), 101-106.

[61] Hogan, WJ; Viegas de Andrade, SR; Winship, DH. Ethanol induced acute esophageal motor dysfunction. *Journal of Applied Physiology,* 1972, 32, 755-760.

[62] Keshavarzian, A; Polepalle, C; Iber, FL; Durkin, M. Esophageal motor disorder in alcoholics: result of alcoholism or withdrawal? *Alcohol Clinical Experimental Research,* 1990, 14, 561-567.

[63] Keshavarzian, A; Polepalle, C; Iber, FL; Durkin, M. Secondary esophageal contractions are abnormal in chronic alcoholics. *Digestive Diseases Sciences,* 1992, 37, 517-522.

[64] Grande, L; Monforte, R; Ros, E; Toledo-Pimentel, V; Estruch, R; Lacima, G; Urbano-Marquez, A; Pera, C. High amplitude contractions in the middle third of the oesophagus: a manometric marker of chronic alcoholism? *Gut,* 1996, 38, 655-662.

[65] Świątkowski, M; Budzyński, J; Kłopocka, M; Ziółkowski, M; Bujak, R; Sinkiewicz, W. Parameters of the functional and morphological status of the upper digestive tract in alcohol-dependent male patients with depression and alexithymia in the context of autonomic nervous system activity and nitric oxide plasma level. *Medical Science Monitor,* 2004, 10, CR68-74.

[66] Wegener, M; Schaffstein, J; Dilger, U; Coenen, C; Wedmann, B; Schmidt, G. Gastrointestinal transit of solid-liquid meal in chronic alcoholics. *Digestive Diseases Sciences,* 1991, 36, 917-923.

[67] Franke, A; Nakchbandi, IA; Schneider, A; Harder, H; Singer, MV. The effect of ethanol and alcoholic beverages on gastric emptying of solid meals in humans. Alcohol Alcoholism, 2005, 40, 187-193.

[68] Dutta, SK; Orestes, M; Vengulekur, S; Kwo, P. Ethanol and human saliva: effect of chronic alcoholism on flow rate, composition, and epidermal growth factor. *American Journal of Gastroenterology, 1992,* 87, 350-354.

[69] Beitman, BD. Panic disorder in patients with angiographically normal coronary arteries. American Journal of Medicine, 1992, 92 (Suppl 5A), S33-S40.

[70] Haug, TT; Mykletun, A; Dahl, AA. Are anxiety and depression related to gastrointestinal symptoms in the general population? *Scandinavian Journal of Gastroenterology*, 2002, 37, 294-298.

[71] Kahrilas, PJ. Diagnosis of symptomatic gastroesophageal reflux disease. *American Journal of Gastroenterology*, 2003, 98 (Suppl), S15-SS23.

[72] Portincasa, P; Moschetta, A; Baldassarre, G; Altomare, DF; Palasciano, G. Pan-enteric dysmotility, impaired quality of life and alexithymia in a large group of patients meeting ROME II criteria for irritable bowel syndrome. *World Journal of Gastroenterology,* 2003, 9, 2293-2299.

[73] Campo, JV; Dahl, RE; Williamson, DE; Birmaher, B; Perel, JM; Ryan, NN. Gastrointestinal distress to serotonergic challenge: a risk marker for emotional disorder? *Journal of the American Academy of Child and Adolescent Psychiatry,* 2003, 42, 1221-1226.

[74] Kłopocka, M; Budzyński, J; Bujak, R; Świątkowski, M; Sinkiewicz, W; Ziółkowski, M. Daily sinus heart rate variability as the indicator of autonomic neural system activity in alcohol dependent male patients during abstinence period. *Alkoholizm i Narkomania,* 2000, 13, 491-501.

[75] Maczka, M; Thor, P; Lorens, K; Konturek, SJ. Nitric oxide inhibits the myoelectric activity of the small intestine in dogs. *Journal of Physiology and Pharmacology,* 1993, 44, 31-42.

[76] Kassim, SK; El Touny, M; El Guinaidy, M; El Moghani, MA; El Mohsen, AA. Serum nitrates and vasoactive intestinal peptide in patients with gastroesophageal reflux disease. *Clinical Biochemistry,* 2002, 35, 641-646.

[77] Namiot, Z; Rourk, RM; Piascik, R; Hetzel, DP; Sarosiek, J; Mc Callum, RW. Interrelationship between esophageal challenge with mechanical and chemical stimuli and salivary protective mechanisms. *American Journal of Gastroenterology,* 1994, 89, 581-587.

[78] Casselbrant, A; Pettersson, A; Fandriks, L. Oesophageal intraluminal nitric oxide facilitates the acid-induced oesophago-salivary reflex. *Scandinavian Journal of Gastroenterology,* 2003, 38, 235-238.

[79] Vrontakis, ME. Galanin: A biologically active peptide. *Current Drug Targets CNS and Neurological Disorders,* 2002, 1, 531-541.

[80] Tache, Y; Martinez, V; Million, M; Wang, L. *American Journal of Physiology-Gastrointestinal and Liver Physiology,* 2001, 280, G173-177.

[81] Scheurer, U; Halter, F. Lower esophageal sphincter in reflux esophagitis. *Scandinavian Journal of Gastroenterology,* 1976, 11, 629-634.

[82] Kłopocka, M; Budzyński, J; Świątkowski, M; Pulkowski, G; Ziółkowski, M. Czynniki wpływające na stężenie czynnika martwicy guza (TNF-alfa) i poziom prób wątrobowych w surowicy u mężczyzn uzależnionych od alkoholu po jego odstawieniu. *Psychiatria Polska,* 2007, 41, 411-425.

[83] Noach, LA; Bosma, NB; Jansen, J; Hoek, FJ; van Deventer, SJ; Tytgat, GN. Mucosal tumor necrosis factor-alpha, interleukin-1 beta, and interleukin-8 production in patients with Helicobacter pylori infection. *Scandinavian Journal of Gastroenterology,* 1994, 29, 425-429.

[84] Yusuf, S; Hawken, S; Ounpuu, S; Dans, T; Avezum, A; Lanas, F; McQueen, M; Budaj, A; Pais, P; Varigos, J; Lisheng, L; INTERHEART Study Investigators. Effect of potentially modifiable risk factors associated with myocardial infarction in 52 countries (the INTERHEART study): case-control study. *Lancet,* 2004, 364, 937-952.

[85] Khot, UN; Khot, MB; Bajzer, CT; Sapp, SK; Ohman, EM; Brener, SJ; Ellis; SG; Lincoff, AM; Topol, EJ. Prevalence of conventional risk factors in patients with coronary heart disease. *JAMA,* 2003, 290, 898-904.

[86] Rizzo, M; Berneis, K. Lipid triad or atherogenic lipoprotein phenotype: a role in cardiovascular prevention? *Journal of Atherosclerosis and Thrombosis,* 2005, 12, 237-239.

[87] O'Keefe, JH; Carter, MD; Lavie, CJ; Bell, DS. The gravity of JUPITER (Justification for the Use of Statins in Primary Prevention: An Intervention Trial Evaluating Rosuvastatin). *Postgrad Med,* 2009, 121, 113-118.

[88] Balbisi, EA. Management of hyperlipidemia: new LDL-C targets for persons at high-risk for cardiovascular events. *Medical Science Monitor,* 2006, 12, RA34-9.

[89] Scandinavian Simvastatin Survival Study Group. Randomized trial of cholesterol lowering in 4444 patients with coronary heart disease: The Scandinavian Simvastatin Survival Study (4S). *Lancet,* 1994, 344, 1383-1389.

[90] Brown, SL. Lowered serum cholesterol and low mood: the links remains unproved. *British Medical Journal,* 1996, 313, 637-638.

[91] Deisenhammer, EA; Lechner-Schoner, T; Kemmler, G; Ober, A; Braidt, E; Hinterhuber, H. Serum lipids and risk factors for attempted suicide in patients with alcohol dependence. *Alcohol Clinical Experimental Research,* 2006, 30, 460-465.

[92] Goldberg, DM; Hahn, SE; Parkes; JG. Beyond alcohol: beverage consumption and cardiovascular mortality. *Clinical Chimica Acta,* 1995, 237, 155-187.

[93] Hannuksela, ML; Liisanantti; MK; Savolainen; MJ. Effect of alcohol on lipids and lipoproteins in relation to atherosclerosis. *Critical Reviews in Clinical Laboratory Sciences,* 2002, 39, 225-283.

[94] Langer, RD; Criqui, MH; Reed, DM. Lipoproteins and blood pressure as biological pathways for effect of moderate alcohol consumption on coronary heart disease. *Circulation,* 1992, 85, 910-915.

[95] Gerlich, MG; Krämer, A; Gmel, G; Maggiorini, M; Lüscher, TF; Rickli, H; Kleger, GR; Rehm, J. Patterns of Alcohol Consumption and Acute Myocardial Infarction: A Case-Crossover Analysis. *Eur Addict Res,* 2009, 15, 143-149.

[96] Budzyński, J; Rybakowski, J; Światkowski, M; Torliński, L; Kłopocka, M; Kosmowski, W; Ziółkowski, M. Naltrexone exerts a favourable effect on plasma lipids in abstinent patients with alcohol dependence. *Alcohol Alcoholism,* 2000, 35, 1-7.

[97] Budzyński, J; Kłopocka, M; Świątkowski, M; Pulkowski, G; Żiółkowki, M. Lipoprotein(a) in alcohol-dependent male patients during a six-month abstinence period. *Alcohol Alcoholism,* 2003, 38, 157-162.

[98] Nikkila, M; Solakivi, T; Lehtimaki, T; Koivula, T; Laippala, P; Astrom, B. Postprandial plasma lipoprotein changes in relation to apolipoprotein E phenotypes and low density lipoprotein size in men with and without coronary artery disease. *Atherosclerosis,* 1994, 106, 149-157.

[99] Slyper, A; Zvereva, S; Schectman, G; Hoffman, RG; Pleuss, J; Walker, JA. Normal postprandial lipemia and chylomicron clearance of offspring of parents with early coronary artery disease. The Journal of Clinical Endocrinological Metabolism, 1998, 83, 1106-1113.

[100] Gotto, AM. Triglyceride as a risk factor for coronary artery disease. *American Journal of Cardiology,* 1998, 82, 22Q-25Q.

[101] Marschang, P; Gotsch, C; Kirchmair, R; Kaser, S; Kahler, CM; Patsch, JR. Postprandial, but not postabsorptive low-density lipoproteins increase the expression of intercellular adhesion molecule-1 in human aortic endothelial cells. *Atherosclerosis,* 2006, 186, 101-106.

[102] Hyson, D; Rutledge, JC; Berglund, L. Postprandial lipemia and cardiovascular disease. *Current Atherosclerosis Reports,* 2003, 5, 437-444.

[103] Syvanne, M; Talmud, PJ; Humphries, SE; Fisher, RM; Rosseneu, M; Hilden, H; Taskinen, MR. Determinans of postprandial lipemia in men with coronary artery disease and low levels of HDL cholesterol. *Journal of Lipid Research,* 1997, 38, 1463-1472.

[104] Dallongeville, J; Tiret, L; Viskis, S; O'Reilly, D; Saava, M; Tsitouris, G; Rosseneu, M; DeBacker, G; Humphries, SE; Beisiegel, U. On behalf of the EARS Group: Effect of apo E phenotype on plasma postprandial triglyceride levels in young male adults with and without a familial history of myocardial infarction: the EARS II study. *Atherosclerosis,* 1999, 145, 381-388.

[105] Lopez-Miranda, J; Perez-Martinez, P; Marin, C; Moreno, JA; Gomez, P; Perez-Jimenez, F. Postprandial lipoprotein metabolism, genes and risk of cardiovascular disease. *Current Opinion in Lipidology,* 2006, 17, 132-138.

[106] Fielding, BA; Reid, G; Grady, M; Humphreys, SM; Evans, K; Frayn, KN. Ethanol with a mixed meal increases postprandial triacylglycerol but decreases postprandial non-esterified fatty acid concentrations. *The British Journal of Nutricion,* 2000, 83, 597-604.

[107] Suter, PM; Gerritsen-Zehnder, M; Hasler, E; Gurtler, M; Vetter, W; Hanseler, E. Effect of alcohol on postprandial lipemia with and without preprandial exercise. *Journal of American Collage of Nutricion,* 2001, 20, 58-64.

[108] Gould, LA; Rossow, JE; Santanello, NC; Heyse, J; Furberg, CD. Cholesterol reduction yields clinical benefit. A new look at old data. *Circulation,* 1995, 91, 2274-2282.

[109] Law, MR; Wald, NJ; Thompson, SG. By how much and how quickly does reduction in serum cholesterol concentration lower risk of ischaemic heart disease? *British Medical Journal,* 1994, 308, 367-372.

[110] Jones, J. Comparative dose efficacy study of atorvastatin versus simvastatin, pravastatin, lovastatin and fluvastatin in patients with hypercholesterolemia (The CURVES Study). *American Journal of Cardiology,* 582-587.

[111] Schrott, X. A multicenter placebo controlled dose ranging study of atorvastatin. *Journal of Cardiovascular Pharmacology and Therapeutics,* 1998, 3, 119-124.

[112] Bryant, HU; Kuta, CC; Story, JA; Yim, GK. Stressand morphine-induced elevations of plasma and tissue cholesterol in mice: reversal by naltrexone. *Biochemical Pharmacology,* 1988, 37, 3777–3780.

[113] Hamed, SA, Nabeshima, T. The high atherosclerotic risk among epileptics: the atheroprotective role of multivitamins. *Journal of Pharmacological Sciences,* 2005, 98, 340-353.

[114] Valle, A; O'connor, DT; Taylor, PW; Zhu, G; Montgomery, GW; Slagboom, PE; Martin, NG; Whitfield, JB. Pseudocholinesterase: Association with the Metabolic Syndrome and Identification of 2 Gene Loci Affecting Activity. *Clinical Chemistry,* 2006, 52, 1014-1020.

[115] Meisinger, C; Doring, A; Schneider, A; Lowel, H. for the KORA Study Group.: Serum gamma-glutamyltransferase is a predictor of incident coronary events in apparently healthy men from the general population. *Atherosclerosis.* 2006, 14, [Epub ahead of print].

[116] Ruttmann, E; Brant, LJ; Concin, H; Diem, G; Rapp, K; Ulmer, H. Vorarlberg Health Monitoring and Promotion Program Study Group.: Gamma-glutamyltransferase as a risk factor for cardiovascular disease mortality: an epidemiological investigation in a cohort of 163,944 Austrian adults. *Circulation,* 2005, 112, 2130-2137.

[117] Baros, AM; Wright, TM; Latham, PK; Miller, PM; Anton, RF. Alcohol consumption, %CDT, GGT and blood pressure change during alcohol treatment. *Alcohol Alcohol,* 2008, 43, 192-197.

[118] Hartung, GH; Lawrence, SJ; Reeves, RS; Foreyt, JP. Effect of alcohol and exercise on postprandial lipemia and triglyceride clearance in men. *Atherosclerosis,* 1993, 100, 33-40.

[119] Gueguen, S; Herbeth, B; Pirollet, P; Paille, F; Siest, G; Visvikis, S. Changes in serum apolipoprotein and lipoprotein profile after alcohol withdrawal: effect of apolipoprotein E polymorphism. *Alcohol Clinical Experimental Research,* 2002, 26, 501-508.

[120] Szmitko, PE; Verma, S. Antiatherogenic potential of red wine: clinician update. *American Journal of Physiology Heart and Circulatory Physiology,* 2005, 288, H2023-2030.

[121] Streppel, MT; Ocké, MC; Boshuizen, HC; Kok, FJ; Kromhout, D. Long-term wine consumption is related to cardiovascular mortality and life expectancy independently of moderate alcohol intake: the Zutphen Study. *J Epidemiol Community Health,* 2009, 63, 534-540.

[122] Das, S; Santani, DD; Dhalla, NS. Experimental evidence for the cardioprotective effects of red wine. *Exp Clin Cardio,* 2007, 12, 5-10.

[123] Opie, LH; Lecour, S. The red wine hypothesis: from concepts to protective signalling molecules. *Eur Heart J,* 2007, 28, 1683-1693.

[124] Koppes, LL; Twisk, JW; Van Mechelen, W; Snel, J; Kemper, HC. Cross-sectional and longitudinal relationships between alcohol consumption and lipids, blood pressure and body weight indices. *Journal of Studies on Alcohol,* 2005, 66,713-721.

[125] Mizia-Stec, K; Zahorska-Markiewicz, B; Mandecki, T; Janowska, J; Szulc, A; Jastrzębska-Maj, E; Gąsior, Z.Hyperlipidaemias and serum cytokines in patients with coronary artery disease. *Acta Cardiologica,* 2003, 58, 9-15.

[126] Rehm, J; Room, R; Graham, K; Monteiro, M; Gmel, G; Sempos, CT. The relationship of average volume of alcohol consumption and patterns of drinking to burden of disease: an overview. *Addiction,* 2003, 98, 1209-1228.

[127] Puddey, IB; Rakic, V; Dimmitt, SB; Beilin, LJ. Influence of pattern of drinking on cardiovascular disease and cardiovascular risk factors--a review. *Addiction,* 1999, 94, 649-663.

[128] Chalasani, N; Aljadhey, H; Kesterson, J; Murray, MD; Hall, SD. Patients with elevated liver enzymes are not at higher risk for statin hepatotoxicity. *Gastroenterology,* 2004, 126, 1287-1292.

[129] Haile, CN; Kosten, TA; Kosten, TR. Pharmacogenetic treatments for drug addiction: alcohol and opiates. *Am J Drug Alcohol Abuse,* 2008, 34, 355-381.

[130] Naruszewicz, M; Johansson, ML; Zapolska-Downar, D; Bukowska, H. Effect of Lactobacillus plantarum 299v on cardiovascular disease risk factors in smokers. *American Journal of Clinical Nutricion,* 2002, 76, 1249-1255.

[131] Gill, HS; Guarner, F. Probiotics and human health: a clinical perspective. *Postgraduate Medical Journal,* 2004, 80, 516-526.

[132] Loguercio, C; Federico, A; Tuccillo, C; Terracciano, F; D'Auria, MV; De Simone, C; Del Vecchio Blanco, C. Beneficial effects of a probiotic VSL#3 on parameters of liver dysfunction in chronic liver diseases. *Journal of Clinical Gastroenterology,* 2005, 39, 540-543.

[133] Vaswani, M; Rao, RV. Biochemical measures in the diagnosis of alcohol dependence using discriminant analysis. *Indian Journal of Medical Sciences,* 2005, 59, 423-430.

[134] Patrono, C; Bachmann, F; Baigent, C; Bode, C; De Caterina, R; Charbonnier, B; Fitzgerald, D; Hirsh, J; Husted, S; Kvasnicka, J; Montalescot, G; Garcia Rodriguez,

LA; Verheugt, F; Vermylen, J; Wallentin, L; Priori, SG; Alonso Garcia, MA; Blanc, JJ; Budaj, A; Cowie, M; Dean, V; Deckers, J; Fernandez Burgos, E; Lekakis, J; Lindahl, B; Mazzotta, G; Morais, J; Oto, A; Smiseth, OA; Morais, J; Deckers, J; Ferreira, R; Mazzotta, G; Steg, PG; Teixeira, F; Wilcox, R; European Society of Cardiology. Expert consensus document on the use of antiplatelet agents. The task force on the use of antiplatelet agents in patients with atherosclerotic cardiovascular disease of the European society of cardiology. *European Heart Journal,* 2004, 25, 166-181.

[135] Wang, MQ; Nicholson, ME; Richardson, MT; Fitzhugh, EC; Reneau, P; Westerfield, CR. The acute effect of moderate alcohol consumption on cardiovascular responses in women. *Journal of Studies on Alcohol,* 1995, 56, 16-20.

[136] Cowan, DH. Effect of alcoholism on hemostasis. *Seminars in Hematology,* 1980, 17, 137-147.

[137] Yazici, M; Kaya, A; Kaya, Y; Albayrak, S; Cinemre, H; Ozhan, H. Lifestyle modification decreases the mean platelet volume in prehypertensive patients. *Platelets,* 2009, 20, 58-63.

[138] Huczek, Z; Kochman, J; Filipiak, KJ; Horszczaruk, GJ; Grabowski, M; Piątkowski, R; Wilczynska, J; Zielinski, A; Meier, B; Opolski, G. Mean platelet volume on admission predicts impaired reperfusion and long-term mortality in acute myocardial infarction treated with primary percutaneous coronary intervention. *Journal of American Collage of Cardiology,* 2005, 46, 284-290.

[139] Conway, DI. Alcohol consumption and the risk for disease. Is there a dose-risk relationship between alcohol and disease? *Evidence Based Dentistry,* 2005, 6, 76-77.

[140] Renaud, SC; Ruf, JC. Effects of alcohol on platelet functions. *Clinical Chimica Acta,* 1996, 246, 77-89.

[141] de Lange, DW; van de Wiel, A. Drink to prevent: review on the cardioprotective mechanisms of alcohol and red wine polyphenols. *Seminars in Vascular Medicine,* 2004, 4, 173-186.

[142] Desai, K; Owen, JS; Wilson, DT; Hutton, RA. Platelet aggregation and plasma lipoproteins in alcoholics during alcohol withdrawal. *Thrombosis and Haemostasis,* 1986, 55, 173-177.

[143] Coccini, T; Castoldi, AF; Gandini, C; Randine, G; Vittadini, G; Baiardi, P; Manzo, L. Platelet monoamine oxidase B activity as a state marker for alcoholism: trend over time during withdrawal and influence of smoking and gender. *Alcohol Alcoholism,* 2002, 37, 566-572.

[144] Kannel, WB. Overview of hemostatic factors involved in atherosclerotic cardiovascular disease. *Lipids,* 2005, 40, 1215-1220.

[145] Trotti, R; Carratelli, M; Barbieri, M; Micieli, G; Bosone, D; Rondanelli, M; Bo, P. Oxidative stress and a thrombophilic condition in alcoholics without severe liver disease. *Haematologica,* 2001, 86, 85-91.

[146] McConnell, MV; Vavouranakis, I; Wu, LL; Vaughan, DE; Ridker, PM. Effects of a single, daily alcoholic beverage on lipid and hemostatic markers of cardiovascular risk. *American Journal of Cardiology,* 1997, 80, 1226-1228.

[147] van Golde, PM; Hart, HCh; Kraaijenhagen, RJ; Bouma, BN; van de Wiel, A. Regular alcohol intake and fibrinolysis. *Netherlanden Journal of Medicine,* 2002, 60, 285-288.

[148] Meade, TW; Chakrabarti, R; Haines, AP; North, WRS; Stirling, Y. Characteristics affecting fibrinolytic activity and plasma fibrinogen concentrations. *British Medical Journal,* 1979, 1, 153-156.

[149] Woodward, M; Lowe, GD; Rumley, A; Tunstall-Pedoe, H; Philippou, H; Lane, DA; Morrison, CE. Epidemiology of coagulation factors, inhibitors and activation markers: The Third Glasgow MONICA Survey. II. Relationships to cardiovascular risk factors and prevalent cardiovascular disease. *British Journal of Haematology,* 1997, 97, 785-97.

[150] Conlan, MG; Folsom, AR; Finch, A; Davis, CE; Marcucci, G; Sorlie, P; Wu, KK. Antithrombin III: association with age, race, sex and cardiovascular disease risk factors. *Thrombosis and Haemostasis,* 1994, 72, 551-556.

[151] Wallestedt, S; Cederblad, G; Korsan- Bengtsen, K; Olsson, R. Coagulation factors and other plasma proteins during abstinence after heavy alcohol consumption in chronic alcoholics. *Scandinavian Journal of Gastroenterology,* 1997, 12, 649- 655.

[152] Kauhanen, J; Kaplan, GA; Goldberg, DD; Cohen, RD; Lakka, TA; Salonen, JT. Frequent hangovers and cardiovascular mortality in middle-aged men. *Epidemiology,* 1997, 8, 310-314.

[153] Ehlers, R; Buttcher, E; Eltzschig, HK; Kazmaier, S; Szabo, S; Helber, U; Hoffmeister, HM. Correlation between ST-T-segment changes with markers of hemostasis in patients with acute coronary syndromes. *Cardiology,* 2002, 98, 40-45.

[154] De Lorenzo, F; Kadziola, Z; Kakkar, VV. Haemostatic factors and risk of coronary heart disease. *Blood Coagulation and Fibrinolysis,* 1999, 10, 113-114.

[155] El-Hazmi, MA. Hematological risk factors for coronary heart disease. *Medical Principles and Practice,* 2002, 11 Suppl 2,56-62.

[156] Freedman, DS; Byers, T; Barboriak, JJ; Flanders, WD; Duncan, A; Yip, R; Meilahn, EN. The relation of prothrombin times to coronary heart disease risk factors among men aged 31-45 years. *American Journal of Epidemiology,* 1992, 136, 513-524.

[157] Landmesser, U; Drexler, H. The clinical significance of endothelial dysfunction. *Current Opinion in Cardiology,* 2005; 20, 547-51.

[158] Constans, J; Conri, C. Circulating markers of endothelial function in cardiovascular disease. *Clinical Chimica Acta,* 2006, 8 [Epub ahead of print]

[159] de Lange, M; de Geus, EJ; Kluft, C; Meijer, P; van Doornen, LJ; Boomsma ,DI; Snieder, H. Genetic influences on fibrinogen, tissue plasminogen activator-antigen and von Willebrand factor in males and females. *Thrombosis and Haemostasis,* 2006, 95, 414-419.

[160] Li, YH; Shi, GY; Wu, HL. The role of thrombomodulin in atherosclerosis: from bench to bedside. *Cardiovascular and Hematological Agents in Medicinal Chemistry,* 2006, 4, 183-187.

[161] Mukamal, KJ; Jadhav, PP; D'Agostino, RB; Massaro, JM; Mittleman, MA; Lipinska, I; Sutherland, PA; Matheney, T; Levy, D; Wilson, PW; Ellison, RC; Silbershatz, H; Muller, JE; Tofler, GH. Alcohol consumption and hemostatic factors: analysis of the Framingham Offspring cohort. *Circulation,* 2001, 104, 1367-1373.

[162] Booyse, FM; Aikens, ML; Grenett, HE. Endothelial cell fibrinolysis: transcriptional regulation of fibrinolytic protein gene expression (t-PA, u-PA, and PAI-1) by low alcohol. *Alcohol Clinical Experimental Research,* 1999, 23, 1119-1124.

[163] Luedemann, C; Bord, E; Qin, G; Zhu, Y; Goukassian, D; Losordo, DW; Kishore, R. Ethanol modulation of TNF-alpha biosynthesis and signaling in endothelial cells: synergistic augmentation of TNF-alpha mediated endothelial cell dysfunctions by chronic ethanol. *Alcohol Clinical Experimental Research,* 2005, 29, 930-938.

[164] Budzyński, J; Kłopocka, M; Świątkowski, M; Pulkowski, G; Ziółkowski, M; Kulwas, A; Kotschy, M. Increased blood coagulation in alcohol dependent male patients during six months abstinence period. *Advances in Clinical and Experimental Medicine,* 2005, 14, 323-331.

[165] Bayraktar, Y; Harmanci, O. Etiology and consequences of thrombosis in abdominal vessels. *World Journal of Gastroenterology,* 2006, 12, 1165-1174.

[166] Rackoff, A; Shores, N; Willner, I. Mesenteric venous thrombosis in a patient with pancreatitis and protein C deficiency. *Southern Medical Journal,* 2005, 98, 232-234.

[167] Agarwal, DP. Cardioprotective effects of light-moderate consumption of alcohol: a review of putative mechanisms. *Alcohol and Alcoholism,* 2002, 37, 409-415.

[168] Brecher, AS; Adamu, MT. Short- and long-term effects of acetaldehyde on plasma. *Alcohol* 2002, 26, 49-53.

[169] Ridker, PM; Vaughan, DE; Stampfer, MJ; Glynn, RJ; Hennekens, CH. Association of moderate alcohol consumption and plasma concentration of endogenous tissue-type plasminogen activator. *JAMA,* 1994, 272, 929-933.

[170] Djousse, L; Pankow, JS; Arnett, DK; Zhang, Y; Hong, Y; Province, MA; Ellison, RC. Alcohol consumption and plasminogen activator inhibitor type 1: the National Heart, Lung, and Blood Institute Family Heart Study. *American Heart Journal,* 2000, 139, 704-709.

[171] Wannamethee, SG; Lowe, GD; Shaper, G; Whincup, PH; Rumley, A; Walker, M; Lennon, L. The effects of different alcoholic drinks on lipids, insulin and haemostatic and inflammatory markers in older men. *Thrombosis and Haemostasis,* 2003, 90, 1080-1087.

[172] Soardo, G; Donnini, D; Varutti, R; Moretti, M; Milocco, C; Basan, L; Esposito, W; Casaccio, D; Stel, G; Catena, C; Curcio, F; Sechi, LA. Alcohol-induced endothelial changes are associated with oxidative stress and are rapidly reversed after withdrawal. *Alcohol Clinical Experimental Research,* 2005, 29, 1889-1898.

[173] Sasaki, A; Kurisu, A; Ohno, M; Ikeda, Y. Overweight/obesity, smoking, and heavy alcohol consumption are important determinants of plasma PAI-1 levels in healthy men. *American Journal of Medical Sciences,* 2001, 322, 19-23.

[174] Pellegrini, N; Pareti, FI; Stabile, F; Brusamolino, A; Simonetti, P. Effects of moderate consumption of red wine on platelet aggregation and haemostatic variables in healthy volunteers. *European Journal of Clinical Nutrition,* 1996, 50, 209-213.

[175] Thorand, B; Baumert, J; Doring, A; Schneider, A; Chambless, L; Lowel, H; Kolb, H; Koenig, W. Association of cardiovascular risk factors with markers of endothelial dysfunction in middle-aged men and women. Results from the MONICA/KORA Augsburg Study. *Thrombosis and Haemostasis,* 2006, 95, 134-141.

[176] Minami, J; Todoroki, M; Yoshii, M; Mita, S; Nishikimi, T; Ishimitsu, T; Matsuoka, H. Effects of smoking cessation or alcohol restriction on metabolic and fibrinolytic variables in Japanese men. *Clinical Science,* 2002, 103, 117-122.

[177] Delahousse, B; Maillot, F; Gabriel, I; Schellenberg, F; Lamisse, F; Gruel, Y. Increased plasma fibrinolysis and tissue-type plasminogen activator/tissue-type plasminogen activator inhibitor ratios after ethanol withdrawal in chronic alcoholics. *Blood Coagulation and Fibrinolysis,* 2001, 12, 59-66.

[178] Kiviniemi, TO; Saraste, A; Lehtimäki, T; Toikka, JO; Saraste, M; Raitakari, OT; Pärkkä, JP; Hartiala, JJ; Viikari, J; Koskenvuo, JW. High dose of red wine elicits enhanced inhibition of fibrinolysis. *Eur J Cardiovasc Prev Rehabil,* 2009, 16, 161-163.

[179] Pawlak, R; Melchor, JP; Matys, T; Skrzypiec, AE; Strickland, S. Ethanol-withdrawal seizures are controlled by tissue plasminogen activator via modulation of NR2B-containing NMDA receptors. *Proceedings of the National Academy of Sciences of the U S A,* 2005, 102, 443-448.

[180] Thatcher, DL; Clark, DB. Cardiovascular risk factors in adolescents with alcohol use disorders. *International Journal of Adolescent Medicine and Health,* 2006, 18, 151-157.

[181] Critchley, J; Capewell, S. Smoking cessation for the secondary prevention of coronary heart disease. *Cochrane Database of Systematic Reviews,* 2004, CD003041.

[182] Shai, I; Rimm, EB; Hankinson, SE; Cannuscio, C; Curhan, G; Manson, JE; Rifai, N; Stampfer, MJ; Ma, J. Lipoprotein (a) and coronary heart disease among women: beyond a cholesterol carrier? *European Heart Journal,* 2005, 26, 1633-1639.

[183] Delarue, J; Husson, M; Schellenberg, F; Tichet, J; Vol, S; Couet, C; Lamisse, F. Serum lipoprotein(a) [Lp(a)] in alcoholic men: effect of withdrawal. *Alcohol,* 1996, 13, 309-314.

[184] Calabresi, L; Gomaraschi, M; Franceschini, G. Endothelial protection by high-density lipoproteins: from bench to bedside. *Arteriosclerosis, Thrombosis and Vascular Biology,* 2003, 23, 1724-1731.

[185] Miller, GJ. Dietary fatty acids and the haemostatic system. *Atherosclerosis,* 2005, 179, 213-227.

[186] Gerlach, M; Blum-Degen, D; Ransmayr, G; Leblhuber, F; Pedersen, V; Riederer, P. Expression, but not activity, of neuronal nitric oxide synthase is regionally increased in the alcoholic brain. *Alcohol and Alcoholism,* 2001, 36, 65-69.

[187] Uzbay, IT; Erden, BF.: Attenuation of ethanol withdrawal signs by high doses of L-arginine in rats. *Alcohol and Alcoholism,* 2003, 38, 213-218.

[188] Okva, K; Lang, A; Pokk, P; Vali, M; Nevalainen, T. Litter has an effect on the behavioural changes caused by the administration of the nitric oxide synthase inhibitor NG-nitro-L-arginine and ethanol in mice. *Prog Neuropsychopharmacol Biol Psychiatry,* 2004, 28, 1171-1179.

[189] Adams, ML; Cicero, TJ. Alcohol intoxication and withdrawal: the role of nitric oxide. *Alcohol,* 1998, 16, 153-158.

[190] Sierksma, A; van der Gaag, MS; Grobbee, DE; Hendriks, HF. Acute and chronic effects of dinner with alcoholic beverages on nitric oxide metabolites in healthy men. *Clinical and Experimental Pharmacology and Physiology,* 2003, 30, 504-506.

[191] Venkov, ChD; Myers, PR; Tanner, MA; Su, M; Vaughan; DE. Ethanol increases endothelial nitric oxide production through modulation of nitric oxide synthase expression. *Thrombosis and Haemostasis,* 1999, 81, 638-642.

[192] Yuksel, N; Uzbay, IT; Karakilic, H; Aki, OE; Etik, C; Erbas, D. Increased serum nitrite/nitrate (NOx) and malondialdehyde (MDA) levels during alcohol withdrawal in alcoholic patients. *Pharmacopsychiatry,* 2005, 38, 95-96.

[193] Budzyński, J; Kłopocka, M; Świątkowski, M; Ziółkowski, M; Pulkowski, G; Kopczyńska, E. Nitric oxide metabolites plasma level in alcohol dependent male patients during six-month abstinence. *Alkoholizm i Narkomania, 2004,* 17, 197-209.

[194] Budzyński, J; Kłopocka, M; Świątkowski, M; Ziółkowski, M; Pulkowski, G; Kopczyńska, E. Can an increase of nitric oxide metabolites concentration after first four weeks of abstinence predict alcohol relapse during the next five months? *Alkoholizm i Narkomania,* 2004, 17, 211-220.

[195] Kahkonen, S; Mechanisms of cardiovascular dysregulation during alcohol withdrawal. *Prog Neuropsychopharmacol Biol Psychiatry,* 2004, 28, 937-941.

[196] Zima, T; Fialova, L; Mestek, O; Janebova, M; Crkovska, J; Malbohan, I; Stipek, S; Mikulikova, L; Popov, P. Oxidative stress, metabolism of ethanol and alcohol-related diseases. *Journal of Biomedical Science,* 2001, 8, 59-70.

[197] Gerlach, M; Blum-Degen, D; Ransmayr, G; Leblhuber, F; Pedersen, V; Riederer, P. Expression, but not activity, of neuronal nitric oxide synthase is regionally increased in the alcoholic brain. *Alcohol and Alcoholism,* 2001, 36, 65-69.

[198] Imhof, A; Froehlich, M; Brenner, H; Boeing, H; Pepys, MB; Koenig, W. Effect of alcohol consumption on systemic markers of inflammation. *Lancet,* 2001, 357, 763-767.

[199] Albert, MA; Glynn, RJ; Ridker, PM. Alcohol consumption and plasma concentration of C-reactive protein. *Circulation.* 2003, 107, 443-447.

[200] Badia, E; Sacanella, E; Fernandez-Sola, J; Nicolas, JM; Antunez, E; Rotilio, D; de Gaetano, G; Urbano-Marquez, A; Estruch, R. Decreased tumor necrosis factor-induced adhesion of human monocytes to endothelial cells after moderate alcohol consumption. *The American Journal of Clinical Nutrition,* 2004, 80, 225-230.

[201] Gonzalez-Quintela, A; Dominguez-Santalla, MJ; Loidi, L; Quinteiro, C; Perez, LF. Relation of tumor necrosis factor (TNF) gene polymorphisms with serum concentrations and in vitro production of TNF-alpha and interleukin-8 in heavy drinkers. *Alcohol,* 2004, 34 273-277.

[202] Fleming, S; Toratani, S; Shea-Donohue, T; Kashiwabara, Y; Vogel, SN; Metcalf, ES. Pro- and anti-inflammatory gene expression in the murine small intestine and liver after chronic exposure to alcohol. *Alcohol Clinical and Experimental Research,* 2001, 25,n579-589.

[203] Poullis, A;, Mendall, MA. Alcohol, obesity, and TNF-alpha. *Gut,* 2001, 49, 313-314.

[204] Sierksma, A; Patel, H; Ouchi, N; Kihara, S; Funahashi, T; Heine, RJ; Grobbee, DE; Kluft, C; Hendriks, HF. Effect of moderate alcohol consumption on adiponectin, tumor necrosis factor-alpha, and insulin sensitivity. *Diabetes Care,* 2004, 27,184-189.

[205] Kim, DJ; Kim, W; Yoon, SJ; Choi, BM; Kim, JS; Go, HJ; Kim, YK; Jeong, J. Effects of alcohol hangover on cytokine production in healthy subjects. *Alcohol*, 2003, 31, 167-170.

[206] Budzyński, J; Kłopocka, M; Ziółkowski, M; Świątkowski, M; Pulkowski, G. Tumour Necrosis Factor- alpha and its relationships to the Biochemical Factors potentially Involved in Atherosclerotic Processes in Alcohol Dependent male Patients after Alcohol Withdrawal. *Advances in Clinical and Experimental Medicine*, 2005, 14, 511-521.

[207] Braun, BL; Wagenaar, AC; Flack, JM. Alcohol consumption and physical fitness among young adults. *Alcoholism, Clinical and Experimental Research*, 1995, 19, 1048-1054.

[208] Klatsky, AL; Gunderson, EP; Kipp, H; Udaltsova, N; Friedman, GD. Higher prevalence of systemic hypertension among moderate alcohol drinkers: an exploration of the role of underreporting. *Journal of Studies on Alcohol*, 2006, 67, 421-428.

[209] Beilin, LJ; Puddey, IB. Alcohol and Hypertension, An Update. *Hypertension*, 2006, 47, 1035-1038.

[210] Kähkönen, S; Bondarenko, BB; Lipsanen, J; Zvartau, EE. Effects of verapamil, an antagonist of L-type calcium channels, on cardiovascular symptoms in alcohol withdrawal. *Neuropsychobiology*, 2008, 58, 123-127.

[211] Ceccanti, M; Sasso, GF; Nocente, R; Balducci, G; Prastaro, A; Ticchi, C; Bertazzoni, G; Santini, P; Attilia, ML. Hypertension in early alcohol withdrawal in chronic alcoholics. *Alcohol and Alcoholism*, 2006, 41, 5-10.

[212] Minami, J; Yoshii, M; Todoroki, M; Nishikimi, T; Ishimitsu, T; Fukunaga, T; Matsuoka, H. Effects of alcohol restriction on ambulatory blood pressure, heart rate, and heart rate variability in Japanese men. *American Journal of Hypertension*, 2002, 15, 125-129.

[213] Kawano, Y; Abe, H; Takishita, S; Omae, T. Effects of alcohol restriction on 24-hour ambulatory blood pressure in Japanese men with hypertension. *American Journal of Medicine*, 1998, 105, 307-311.

[214] Tobe, SW; Soberman, H; Kiss, A; Perkins, N; Baker, B. The effect of alcohol and gender on ambulatory blood pressure: results from the Baseline Double Exposure study. *American Journal of Hypertension*, 2006, 19, 136-139.

[215] Minami, J; Todoroki, M; Ishimitsu, T; Yamamoto, H; Abe, S; Fukunaga, T; Matsuoka, H. Effects of alcohol intake on ambulatory blood pressure, heart rate, and heart rate variability in Japanese men with different ALDH2 genotypes. *Journal of Human Hypertension*, 2002, 16, 345-351.

[216] Husain, K; Ortiz, MV; Lalla, J. Physical training ameliorates chronic alcohol-induced hypertension and aortic reactivity in rats. *Alcohol and Alcoholism*, 2006, 41, 247-253.

[217] Sakuta, H; Suzuki, T; Yasuda, H; Ito, T. Gamma-glutamyl transferase and metabolic risk factors for cardiovascular disease. *Internal Medicine*, 2005, 44, 538-541.

[218] Yamada, Y; Noborisaka, Y; Ishizaki, M; Tsuritani, I; Honda, R; Yamada, S. Alcohol consumption, homeostasis model assessment indices and blood pressure in middle-aged healthy men. *Journal of Human Hypertension*, 2004, 18, 343-350.

[219] Jae, SY; Fernhall, B; Heffernan, KS; Kang, M; Lee, MK; Choi, YH; Hong, KP; Ahn, ES; Park, WH. Exaggerated blood pressure response to exercise is associated with carotid atherosclerosis in apparently healthy men. *Journal of Hypertension,* 2006, 24, 881-887.

[220] Tsumura, K; Hayashi, T; Hamada, C; Endo, G; Fujii, S; Okada, K. Blood pressure response after two-step exercise as a powerful predictor of hypertension: the Osaka Health Survey. *Journal of Hypertension,* 2002, 20, 1507-1512.

[221] Singh, JP; Larson, MG; Manolio, TA; O'Donnell, CJ; Lauer, M; Evans, JC; Levy, D. Blood pressure response during treadmill testing as a risk factor for new-onset hypertension. *The Framingham heart study. Circulation,* 1999, 99, 1831-1836.

[222] Miyai, N; Arita, M; Morioka, I; Takeda, S; Miyashita, K. Ambulatory blood pressure, sympathetic activity, and left ventricular structure and function in middle-aged normotensive men with exaggerated blood pressure response to exercise. *Medical Science Monitor,* 2005, 11, CR478-484.

[223] Budzyński, J; Kłopocka, M; Bujak, R; Świątkowski, M; Pulkowski, G;, Sinkiewicz, W. Autonomic nervous function in Helicobacter pylori-infected patients with atypical chest pain studied by analysis of heart rate variability. *European Journal of Gastroenterology and Hepatology,* 2004, 16, 451-457.

[224] Janszky, I; Ericson, M; Blom, M; Georgiades, A; Magnusson, JO; Alinagizadeh, H; Ahnve, S. Wine drinking is associated with increased heart rate variability in women with coronary heart disease. *Heart,* 2005, 91, 314-318.

[225] Koskinen, P; Virolainen, J; Kupari, M. Acute alcohol intake decreases short-term heart rate variability in healthy subjects. *Clinical Sciences,* 1994, 87, 225–230.

[226] Rossinen, J; Partanen, J; Koskinen, P; Toivonen, L; Kupari, M; Nieminen, MS. Acute heavy alcohol intake increases silent myocardial ischaemia in patients with stable angina pectoris. *Heart,* 1996, 75, 563-567.

[227] Bennett, AJ; Sponberg, AC; Graham, T; Suomi, SJ; Higley, JD; De Petrillo, PB. Initial ethanol exposure results in decreased heart rate variability in ethanol-naive rhesus monkeys. *European Journal of Pharmacology,* 2001, 433,169–172.

[228] Malpas, SC; Whiteside, EA; Maling, TJ; Heart rate variability and cardiac autonomic function in men with chronic alcohol dependence. *British Heart Journal,* 1991, 65, 84–88.

[229] De Petrillo, PB; White, KV; Liu, M; Hommer, D; Goldman, D. Effects of alcohol use and gender on the dynamics of EKG time-series data. *Alcoholism, Clinical and Experimental Research,* 1999, 23,745–750.

[230] Kłopocka, M; Budzyński, J; Bujak, R; Świątkowski, M; Sinkiewicz, W; Ziółkowski, M. Daily sinus heart rate variability as the indicator of autonomic neural system activity in alcohol dependent male patients during abstinence period. *Alkoholizm i Narkomania,* 2000, 13, 491-501.

[231] Minami, J; Ishimitsu, T; Matsuoka, H. Effects of smoking cessation on blood pressure and heart rate variability in habitual smokers. *Hypertension,* 1999, 33, 586-590.

[232] Heitzler, VN; Eremic, Z. The effect of excessive alcohol consumption on the heart function and working capacity of manual workers. Acta Medica Austriaca, 1998, 25, 96-100.

[233] Capodaglio, EM; Vittadini, G; Bossi, D; Sverzellati, S; Facioli, M; Montomoli, C; Dalla Toffola, E. A functional assessment methodology for alcohol dependent patients undergoing rehabilitative treatments. *Disabilily and Rehabilitation,* 2003, 25, 1224-1230.

[234] Hartung, GH; Kohl, HW; Blair, SN; Lawrence, SJ; Harrist, RB. Exercise tolerance and alcohol intake. Blood pressure relation. *Hypertension,* 1990, 16, 501-507.

[235] Sulander, T; Martelin, T; Rahkonen, O; Nissinen, A; Uutela, A. Associations of functional ability with health-related behavior and body mass index among the elderly. *Archives of Gerontology and Geriatrics,* 2005, 40, 185-199.

[236] El-Sayed, MS; Ali, N; El-Sayed Ali, Z. Interaction between alcohol and exercise: physiological and haematological implications. *Sports Medicine,* 2005, 35, 257-269.

[237] Ratti, L; Pozzi, M. The pulmonary involvement in portal hypertension: portopulmonary hypertension and hepatopulmonary syndrome. *Gastroenterology and Hepatology,* 2006, 29, 40-50.

[238] Gowda, RM; Khan, IA; Vasavada, BC; Sacchi, TJ. Alcohol-triggered acute myocardial infarction. *American Journal of Therapeutics,* 2003, 10, 71-72.

[239] Rossinen, J; Viitasalo, M; Partanen, J; Koskinen, P; Kupasi, M; Nieminen, MS. Effects of acute alcohol ingestion on heart rate variability in patients with documented coronary artery disease and stable angina pectoris.*The American Journal of Cardiology,* 1997, 79, 487–491.

[240] Gazzieri, D; Trevisani, M; Tarantini, F; Bechi, P; Masotti, G; Gensini, GF; Castellani, S; Marchionni, N; Geppetti, P; Harrison, S. Ethanol dilates coronary arteries and increases coronary flow via transient receptor potential vanilloid 1 and calcitonin gene-related peptide. *Cardiovascular Research,* 2006, 70, 589-599.

[241] Itoh, K; Osada, N; Inoue, K; Samejima, H; Seki, A; Omiya, K; Miyake, F. Relationship between exercise intolerance and levels of neurohormonal factors and proinflammatory cytokines in patients with stable chronic heart failure. *International Heart Journal, 2005,* 46, 1049-1059.

[242] Cicoira, M; Bolger, AP; Doehner, W; Rauchhaus, M; Davos, C; Sharma, R; Al-Nasser, FO; Coats, AJ; Anker, SD. High tumour necrosis factor-alpha levels are associated with exercise intolerance and neurohormonal activation in chronic heart failure patients. *Cytokine,* 2001, 15, 80-86.

[243] Yamada, Y; Noborisaka, Y; Suzuki, H; Ishizaki, M; Yamada, S. Alcohol consumption, serum gamma-glutamyltransferase levels, and coronary risk factors in a middle-aged occupational population. *Journal of Occupational Health,* 2003, 45, 293-299.

[244] Pfeiffer, M; Ludwig, T; Wenk, C; Colombani, PC. The influence of walking performed immediately before meals with moderate fat content on postprandial lipemia. *Lipids in Health and Disease,* 2005, 4, 24.

[245] Corrao, G; Bagnardi, V; Zambon, A; La Vecchia, C. A meta-analysis of alcohol consumption and the risk of 15 diseases. *Preventive Medicine,* 2004, 38, 613-619.

[246] Englund Ogge, L; Brohall, G; Behre, CJ; Schmidt, C; Fagerberg, B. Alcohol consumption in relation to metabolic regulation, inflammation, and adiponectin in 64-year-old Caucasian women: a population-based study with a focus on impaired glucose regulation. *Diabetes Care,* 2006, 29, 908-913.

[247] Pitsavos, C; Makrilakis, K; Panagiotakos, DB; Chrysohoou, C; Ioannidis, I; Dimosthenopoulos, C; Stefanadis, C; Katsilambros, N. The J-shape effect of alcohol intake on the risk of developing acute coronary syndromes in diabetic subjects: the CARDIO2000 II Study. *Diabetic Medicine,* 2005, 22, 243-248.

[248] Yoon, YS; Oh, SW; Baik, HW; Park, HS; Kim, WY. Alcohol consumption and the metabolic syndrome in Korean adults: the 1998 Korean National Health and Nutrition Examination Survey. *American Journal of Clinical Nutrition,* 2004, 80, 217-224.

[249] Zilkens, RR; Burke, V; Watts, G; Beilin, LJ; Puddey, IB. The effect of alcohol intake on insulin sensitivity in men: a randomized controlled trial. *Diabetes Care,* 2003, 26, 608-612.

[250] Gursoy, S; Baskol, M; Ozbakir, O; Guven, K; Kelestimur, F; Yucesoy, M. Hypothalamo-pituitary gonadal axis in men with chronic hepatitis. *Hepatogastroenterology,* 2004, 51, 787-790.

[251] Iturriaga, H; Valladares, L; Hirsch, S; Devoto, E; P'erez, C; Bunout, D; Lioi, X; Petermann, M. Effects of abstinence on sex hormone profile in alcoholic patients without liver failure. *Journal of Endocrinological Investigation,* 1995, 18, 638-644.

[252] Emanuele, NV; LaPaglia, N; Steiner, J; Kirsteins, L; Emanuele, MA; Effect of chronic ethanol exposure on female rat reproductive cyclicity and hormone secretion. *Alcoholism, Clinical and Experimental Research,* 2001, 25, 1025-1029.

[253] Simon, FR; Fortune, J; Iwahashi, M; Sutherland, E. Sexual dimorphic expression of ADH in rat liver: importance of the hypothalamic-pituitary-liver axis. *American Journal of Physiology and Gastrointestinal Liver Physiology,* 2002, 283, G646-655.

[254] Mowat, NA; Edwards, CR; Fisher, R; McNeilly, AS; Green, JR; Dawson, AM. Hypothalamic-pituitary-gonadal function in men with cirrhosis of the liver. *Gut,* 1976, 17, 345-350.

In: Substance Withdrawal Syndrome
Editors: J. P. Rees and O. B. Woodhouse

ISBN 978-1-60692-951-3
© 2009 Nova Science Publishers, Inc.

Chapter VII

The Effects of Acute, Chronic and Withdrawal from Chronic Ethanol on Emotional Learning[*]

Danielle Gulick and Thomas J. Gould
Department of Psychology, Neuroscience Program,
Temple University, Philadelphia, PA 19122

Abstract

Alcohol is the most commonly used and abused recreational drug, and one effect of ethanol administration, regardless of whether it is acute or chronic, is the disruption of learning and memory. Although recent studies have demonstrated that ethanol does not produce global deficits but, rather, acts on specific substrates to alter neural function, our understanding of the effects of ethanol on cognitive processes remains incomplete. The studies discussed herein offer support for the specificity of the effects of ethanol on learning-related processes and examine how these effects vary with both the task and the phase of ethanol administration examined. Acute ethanol impairs emotional learning as measured by standard contextual and cued fear conditioning, as well as trace fear conditioning and passive avoidance. However, the effects of acute ethanol on these tasks are influenced by multiple factors, such as genetics and age. Furthermore, as ethanol administration transitions into chronic and withdrawal from chronic ethanol, the pattern of impairments in emotional learning changes. This suggests that acute, chronic, and withdrawal from chronic ethanol differentially alter behavior and therefore may also differentially alter neuronal function. Thus, the current review compares and contrasts the effects of acute, chronic, and withdrawal from chronic ethanol within fear conditioning and passive avoidance tasks, and across these two models of aversive/emotional learning.

---

[*] A version of this chapter was also published as a chapter in *Cognitive Sciences, Volume 4, Issue 1*, edited by Miao-Kun Sun, published by Nova Science Publishers, Inc. It was submitted for appropriate modifications in an effort to encourage wider dissemination of research.

Keywords: Alcohol, Addiction, Learning and Memory, Hippocampus, Genetics.

Introduction

Despite the well-known deficits in cognition and locomotion caused by both acute and chronic administration of ethyl alcohol (ethanol), approximately 17.6 million adult Americans abuse alcohol on a regular basis (National Institute on Alcohol Abuse and Alcoholism (NIAAA), 2004). Ethanol has an extremely low potency compared to other drugs of abuse, yet 10% of the adult male population in the United States drinks heavily enough to be diagnosed as alcoholic (Crabbe, 1997). Furthermore, this is likely an underestimate of the frequency of alcohol abuse; although the deficits associated with ethanol use are easily identifiable, alcoholism is rarely diagnosed, and few alcoholics seek treatment (for review, Pihl and Peterson, 1995). Successful cessation is associated with immediate improvements in cognitive function, yet the current options for treatment are ineffective; alcoholics are equally likely to successfully quit drinking regardless of whether they are in treatment programs or not (Cutler and Fishbain, 2005). In order to develop more effective therapies, it is important to understand the neural and behavioral changes associated with alcohol abuse.

Whereas individuals may initially consume ethanol for beneficial effects such as reductions in anxiety, neural adaptations occur with chronic use leading to changes in the behavioral effects of ethanol, such as the development of tolerance. In addition, changes in cognitive function occur with alcohol consumption. The cognitive impairments associated with acute and chronic alcohol abuse range from short-term memory loss and learning deficits to blackouts and the permanent inability to form new memories (Ryback, 1971; Wilkinson and Poulos, 1987). Furthermore, withdrawal from chronic ethanol also produces cognitive deficits (Borlikova et al., 2006; Markel et al., 1986; Ripley et al., 2003). Understanding the mechanisms that underlie the cognitive impairments associated with acute, chronic, and withdrawal from chronic ethanol may lead to better treatments for the impairing effects of both acute ethanol intoxication and chronic ethanol abuse.

Initially, it was believed that ethanol created a general depression in the central nervous system, producing a nonspecific disruption in cognitive processing (Himwich, 1932; Wallace, 1932). According to this theory, ethanol-induced performance deficits in tasks that rely on learning or memory were merely one aspect of a generalized neural dysfunction. However, more recent work suggests that the effects of ethanol on learning are highly specific. For example, ethanol has minimal impact on recall of learned information; instead, ethanol impairs the acquisition of learning in many paradigms (Birnbaum et al., 1978; Givens, 1995; Gould, 2003; Higgins et al., 1992), thus producing 'blackouts' for experiences during intoxication.

Ethanol-induced learning deficits have been demonstrated in a wide range of tasks, and understanding the effects of ethanol on learning is an essential step in developing treatments that deal with the many symptoms of alcoholism. This review will focus on emotional learning and, within this field, on aversive classical and instrumental conditioning. Learning how to predict and thus avoid aversive events is essential to the survival of all organisms, and aversive learning can be studied by examining the associations that are formed between environmental stimuli and aversive events. Although these associations are experience-dependent, responses to aversive stimuli are innate; both rats and mice that have been raised entirely in laboratory environments are averse to cues signaling the presence of a predator (Blanchard and Blanchard, 1977; Dell'Omo and Alleva, 1994). Aversive learning, which may reflect or model emotional learning, is seen in all species and is rapidly acquired, making it easy to study in a laboratory setting and externally valid in translation to human research. In addition to being acquired in as little as a single trial, aversive learning is also long-lasting, making it ideal for studying the substrates underlying both short-term and long-term memory.

The two tasks discussed herein are examples of Pavlovian (classical) and instrumental (operant) learning tasks, namely fear conditioning and passive avoidance, that are impaired by pre-training or chronic administration of ethanol (Bammer and Chesher, 1982; Gould, 2003; Melis et al., 1996). Thus, fear conditioning and passive avoidance are useful models for identifying the behavioral and neural correlates of the effects of ethanol on learning. Fear conditioning tests both contextual learning, in which contextual features are associated with an unconditioned stimulus (US) foot shock, and cued learning, in which a discrete conditioned stimulus (CS) cue is associated with the US (Fendt and Fanselow, 1999; Logue et al., 1997; Phillips and LeDoux, 1992). In standard contextual and cued fear conditioning, the animal is placed in a novel context and then exposed to a previously neutral auditory CS that co-terminates with the US; this leads to both context-US and CS-US associations. Both short-term and long-term memory can be tested for contextual and cued learning. In another type of fear conditioning, trace fear conditioning, the CS terminates for a period of time before the presentation of the US (McEchron et al., 1998). In order to learn the association between the CS and the US when there is a delay separating them, the subject must maintain a memory trace of the CS in working memory until presentation of the US. Thus, acquisition of trace fear conditioning may model some aspects of working memory (Carter et al., 2003) that are not recruited by standard fear conditioning. The use of fear conditioning allows investigators to look at multiple types of learning and memory, such as contextual learning, cued learning, and working memory.

In passive avoidance, the animal is placed either on a platform or in one of a connected pair of chambers. Upon stepping down from the platform (step-down avoidance) or moving into the second chamber (inhibitory avoidance), the animal is exposed to an inescapable foot shock. Testing consists of returning the animal to the platform or initial chamber and measuring the latency to step down or into the second chamber (Alkana and Parker, 1979; Bammer and Chesher, 1982). Although there are similarities in the stimuli, behaviors, and neural substrates associated with passive avoidance and the various forms of fear conditioning, there are also differences in the neural substrates underlying these tasks (Wilensky et al., 2000). Thus, both passive avoidance and fear conditioning allow examination of the effects of ethanol on aversive learning and, because some neural substrates involved in these tasks differ, this examination may facilitate identification of the substrates altered by ethanol.

Although the anxiolytic and rewarding properties of ethanol are major factors in addiction, ethanol-associated changes in cognitive processes are also a hallmark of alcohol abuse. In the following sections, we will review the brain areas involved in the effects of ethanol on aversive learning. In addition, we will examine how the acute, chronic, and withdrawal effects of ethanol alter aversive learning, and how methodological differences between studies may influence results. Within our discussion of each phase of ethanol administration, we will review the differential effects of ethanol on fear conditioning and passive avoidance and examine how these differences may inform us about the effects of ethanol on learning. Finally, we will discuss the effects of ethanol on specific neurotransmitter systems as a model for the cellular changes that may underlie ethanol-induced learning deficits.

Brain Areas Involved in the Modulation of Learning by Ethanol

The brain regions involved in fear conditioning, which include the hippocampus, amygdala and prefrontal cortex, have been well-characterized (for review, Fendt and Fanselow, 1999). Although less is known about the substrates of passive avoidance, research suggests that the amygdala and hippocampus are also essential for this task (Izquierdo et al., 2006). In both tasks, the hippocampus encodes contextual information (Fanselow, 2000; Martinez et al., 2002; Phillips and LeDoux, 1992; Rudy et al., 2002) and the amygdala is the site where fear-related memories are formed (LeDoux, 2003; Nader et al., 2001; Rodrigues et al., 2004). In addition, the prefrontal cortex mediates the attentional aspects of learning and may underlie attention to conditioned and unconditioned stimuli during training in both tasks (for review, Faw, 2003). Finally, aversive learning is associated with an increase in striatal activity that may reflect anticipation for upcoming events; the striatum may increase attention to predictive stimuli (Matsushima et al., 2003; McNally and Westbrook, 2006) and, thus, may signal to animals that the foot-shock is imminent.

Even though passive avoidance and fear conditioning involve many of the same neural areas, the functions of these areas may differ between tasks. Specifically, the amygdala may be differentially involved in fear conditioning compared to passive avoidance; Wilensky and colleagues (2000) have demonstrated that training day inactivation of the basolateral nucleus of the amygdala inhibits acquisition of fear conditioning but not passive avoidance, while post-training inactivation of the basolateral amygdala alters consolidation of passive avoidance without altering fear conditioning. Thus, understanding the different ways in which ethanol acts in these areas to alter learning may aid in understanding the cognitive changes that occur with alcohol abuse.

Acquisition of aversive learning is consistently altered by ethanol treatment (Givens, 1995; Higgins et al., 1992; Ripley et al., 2003) and this effect may be due to the actions of ethanol in the brain areas discussed above. Ethanol disrupts excitatory activity in the hippocampus (Schummers and Browning, 2001) and amygdala (Roberto et al., 2006), and binge drinking-induced changes in these areas have been implicated in ethanol-induced memory deficits (Stephens et al., 2005). These areas are not independent; instead, they have reciprocal connections that provide feedback for modulation of memory processing. Thus, ethanol may alter activity in one of these structures or may alter the communication between them. It has been suggested that changes in signaling through the pathway connecting the amygdala and hippocampus may underlie some of the ethanol-induced deficits in learning.

For example, Abe and colleagues (2004) have demonstrated that ethanol potentiates GABAergic inhibition of synaptic transmission from the basolateral nucleus of the amygdala to the dentate gyrus of the hippocampus. Thus, the effects of ethanol on aversive learning may be due to changes in the hippocampus and the amygdala, as well as signaling from the amygdala to the hippocampus; this dual process could create additive effects of ethanol on hippocampal function.

The ability of ethanol to act on multiple targets within a single system may also be a factor in the potent effects of ethanol on aversive learning. For example, hippocampus-dependent contextual fear conditioning is particularly sensitive to the impairing effects of ethanol, but cued fear conditioning, a hippocampus-independent form of learning, is impaired by higher doses of ethanol (Gould, 2003; Popke et al., 2000). Furthermore, a hippocampus-dependent form of cued conditioning, trace fear conditioning, also shows greater ethanol-induced deficits than standard cued fear conditioning (Weitemier and Ryabinin, 2003). There are two possible explanations for the greater effects of ethanol on hippocampus-dependent learning processes. It may be that hippocampal substrates underlying learning are more sensitive to the effects of ethanol, while similar substrates in other brain areas are affected to a lesser degree. Alternatively, the greater effects of ethanol on contextual and trace fear conditioning may be due to the dependence of these forms of learning on both the hippocampus and amygdala (Buchel et al., 1999; Logue et al., 1997; Phillips and LeDoux, 1992). As discussed, both hippocampal and amygdalar function are altered by ethanol (Stephens et al., 2005), and the additive effects of ethanol in these areas may lead to the greater deficits seen in contextual and trace fear conditioning compared to cued fear conditioning.

Ethanol may also act in the striatum and prefrontal cortex to alter learning (Vertes, 2006). Ethanol alters striatal neurotransmitter release (Heinz et al., 2004), and it may be that ethanol-induced changes in neurotransmitter release alter signaling from the striatum that is required for anticipatory attention during associative conditioning tasks. Additionally, the prefrontal cortex is involved in attention (for review, Knudsen, 2007) and has been shown to be especially vulnerable to the cellular damage associated with chronic ethanol use (Fadda and Rossetti, 1998). Therefore, although the effects of ethanol on hippocampal and amygdalar function have received a great deal of attention (Koob, 2004; McBride, 2002), ethanol-induced changes in other, interconnected regions may also disrupt learning (Givens and McMahon, 1997; Lyon et al., 1975; Rezvani and Levin, 2003). Thus, the acute, chronic, and the post-chronic effects of ethanol in any of these brain areas may produce changes in learning and memory. However, because there are differences in the brain regions (Ambrogi Lorenzini et al., 1991; Wilensky et al., 2000) and molecular substrates (Korte, 2001; Tinsley et al., 2004) involved in fear conditioning and passive avoidance, ethanol may differentially alter learning in these tasks.

Effects of Acute Ethanol on Aversive Learning

In the following sections, we will first discuss the effects of acute ethanol on acquisition, consolidation, and recall of fear conditioning. We will compare these effects across contextual, cued, and trace fear conditioning as well as across low and high doses of ethanol. We will then discuss the effects of acute ethanol on acquisition, consolidation, and recall of passive avoidance. Finally, we will examine factors, such as development and genetics, that influence the effects of acute ethanol on these tasks.

Standard Fear Conditioning

One of the major effects of ethanol on cognition, whether administered acutely or chronically, is the dose-dependent impairment of learning and memory (Table 1). In fear conditioning, acute ethanol administration produced impairments in contextual and cued fear conditioning by decreasing acquisition of learning (Gould and Lommock, 2003; Gulick and Gould, 2007; Gulick and Gould, 2008b; Melia et al., 1996). Because ethanol blocked acquisition of learning during the training session itself, ethanol-induced learning deficits were visible at 4 hours, 24 hours, and 1 week after training (Gould and Lomock, 2003; Gulick and Gould, 2007). This effect persisted even when ethanol was administered on training and testing days, suggesting that ethanol-induced deficits are not state-dependent (Gould and Lommock, 2003). However, a higher dose of acute ethanol was needed to impair fear conditioning if drug administration occured on both training and testing days compared to training day-only administration (Gould, 2003), suggesting that there may be some effects of ethanol on testing day when ethanol has been administered on training day as well.

A number of studies have demonstrated that ethanol has less of an impact on consolidation and recall of learned information compared to acquisition of information (Ripley et al., 2003; Stephens et al., 2001). Research has demonstrated that a dose of ethanol that impairs learning when administered before training does not alter contextual or cued fear conditioning when administered after training (Gulick and Gould, 2007). Furthermore, Gould (2003) has shown that testing day-only administration of acute ethanol did not disrupt fear conditioning. Taken together, these results suggest that during learning, acute ethanol largely disrupts acquisition.

Low doses of ethanol have been shown to produce stimulatory effects in the brain (Gessa et al., 1986; Lima-Landman and Albuquerque, 1989) and, thus, could enhance learning. Furthermore, ethanol has biphasic effects on glutamatergic receptors that may underlie learning, enhancing activity at low doses and inhibiting it at high doses (Lima-Landman and Albuquerque, 1989). Therefore, it is not surprising that ethanol also has biphasic effects on learning in multiple conditioning tasks (Gulick and Gould, 2007; Gulick and Gould, 2008a; Hernandez et al., 1985; Hernandez and Powell, 1986; Hernandez and Valentine, 1990). If low doses of ethanol can enhance associative learning, then these doses may contribute to addiction by facilitating the formation of associations between positive drug effects and the environmental cues that signal drug use. Later re-exposure to the context in which ethanol was consumed may trigger the learned associations and initiate drug-seeking behavior. In support of this, studies have demonstrated that animals develop a conditioned preference for contexts in which they have received ethanol (Cunningham and Noble, 1992; Reid et al., 1985).

Table 1. Effects of Ethanol Treatment on Aversive Learning

Treatment	Trace Conditioning	Contextual Conditioning	Cued Conditioning	Passive Avoidance
High Doses(1.0+ g/kg acute; variable chronic)				
Acute	Impaired Acquisition[r]	Impaired Acquisition[f,k,l]	Impaired Acquisition[a,h]	Impaired[h,i,o]
Chronic	???	???	???	Impaired[c,a,j,l]
Short-term Single Withdrawal	???	No Effect[h]	No Effect[h,p]	Impaired Acquisition and/or Retrieval[s,q]
Short-term Multiple Withdrawal	???	No Effect[h,p]	Impaired with 2+ WDs[h,l,p]	No Effect[h]
Long-term Withdrawal	???	Impaired[d]	No Effect[d]	Variable[c,m,q]
Low Doses (0.25 g/kg acute)				
Acute	???	Enhanced Acquisition[h]	Enhanced Acquisition[h]	???
Chronic	???	???	???	???
Withdrawal	???	???	???	???

Sources:

a Bammer and Chester, 1982; b Borlikova et al., 2006; c Casamenti et al., 1993; d Celerier et al., 2000;
e Celik et al., 2005; f Gould, 2003; g Gould and Lommock, 2003; h Gulick and Gould, 2007a;
i Holloway, 1976; j Kuzmenka-Leska et al., 1999; k Markel et al., 1986; l Melia et al., 1996; m Melis et al., 1996;
n Popovic et al., 2004; o Rezayof et al., 2007; p Ripley et al., 2003; q Snell and Harris, 1979;
r Weitemier and Ryabinin, 2003.

Trace Fear Conditioning

Another form of fear conditioning disrupted by ethanol is trace fear conditioning. In trace fear conditioning, there is a delay between the termination of the CS and the onset of the US. In order to learn the association between the CS and the US when there is a delay separating them, animals must keep the CS in working memory. Trace cued fear conditioning is more sensitive to the effects of ethanol than standard cued fear conditioning (Weitemier and Ryabinin, 2003) and there are multiple potential explanations for the differential impact of ethanol on standard and trace cued conditioning. Cued learning may be more sensitive to impairment by ethanol in trace conditioning because the association between the tone and shock is weakened by the delay between them or because these tasks rely on different neural substrates. In support of the latter, Wagner and Hunt (2006) have demonstrated that brief exposure to ethanol (over a period of 5 days; far less than the typical chronic ethanol treatment) impaired trace, but not standard, cued fear conditioning in neonatal rats. This suggests that sensitivities to the effects of ethanol on trace and standard cued fear conditioning develop independently of each other and may be due to the effects of ethanol on separate systems. One region that may be involved in the differential sensitivities of these tasks to ethanol is the hippocampus, which is necessary for trace fear conditioning but not standard cued fear conditioning. Furthermore, Knight and colleagues (2006) demonstrated that awareness – an aspect of cognition mediated by the prefrontal cortex – is necessary for trace, but not standard, cued fear conditioning and, therefore, the effects of ethanol in the prefrontal cortex could produce greater disruption of trace fear conditioning. Thus, the recruitment of different brain regions in trace versus standard cued fear conditioning may make trace conditioning more sensitive to the effects of ethanol.

Acute ethanol clearly disrupts contextual fear conditioning (Gould and Lommock, 2003; Gulick and Gould, 2007) but the disruptive effects of ethanol may depend on the paradigm being used. For example, contextual fear conditioning was less impaired by acute ethanol administration during trace versus standard conditioning (Weitemier and Ryabinin, 2003). The cause underlying the differential effects of ethanol on contextual learning in standard and trace fear conditioning is unclear. These differences may be due to the actions of ethanol in different brain areas or to distinct effects of ethanol in the hippocampus. In support of the latter possibility, there is evidence that trace and standard fear conditioning recruit different hippocampal substrates. In standard contextual fear conditioning, the hippocampus is necessary to learn the context-shock association (Phillips and LeDoux, 1992). In trace fear conditioning, the hippocampus is still necessary to learn contextual associations; in addition, the hippocampus is recruited to maintain an association between temporally dissociated events (Knight et al., 2004; McEchron et al., 1998; McEchron and Disterhoft, 1999). As suggested by Weitemier and Ryabinin (2003), the requirement of the hippocampus to keep the CS in short-term memory until the US presentation may alter hippocampal processing of contextual information. If this is the case, then there should be differences in hippocampal activity in trace versus standard fear conditioning. In support, studies have shown that trace cued fear conditioning develops after contextual fear conditioning (Barnet and Hunt, 2005; Moye and Rudy, 1987), and that there is differential activity of hippocampal cholinergic, glutamatergic, and GABAergic systems in trace versus standard fear conditioning (Hunt and

Richardson, 2007; Wanisch et al., 2005; Wiltgen et al., 2005). Further research is needed to identify if these changes are responsible for the differential effects of ethanol on contextual learning in trace versus standard fear conditioning paradigms.

Passive Avoidance

Compared to fear conditioning, fewer studies have examined the acute effects of ethanol on passive avoidance. Nonetheless, those studies that have been conducted demonstrate that there are similar impairing effects of acute ethanol on fear conditioning and passive avoidance. These impairing effects may depend upon when ethanol is administered; administration before training may have different effects than administration after training or before recall. Studies have consistently shown that ethanol administered before training impairs passive avoidance learning in both rats and mice (Bammer and Chesher, 1982; Holloway, 1972; Rezayof et al., 2007). These results suggest that ethanol may impair acquisition, but do not rule out the possibility that ethanol may be altering consolidation of passive avoidance; furthermore, ethanol administration before training does not speak to the effects of ethanol on recall.

Unlike the results found with pre-training administration of ethanol, variable effects of ethanol on passive avoidance have been demonstrated following post-training administration. Alkana and Parker (1979) found that post-training administration of an acquisition-impairing dose of ethanol actually enhanced passive avoidance. However, Castellano and Pavone (1988) found that a dose range of ethanol similar to that used in the Alkana and Parker study impaired passive avoidance when administered post-training. Finally, Naylor and colleagues (2001) found no effect of post-training ethanol on passive avoidance conditioning, even though they also used a similar dose range. The differences between these studies may be due to differences in shock level and length of presentation of both the CS and the US. However, changes in shock intensity within the range used by these studies do not have a significant effect on conditioning (Bammer and Chesher, 1982), and all three studies saw similar levels of conditioning in controls, suggesting that there may be some as-yet unidentified explanation for the differential effects of post-training ethanol on passive avoidance in these studies. One possibility is that environmental factors may influence the effects of ethanol on passive avoidance. For example, Colbern and colleagues (1986) found that post-training administration of ethanol enhanced training if animals were returned to their home cage, but not if they were placed in a novel environment. Whereas it is clear that acute ethanol disrupts acquisition of passive avoidance, more research is needed on the effects of ethanol on consolidation of passive avoidance.

There is limited support for an effect of ethanol on recall of passive avoidance. Holloway (1972) found greater impairing effects of ethanol (2.0 g/kg) administered before training, but also found some impairment in avoidance behavior when ethanol was administered before testing. The testing day effect of ethanol may be explained in terms of anxiolysis, which could diminish fear and, thus, decrease the freezing response. This suggests that ethanol may disrupt performance in the passive avoidance test without directly altering recall. Interestingly, Holloway (1972) also found less impairment when ethanol was administered on both days compared to administration on only one day, suggesting a role of state dependence in the effects of ethanol on passive avoidance. In addition, state-dependent effects are seen in passive avoidance for lower doses of ethanol; a moderate dose of 0.5 g/kg ethanol impaired learning when administered before training but not when administered before training and testing (Rezayof et al., 2007). Nonetheless, Bammer and Chesher (1982) found no such state-dependency in passive avoidance conditioning using the same dose range as in the aforementioned studies. Thus, although state-dependency may play a role in the effects of ethanol on memory, ethanol also produces robust deficits in the acquisition of learning.

Factors Influencing the Effects of Ethanol on Aversive Learning

The effects of ethanol on aversive learning depend upon both the developmental state and the genetic background of the animal model being studied. There are differences in the sensitivity to ethanol between adolescent and adult animals, suggesting that there may be developmental changes in the way that the brain responds to ethanol treatment. Adolescent rats are less sensitive than adult rats to many of the impairing effects of ethanol (Silveri and Spear, 1998). For example, Land and Spear (2004) have demonstrated that adolescent rats were less impaired by ethanol in acquisition of both contextual and cued fear conditioning compared to adults, despite comparable blood alcohol levels across groups. Similarly, Hefner and Holmes (2006) found that adult mice were more susceptible to the effects of ethanol on contextual and cued fear conditioning compared to early adolescent and peri-adolescent mice. Thus, it appears that sensitivity to the effects of ethanol on learning increases with age. Reduced aversive effects of ethanol during adolescence may increase consumption during this period of high susceptibility to substance abuse (Carpenter-Hyland and Chandler, 2007; Crews et al., 2007).

Genetics are another factor that has been demonstrated to influence the effects of ethanol on multiple behaviors, including learning. There are many inter-strain differences in behavioral responses to ethanol treatment and understanding these genetic differences may aid in identifying risk factors in the development of alcoholism. For instance, different inbred strains of mice show different degrees of sensitivity, and even converse behavioral responses, to the effects of ethanol on locomotion (Crabbe et al., 1994; Crabbe et al., 2006; Crawley et al., 1997); some mouse strains, such as SWR/J, showed enhanced locomotor activity in response to 2 mg/kg ethanol, while other strains, such as AKR/J, showed depressed locomotion in response to the same dose (Crabbe et al., 1994). The influence of genetics is not limited to the effects of ethanol on locomotion but is also seen in the effects of ethanol on learning. Shapiro and Riley (1980) demonstrated that mice bred selectively for differential sensitivity to the motor-impairing effects of ethanol also showed differential levels of passive avoidance conditioning. Specifically, animals bred for high sensitivity to the effects of ethanol on locomotion showed better acquisition of avoidance learning (Shapiro and Riley, 1980). These results suggest a genetic correlation between sensitivity to the effects of ethanol on locomotion and aversive learning. Thus, studies examining the influences of genetics and development on ethanol-induced changes in learning will aid in identifying critical risk factors in the effects of alcohol on learning-related processes.

Summary

The combined research into the effects of acute ethanol on fear conditioning and passive avoidance has demonstrated robust impairments in acquisition of aversive learning, as well as some less-clear effects when ethanol is administered after training that may reflect changes in consolidation. The effects of acute ethanol on learning are complex, as task parameters, dose, developmental state, and genetics influence outcomes.

In addition, it is still unclear if acute ethanol similarly affects fear conditioning and passive avoidance, as no studies have directly compared the effects of ethanol on these tasks. Further work is needed to identify whether there are differential effects of ethanol on these tasks and on the underlying neural substrates.

Effects of Chronic Ethanol and Withdrawal from Chronic Ethanol on Aversive Learning

As discussed, acute ethanol disrupts learning. One important issue is whether the same effects are seen across acute ethanol administration, chronic ethanol administration, and withdrawal from chronic ethanol. If acute, chronic, and withdrawal from chronic ethanol differentially affect learning, this could suggest that these states of ethanol administration are also differentially altering the underlying neural substrates of learning, and understanding these differences will facilitate development of treatments for alcohol abuse. However, when comparing studies using chronic ethanol and withdrawal from chronic ethanol protocols, it is important to compare studies that examine similar time-points in ethanol treatment. For example, some studies examining the effects of chronic ethanol on learning have tested animals during chronic administration, while others have withdrawn animals from ethanol and then tested them either immediately after withdrawal or after enough time has passed for withdrawal symptoms to have diminished.

These different time-points, during and after chronic administration, may differentially affect both the behavior and the neural substrates of the behavior. Indeed, it has been shown that chronic ethanol induces changes in NMDA and GABA receptor subunit expression, but most ethanol-induced changes in protein synthesis disappeared after withdrawal (Sheela Rani and Ticku, 2006), suggesting that the effects of ethanol after withdrawal may differ from those of chronic ethanol treatment.

If the molecular changes that underlie the effects of chronic ethanol return to baseline levels after withdrawal, then it is essential to study the effects of chronic ethanol treatment during the drug administration phase separately from the post-withdrawal effects of ethanol. Thus, in this review, studies examining the chronic effects of ethanol will be discussed in terms of when testing occurs – during chronic administration, during the initial withdrawal period, after multiple withdrawals, or after a long period of abstinence. Because of this, when talking about chronic treatment, we will describe both the dose and treatment duration.

Effects of Chronic Ethanol on Aversive Learning

Passive Avoidance

Despite the different lengths of ethanol administration (1-6 months) used, there is a general impairment in passive avoidance induced by chronic ethanol when training and testing occur during ethanol administration. Markel and colleagues (1986) found that 28 days of chronic ethanol (~1.7 g/kg/day) consumption resulted in similar impairments of passive avoidance when conditioning occurred during day 10, 20, or 28 of chronic ethanol consumption. Interestingly, they also found an increase in pain sensitivity with chronic ethanol treatment, as opposed to the decreased sensitivity found with acute treatment. Logically, increased sensitivity to shock should increase conditioning in a passive avoidance task (Bammer and Chesher, 1982), so the persistent impairments in passive avoidance in the studies discussed herein suggest that the impairing effects of chronic ethanol are robust. Conversely, Sasaki and colleagues (1995) found no effect of ethanol (~8 mL/day of 15% EtOH) on passive avoidance after 20 weeks of chronic ethanol consumption. However, methodological differences such as shock level and dose of ethanol compared to the other studies discussed in this review could account for differences between studies. Farr and colleagues (2005) used comparable shock levels to those used in other studies and found that 8, but not 4, weeks of chronic ethanol (20% by volume) consumption impaired passive avoidance, suggesting that there is a minimum time for the development of chronic effects of ethanol on cognition. Thus, whereas both acute and chronic ethanol disrupt passive avoidance, the acute effects and the chronic effects of ethanol on passive avoidance may differ because deficits do not appear immediately in the chronic treatment paradigm.

Whereas the behavioral effects of chronic ethanol treatment on passive avoidance may not emerge immediately, some changes in underlying cellular and molecular processes may begin early in treatment and, over time, may become sufficient to disrupt behavior. For example, Nixon and Crews (2002) have demonstrated that a 4-day binge ethanol (~9.3 g/kg/day) protocol is enough to decrease the survival of neural progenitor cells in the hippocampus, but changes in receptor density only occur after 6 weeks or longer of chronic ethanol administration (for review, Matthews and Morrow, 2000). Similar chronic ethanol-induced changes may occur in additional brain areas. Santucci and colleagues (2004) showed that 26 days of chronic ethanol (~16 g/kg/day) administration produced a decrease in cortical volume that persisted for 6 months after cessation of ethanol treatment; although this does not address the time-point at which the chronic effects of ethanol develop, it does suggest that chronic ethanol alters multiple neural substrates.

Fear Conditioning

Although many studies have examined the effects of chronic ethanol on passive avoidance, the effects of chronic ethanol on fear conditioning have yet to be examined; thus, task-dependent differences in the cognitive effects of chronic ethanol cannot be examined within the scope of the current review.

Effects of Withdrawal from Chronic Ethanol on Aversive Learning

Studies of the effects of withdrawal from chronic ethanol on aversive learning have used a range of paradigms that may model different aspects of ethanol withdrawal. For example, some studies have used a paradigm in which chronic ethanol is followed by a single withdrawal episode, while other studies have used repeated withdrawal episodes, and a third group of studies have examined the effects of withdrawal from ethanol after withdrawal symptoms have dissipated. A single withdrawal episode may model the effects of ethanol in abstaining alcoholics, while repeated withdrawal episodes during chronic administration may model the effects of binge drinking. Furthermore, changes in learning that remain after withdrawal symptoms dissipate may reflect long-lasting deficits and changes in underlying neural substrates. Thus, the remainder of this review will examine the short-term effects of withdrawal from chronic intermittent ethanol exposure and chronic continuous ethanol exposure, and the long-term effects of withdrawal from chronic ethanol.

Chronic Intermittent Ethanol and Withdrawal

Fear Conditioning

Fear conditioning has been shown to be particularly sensitive to repeated withdrawal episodes. Repeated withdrawal episodes (30 days of ~17.5 g/kg/day, with two 3-day withdrawals, starting at days 11 and 21) produced task-dependent impairments in fear conditioning (Ripley et al., 2003; Stephens et al., 2001) when conditioning occurred 12 days after the last withdrawal from ethanol, although a single withdrawal episode had no significant effect on fear conditioning at this time-point. Furthermore, fear conditioning was also impaired in human binge drinkers (Stephens et al., 2005). Interestingly, repeated withdrawal-induced deficits were specific for cued fear conditioning but not contextual fear conditioning (Borlikova et al., 2006; Ripley et al., 2003; Stephens et al., 2001; Stephens et al., 2005). In addition, associations that were formed before ethanol administration were not impaired by repeated withdrawal episodes, but new learning was impaired (Ripley et al., 2003). Whereas it is unclear why repeated episodes, but not a single episode, disrupt cued fear conditioning, these repeated withdrawal episodes may differentially alter brain areas involved in cued versus contextual fear conditioning. Borlikova and colleagues (2006) suggest that the behavioral changes seen after withdrawal from chronic intermittent ethanol may be due to changes in cortical activity, but it remains to be determined if these changes are responsible for the differential effects of ethanol on cued versus contextual fear conditioning as well. Thus, whereas acute ethanol impairs both contextual and cued fear conditioning, multiple withdrawal experiences impair only cued fear conditioning, suggesting that these ethanol treatments may differentially impact the neural substrates involved in fear conditioning.

Passive Avoidance

In addition to having selective effects on cued fear conditioning, repeated withdrawal episodes did not alter passive avoidance (Celik et al., 2005; Popovic et al., 2004; Snell and Harris, 1979). This is in contrast to the acute effects of ethanol on passive avoidance, in which learning is disrupted. The results of these studies demonstrate that the effects of withdrawal from chronic intermittent ethanol on contextual fear conditioning, cued fear conditioning, and passive avoidance are distinct across tasks and differ from the acute effects of ethanol.

Effects of Single Withdrawal from Chronic Ethanol

Passive Avoidance

The effects of a single withdrawal episode on passive avoidance and fear conditioning are different than the effects of repeated withdrawal episodes. However, the time-course for the expression of deficits due to a single withdrawal from chronic ethanol varies across studies, making comparisons difficult. Celik and colleagues (2005) found impairments in passive avoidance 72 hours after withdrawal from 28 days of chronic ethanol (~13 g/kg/day). However, they found no impairment in passive avoidance at an early (24 hr) stage of withdrawal. The lack of withdrawal effects at 24 hours may be due to a delay in the molecular changes that occur in the transition from chronic effects to withdrawal effects. However, Snell and Harris (1979) found that withdrawal from 5 days of chronic oral ethanol administration (5% by volume) was enough to impair passive avoidance at 5 hours and at 5 days, but not at 2 weeks, post-withdrawal. In addition, animals on a chronic ethanol (~15g/kg/day) diet for 9 weeks, followed by 12 hours of withdrawal, were impaired in passive avoidance (Kuziemka-Leska et al., 1999). Thus, all three studies demonstrated that a single withdrawal episode disrupts passive avoidance; however, further work is needed to clarify why there are differences in the time-points at which the deficits occur. Finally, single withdrawal episodes differentially affect passive avoidance and fear conditioning, as a single episode was not enough to impair fear conditioning (Stephens et al., 2001); however, conditioning was only examined 12 days post-withdrawal, and thus more time-points for fear conditioning should be examined.

Post-withdrawal Effects of Ethanol on Aversive Learning

As already discussed, many studies that use a chronic ethanol treatment paradigm actually test after the somatic signs of withdrawal have disappeared. The chronic effects of ethanol may persist after withdrawal, but molecular evidence argues against this possibility, as most chronic ethanol-induced changes in levels of glutamate and GABA receptor subunit mRNA returned to baseline levels after withdrawal (Sheela Rani and Ticku, 2006).

Furthermore, it is unclear whether the cognitive and somatic symptoms of withdrawal persist for an equal length of time, and testing after the cessation of somatic withdrawal signs may not actually reflect the post-withdrawal effects of ethanol on cognition. Thus, the post-withdrawal effects of ethanol are discussed here as independent from the chronic effects of ethanol.

Fear Conditioning

Only one study has examined the post-withdrawal effects of ethanol on fear conditioning. Celerier and colleagues (2000) demonstrated that chronic oral ethanol consumption (12% by volume) severely impaired contextual fear conditioning without altering cued fear conditioning 4 weeks after cessation of an 11-month treatment. This is in sharp contrast to acute ethanol administration, in which contextual and cued conditioning were both sensitive to the impairing effects of ethanol (Gould, 2003; Gulick and Gould, 2007), and to the results from studies looking at multiple withdrawal episodes, which impaired only cued conditioning (Borlikova et al., 2006; Ripley et al., 2003; Stephens et al., 2001). One possible explanation for the dissociable effects of immediate withdrawal and long-term withdrawal from ethanol on fear conditioning may be the length of chronic treatment. The Celerier study (2000) administered ethanol for 11 months, while the Stephens study (2001), as aforementioned, administered ethanol for only one month. In addition, it is possible that long-term compensatory changes develop slowly in the neural substrates of learning that are altered by ethanol, producing behavioral effects long after the initial withdrawal episode. However, this possibility requires further research.

Passive Avoidance

The results from studies that examined the effects of chronic ethanol on passive avoidance after somatic withdrawal symptoms had disappeared (i.e. after at least one week of withdrawal from chronic ethanol) show variable results. Two studies have found deficits in passive avoidance after an extended period of withdrawal from chronic ethanol treatment. Animals that consumed ethanol (20% by volume) for 3 or 6 months, followed by 4 weeks without ethanol, were impaired in passive avoidance, although there was some recovery in the 3-month ethanol group (Casamenti et al., 1993). Similarly, Melis and colleagues (1996) withdrew rats after 36 weeks of chronic ethanol (~9 g/kg/day) consumption and then tested them in passive avoidance 15 days later and found a significant impairment of passive avoidance in ethanol-treated rats. However, Fadda and colleagues (1999) used a paradigm that achieved similar blood alcohol levels as Melis and colleagues (1996), and found no impairment in passive avoidance after ethanol treatment. Differences in methodology may explain the variability of these results. For example, a major difference between these two studies is that Melis and colleagues used a forced-consumption paradigm (ethanol was the only liquid available) while Fadda and colleagues used a drink-choice paradigm (ethanol and water were both available). Thus, it may be that consumption choice plays a role in the effects of chronic ethanol treatment on learning. In fact, studies have shown that passive administration and self-administration produced different drug effects (Donny et al., 2000; Greenwald and Roehrs, 2005). However, Santucci and colleagues (2004) used a forced-consumption paradigm to administer 26 days of ethanol (~16 g/kg/day) and found no effect of ethanol treatment on passive avoidance at 17 days after withdrawal. This suggests that drink choice may not be the factor contributing to the differences in the results between the Melis (1996) and Fadda (1999) studies. Finally, as discussed earlier, Snell and Harris (1979) administered 5 days of chronic ethanol (5% by volume) and found no effect at two weeks after withdrawal despite seeing an effect at earlier time-points. Both the duration of ethanol treatment and the time-point after treatment at which testing occurs may influence the effects of long-term withdrawal from ethanol on cognitive processes, but more research is needed to identify how these factors contribute to ethanol-induced deficits in learning. Furthermore, because deficits in passive avoidance are seen with immediate withdrawal and long-term withdrawal, it remains to be determined if the deficits found after an extended withdrawal are a continuation of the same deficits associated with immediate withdrawal, or if they represent unique deficits.

Cellular Processes Underlying Ethanol-Induced Memory Deficits

As exemplified by results from behavioral studies, ethanol has complex effects on learning and memory. These complexities may reflect the many cellular and molecular substrates altered by ethanol. Thus, one way to further understand the behavioral effects of ethanol on learning and memory is to examine cellular processes of learning and memory that are altered by acute, chronic, and withdrawal from chronic ethanol treatment. Three neurotransmitters commonly implicated in learning and memory processes (for review, Myhrer, 2003) that may also be involved in the effects of ethanol on learning are glutamate, gamma-aminobutyric acid (GABA), and acetylcholine (Beracochea et al., 1986; Peris et al., 1997a; Schummers and Browning, 2001). Glutamate is the primary excitatory neurotransmitter in the brain and GABA is the primary inhibitory neurotransmitter in the brain. Unlike GABA and glutamate, acetylcholine is a modulatory neurotransmitter that can alter signaling in both GABAergic and glutamatergic systems (Ge and Dani, 2005; Yamazaki et al., 2005). As mentioned, these neurotransmitter systems underlie learning in the hippocampus and related structures (Myhrer, 2003). Furthermore, all three neurotransmitters are involved in the behavioral effects of acute and chronic ethanol (Nevo and Hamon, 1995).

As reviewed, acute ethanol disrupts both fear conditioning and passive avoidance (Bammer and Chesher, 1982; Gould, 2003; Melis et al., 1996). It is possible that changes in GABAergic, glutamatergic, and/or acetylcholinergic signaling modulate these effects. Administration of GABA receptor agonists disrupts both fear conditioning (Muller et al., 1997) and passive avoidance (Tohyama et al., 1991), and administration of glutamate antagonists also disrupts fear conditioning (Gould et al., 2002) and passive avoidance (Jafari-Sabet, 2006). Finally, cholinergic antagonists impair contextual fear conditioning (Gale et al., 2001; Vago and Kesner, 2007) and passive avoidance (Riekkinen et al., 1993). Acute ethanol potentiates GABA receptor-mediated activity (Suzdak and Paul, 1987) and inhibits glutamate receptor-mediated activity (Woodward et al., 2006; Yang et al., 1996); the summative effect of ethanol on these receptors is a depression of neural activity (Schummers et al., 1997; Schummers and Browning, 2001). Ethanol can also potentiate acetylcholinergic signaling (Forman and Zhou, 1999), which then alters the release of both GABA and glutamate (Wonnacott, 1997). Thus, ethanol may act on these neurotransmitter systems to alter learning. GABA antagonists block the impairing effects of ethanol on passive avoidance (Castellano and Pavone, 1988), while deletion of specific acetylcholine receptor subunits can decrease sensitivity to the memory-impairing effects of ethanol (Wehner et al., 2004). In addition, co-administration of ethanol and a sub-threshold dose of the glutamate antagonist MK-801 enhances the impairing effects of ethanol on passive avoidance (Aversano et al., 2002). This impairment is reversed by administration of GABA antagonists, suggesting that ethanol may facilitate interactions between GABAergic and glutamatergic processes. Further research is needed to compare the interactive effects of acute ethanol and all three neurotransmitter systems on fear conditioning and passive avoidance.

Like acute ethanol treatment, chronic ethanol alters learning. Whereas acute ethanol may modulate neurotransmitter receptor function, chronic ethanol produces changes in receptor density as well as receptor function. For example, chronic ethanol inhibits glutamate receptors, producing both a decrease in activity and a subsequent up-regulation of these receptors (Grant et al., 1990; Sanna et al., 1993; Snell et al., 1993). Because glutamate is critically involved in learning (Gould et al., 2002; Jafari-Sabet, 2006), perturbation of this system by chronic ethanol could contribute to learning deficits. Chronic ethanol also increases GABA receptor activity, leading to receptor desensitization and tolerance, and alters the subtypes of GABA receptors that are expressed (Grobin et al., 1998; Mhatre and Ticku, 1992; Sanna et al., 1993). Since these receptor subtypes have differential roles in cognition (Rudolph and Mohler, 2006), ethanol-induced changes in expression may also alter learning. In addition, chronic ethanol-associated neural changes, such as a decrease in GABA receptor sensitivity (Littleton and Little, 1994; Samson and Harris, 1992), that are associated with behavioral and cellular measures of tolerance (Allan and Harris, 1987; Grobin et al., 1998) may also contribute to ethanol-associated changes in learning-related processes. Finally, chronic ethanol decreases cholinergic function in many brain areas, and these changes have been linked to memory deficits associated with chronic ethanol consumption in multiple learning tasks (Arendt et al., 1989; Beracochea et al., 1986), although no studies have yet examined if the same changes alter fear conditioning or passive avoidance.

There are differences in the neural changes associated with chronic ethanol consumption and chronic intermittent ethanol consumption, just as there are differences in the behavioral effects of these treatments. Chronic and chronic intermittent ethanol produce differential up- and down-regulation of GABA and glutamate receptor subunits (Sheela Rani and Ticku, 2006), and these effects may be associated with different neural changes. For example, chronic intermittent ethanol compared to chronic ethanol has less of an effect on GABA receptor subunit expression but a greater effect on some glutamate receptor subunits (for review, Faingold et al., 1998; Sheela Rani and Ticku, 2006). Nonetheless, some GABA receptors are still up-regulated by chronic intermittent ethanol and GABA release is increased in the hippocampus (Peris et al., 1997b), which could produce changes in learning. It is unclear, however, if similar changes occur in other brain regions. Although chronic intermittent ethanol disrupts fear conditioning, it disrupts hippocampus-independent cued fear conditioning but not hippocampus-dependent passive avoidance and contextual fear conditioning (Popovic et al., 2004; Roberto et al., 2002; Stephens et al., 2001). Thus, the actions of chronic intermittent ethanol in other brain regions may underlie the behavioral changes associated with this treatment. Further examination of how chronic intermittent ethanol alters neurotransmitter release in brain regions other than the hippocampus will be essential in understanding the effects of ethanol on learning.

Withdrawal from chronic ethanol produces learning and memory deficits in fear conditioning and passive avoidance (Casamenti et al., 2003; Stephens et al., 2001). These deficits associated with withdrawal from chronic ethanol may be due to residual neural changes that are unmasked when chronic ethanol treatment ceases. For example, glutamate receptors increase in density but decrease in activation during chronic ethanol treatment; once ethanol is removed, the receptors rapidly return to a higher activation level, but more time is required for down-regulation of receptors (Hendricson et al., 2007). In addition, GABA receptors have reduced efficacy following chronic ethanol treatment (Kang et al., 1996); as a result, GABAergic inhibition is decreased when ethanol is removed, although these effects may vary between brain regions (for review, Weiner and Valenzuela, 2006). Both of these changes produce neuronal hyperexcitability, and this hyperexcitability is associated with the neural and behavioral symptoms of ethanol withdrawal (Little, 1999; Grant et al., 1990). Hyperexcitability produces indiscriminate neural activation; since learning requires the activation of specific neural networks, this over-activation may disrupt learning. Withdrawal from chronic ethanol also decreases acetylcholinergic function, and this decrease is associated with long-lasting deficits in passive avoidance (Casamenti et al., 1993), although it is unclear whether this deficit represents persistence of the chronic ethanol-induced deficit, or whether it represents a unique effect of ethanol withdrawal. Together, the studies reviewed suggest that the effects of acute ethanol, chronic ethanol, and withdrawal from chronic ethanol on glutamate-, GABA-, and acetylcholine-mediated processes may contribute to the ethanol-induced deficits in fear conditioning and passive avoidance, but more work is needed to link the variable effects of ethanol treatments on different types of learning to specific neural processes.

Conclusions

Alcohol abuse is a major societal issue, and one problem associated with acute and chronic alcohol consumption is disrupted cognition. Nonetheless, our understanding of the effects of ethanol on cognitive processes remains incomplete. Developments in the field of alcohol research have demonstrated that, contrary to initial theories, ethanol does not produce global deficits; rather, ethanol acts on specific substrates to alter neural function. The studies reviewed herein offer evidence for the specificity of the effects of ethanol on learning-related processes. These effects vary not only across learning tasks, but also vary within tasks with the phase of ethanol administration. Acute ethanol impairs both standard contextual and cued fear conditioning, as well as trace fear conditioning and passive avoidance; whereas the effects of chronic ethanol on fear conditioning are unknown, chronic ethanol also impairs passive avoidance. The effects of acute ethanol on passive avoidance may differ from the effects of chronic ethanol because shorter chronic treatments do not disrupt passive avoidance but extended treatments do. Withdrawal from chronic ethanol also disrupts learning. A single immediate withdrawal episode impairs passive avoidance without altering fear conditioning, although only one time-point was examined, while multiple withdrawal episodes impair cued fear conditioning without altering contextual fear conditioning or passive avoidance. Finally, long-term withdrawal from ethanol impairs contextual fear conditioning but leaves cued fear conditioning intact; the effects of long-term withdrawal on passive avoidance are variable and depend on the protocol being employed (Table 1). Thus, the duration of ethanol treatment and the duration of withdrawal from chronic treatment may differentially influence learning and underlying neural substrates. In addition, as reviewed, other factors such as genetics and age can influence the effects of ethanol on learning-related processes even within a single task. Understanding how genetics, age, and duration of ethanol treatment interact to alter both learning and its underlying neural substrates will be important for understanding and treating alcohol abuse and alcoholism.

References

Abe, K. and Misawa, M. GABAA receptor-mediated inhibition by ethanol of long-term potentiation in the basolateral amygdala-dentate gyrus pathway in vivo. *Neuroscience*, 125(1): 113-117, 2004.

Alkana, R.L. and Parker, E.S. Memory facilitation by post-training injection of ethanol. *Psychopharm*, 66(2): 117-119, 1979.

Allan, A.M. and Harris, R.A. Involvement of neuronal chloride channels in ethanol intoxication, tolerance, and dependence. *Rec. Dev. Alcohol* 5: 313-325. 1987.

Ambrogi Lorenzini, C., Bucherelli, C., Giachetti, A., Mugnai, L. and Tassoni, G. Effects of nucleus basolateralis amygdalae neurotoxic lesions on aversive conditioning in the rat. *Physiol. Behav.*, 49(4): 765-770, 1991.

Arendt, T., Allen, Y., Marchbanks, R.M., Schugens M.M., Sinden, J., Lantos, P.L. and Gray, J.A. Cholinergic system and memory in the rat: effects of chronic ethanol, embryonic basal forebrain brain transplants and excitotoxic lesions of cholinergic basal forebrain projection system. *Neuroscience* 33(3): 435-462, 1989.

Aversano, M., Ciamei, A., Cestari, V., Passino, E., Middei, S. and Castellano, C. Effects of MK-801 and ethanol combinations on memory consolidation in CD1 mice: involvement of GABAergic mechanisms. *Neurobio Learn. Mem.* 77(3): 327-337, 2002.

Bammer, G. and Chesher, G.B. An analysis of some effects of ethanol on performance in a passive avoidance task. *Psychopharm*, 77: 66-73, 1982.

Barnet, R.C. and Hunt, P.S. Trace and long-delay fear conditioning in the developing rat. *Learn Behav.*, 33(4): 437-443, 2005.

Beracochea, D., Durkin, T.P. and Jaffard, R. On the involvement of the central cholinergic system in memory deficits induced by long term ethanol consumption in mice. *Pharmacol Biochem Behav* 24(3): 519-524, 1986.

Birnbaum, I.M., Parker, E.S., Hartley, J.T. and Noble, E.P. Alcohol and memory: retrieval processes. *J. Verb. Learn Verb Behav*, 17: 325-335, 1978.

Blanchard, R.J. and Blanchard, D.C. Aggressive behavior in the rat. *Behav Biol*, 21(2): 197-224, 1977.

Borlikova, G.G., Elbers, N.A. and Stephens, D.N. Repeated withdrawal from ethanol spares contextual fear conditioning and spatial learning but impairs negative patterning and induces over-responding: evidence for effect on frontal cortical but not hippocampal function? *Euro. J. Neurosci.*, 24(1): 205-216, 2006.

Buchel, C., Dolan, R.J., Armony, J.L. and Friston, K.J. Amygdala-hippocampal involvement in human aversive trace conditioning revealed through event-related functional magnetic resonance imaging. *J. Neurosci.* 19(24): 10869-76, 1999.

Carpenter-Hyland, E.P. and Chandler, L.J. Adaptive plasticity of NMDA receptors and dendritic spines: Implications for enhanced vulnerability of the adolescent brain to alcohol addiction. *Pharmacol. Biochem. Behav.* 86(2): 200-208, 2007.

Carter, R.M., Hofstotter, C., Tsuchiya, N. and Koch, C. Working memory and fear conditioning. *PNAS,* 100(3): 1399-1404, 2003.

Casamenti, F., Scali, C., Vannucchi, M.G., Bartolini, L. and Pepeu, G. Long-term ethanol consumption by rats: effect on acetylcholine release in vivo, choline acetyltransferase activity, and behavior. *Neurosci,* 56(2): 465-471, 1993.

Castellano, C. and Pavone, F. Effects of ethanol on passive avoidance behavior in the mouse: involvement of GABAergic mechanisms. *Pharmacol. Biochem. Behav.*, 29(2): 321-324, 1988.

Celerier, A., Ognard, R., Decorte, L. and Beracochea, D. Deficits of spatial and non-spatial memory and of auditory fear conditioning following anterior thalamic lesions in mice: comparison with chronic alcohol consumption. *Euro. J. Neuro*, 12: 2575-2584, 2000.

Celik, T., Cakir, E., Kayir, H., Bilgi, C. and Uzbay, I.T. The effects of chronic ethanol consumption and withdrawal on passive avoidance task and serum cholinesterase level in rats. *Prog. Neuropsychopharmacol Biol. Psychiatry*, 29(4): 505-509, 2005.

Colbern, D.L., Sharek, P. and Zimmermann, E.G. The effect of home or novel environment on the facilitation of passive avoidance by post-training ethanol. *Behav Neural Biol*, 46(1): 1-12, 1986.

Crabbe, J.C. Where does alcohol act in the brain? *Mol Psych*, 2: 17-20, 1997.

Crabbe, J.C., Gallaher, E.S., Phillips, T.J., Belknap, J.K. Genetic determinants of sensitivity to ethanol in inbred mice. *Behav. Neurosci.*,108(1): 186-95, 1994.

Crabbe, J.C., Phillips, T.J., Harris, R.S., Arends, M.A. and Koob, G.F. Alcohol-related genes: contributions from studies with genetically engineered mice. *Add. Bio*, 11(3-4): 195-269, 2006.

Crawley, J.N., Belknap, J.K., Collins, A., Crabbe, J.C., Frankel, W., Henderson, N., Hitzemann, R.J., Maxson, S.C., Miner, L.L., Silva, A.J., Wehner, J.M., Wynshaw-Boris, A. and Paylor, R. Behavioral phenotypes of inbred mouse strains: implications and recommendations for molecular studies. *Psychopharm*, 132 (2): 107-124, 1997.

Crews, F., He, J. and Hodge, C. Adolescent cortical development: A critical period of vulnerability for addiction. *Pharmacol Biochem. Behav.*, 86(2): 189-199, 2007.

Cunningham, C.L. and Noble, D. Conditioned activation induced by ethanol: role in sensitization and conditioned place preference. *Pharmacol. Biochem. Behav.* 43(1): 307-13, 1992.

Cutler, R.B. and Fishbain, D.A. Are alcoholism treatments effective? The project MATCH data. *BMC Pub Health*, 5: 75-86, 2005.

Dell'Omo, G. and Alleva, E. Snake odor alters behavior, but not pain sensitivity in mice. *Physiol. Behav.*, 55(1): 125-128, 1994.

Donny, E.C., Caggiula, A.R., Rose, C., Jacobs, K.S., Mielke, M.M. and Sved, A.F. Differential effects of response-contingent and response-independent nicotine in rats. *Eur J. Pharmacol.*, 402(3): 231-240, 2000.

Fadda, F. and Rossetti, Z.L. Chronic ethanol consumption: from neuroadaptation to neurodegeneration. *Prog. in Neurobio*, 56: 385-431, 1998.

Fadda, F., Cocco, S., Stancampiano, R. and Rossetti, Z.L. Long-term voluntary ethanol consumption affects neither spatial nor passive avoidance learning, nor hippocampal acetylcholine release in alcohol-preferring rats. *Behav. Brain Res.*, 103(1): 71-76, 1999.

Faingold, C.L., N'Gouemo, P. and Riaz, A. Ethanol and n eurotransmitter interactions--from molecular to integrative effects. *Prog. Neurobiol.* 55(5): 509-535, 1998.

Fanselow, M.S. Contextual fear, gestalt memories, and the hippocampus. *Behav. Brain Res.*, 110(1-2): 73-81, 2000.

Farr, S.A., Scherrer, J.F., Banks, W.A., Flood, J.F. and Morley, J.E. Chronic ethanol consumption impairs learning and memory after cessation of ethanol. *Alc. Clin. Exp. Res,* 29 (6): 971-982, 2005.

Faw B. Pre-frontal executive committee for perception, working memory, attention, long-term memory, motor control, and thinking: a tutorial review. *Conscious Cogn*, 12(1): 83-139, 2003.

Fendt, M. and Fanselow, M.S. The neuroanatomical and neurochemical basis of conditioned fear. *Neurosci Biobehav Rev*, 23: 743-760, 1999.

Forman, S.A. and Zhou, Q. Novel modulation of a nicotinic receptor channel mutant reveals that the open state is stabilized by ethanol. *Mol Pharm*, 55: 102-108, 1999.

Gale, G.D., Anagnostaras, S.G. and Fanselow, M.S. Cholinergic modulation of pavlovian fear conditioning: effects of intrahippocampal scopolamine infusion. *Hippocampus* 11(4): 371-376, 2001.

Ge, S. and Dani, J.A. Nicotinic acetylcholine receptors at glutamate synapses facilitate long-tem depression or potentiation. *J Neuro*, 25(26): 6084-6091, 2005.

Gessa, G.L., Muntoni, F., Collu, M., Vargiu, L. and Mereu, G. Low doses of ethanol activate dopaminergic neurons in the ventral tegmental area. *Brain Res*, 348: 201-203, 1985.

Givens, B. Low doses of ethanol impair spatial working memory and reduce hippocampal theta activity. *Alc Clin Exp Res*, 19 (3): 763-767, 1995.

Givens, B. and McMahon, K. Effects of ethanol on nonspatial working memory and attention in rats. *Behav Neuro*, 111(2): 275-282, 1997.

Gould, T.J. Ethanol disrupts fear conditioning in C57BL/6J mice. *J Psychopharm*, 17(1): 77-81, 2003.

Gould, T.J., McCarthy, M.M. and Keith, R.A. MK-801 disrupts acquisition of contextual fear conditioning but enhances memory consolidation of cued fear conditioning. *Behav. Pharmacol.* 13(4): 287-294, 2002.

Gould, T.J. and Lommock, J.A. Nicotine enhances contextual fear conditioning and ameliorates ethanol-induced deficits in contextual fear conditioning. *Behav. Neuro*, 117 (6): 1276-1282, 2003.

Grant, K.A., Valverius, P., Hudspith, M. and Tabakoff, B. Ethanol withdrawal seizures and the NMDA receptor complex. *Eur. J. Pharm.*, 176: 289-296, 1990.

Greenwald, M.K. and Roehrs, T.A. Mu-opioid self-administration vs. passive administration in heroin abusers produces differential EEG activation. *Neuropsychpharm*, 30(1): 212-221, 2005.

Grobin, A.C., Matthews, D.B., Devaud, L.L. and Morrow, A.L. The role of GABA(A) receptors in the acute and chronic effects of ethanol. *Psychopharm* 139(1-2): 2-19, 1998.

Gulick, D. and Gould, T.J. Acute ethanol has biphasic effects on short- and long-term memory in both foreground and background contextual fear conditioning in C57BL/6 mice. *Alc Clin Exp Res*, 31(9): 1528-1537, 2007 .

Gulick D. and Gould T.J. Interactive effects of ethanol and nicotine on learning in C57BL/6J mice depend on both dose and duration of treatment. *Psychopharm,* 196(3): 483-495, 2008a.

Gulick, D. and Gould, T.J. Varenicline Ameliorates Ethanol-Induced Deficits in Learning in C57BL/6 Mice. *Neurobio Learn Mem,* in press.

Hefner K. and Holmes A. An investigation of the behavioral actions of ethanol across adolescence in mice. *Psychopharm*, 191(2): 311-322, 2006.

Heinz, A., Siessmeier, T., Wrase, J., Hermann, D., Klein, S., Grusser, S.M., Flor, H., Braus, D.F., Buchholz, H.G., Grunder, G., Schreckenberger, M., Smolka, M.N., Rosch, F., Mann, K. and Bartenstein, P. Correlation between dopamine D(2) receptors in the ventral striatum and central processing of alcohol cues and craving. *Am. J. Psychiatry*, 161(10): 1783-1789, 2004.

Hendricson, A.W., Maldve, R.E., Salinas, A.G., Theile, J.W., Zhang, T.A., Diaz, L.M. and Morrisett, R.A. Aberrant synaptic activation of N-methyl-D-aspartate receptors underlies ethanol withdrawal hyperexcitability. *J. Pharmacol. Exp. Ther.,* 321(1): 60-72, 2007.

Hernandez, L.L. and Powell, D.A. Ethanol enhancement of Pavlovian conditioning: comparison with instrumental conditioning. *Psychopharm*, 88: 75-81, 1986.

Hernandez, L.L., Valentine, J.D. and Powell, D.A. Ethanol enhancement of Pavlovian conditioning. *Behav. Neurosci.,* 100(4): 494-503, 1986.

Hernandez, L.L. and Valentine, J.D. Mild ethanol intoxication may enhance pavlovian conditioning. *Drug Dev. Res.,* 20: 155-167, 1990.

Higgins, S.T., Rush, C.R., Hughes, J.R., Bickel, W.K., Lynn, M. and Capeless, M.A. Effects of cocaine and alcohol, alone and in combination, on human learning and performance. *J Exp. An. Behav.*, 58 (1): 87-105, 1992.

Himwich, H.E. The physiological action of alcohol. Emerson H. (Ed.), *Alcohol and Man*, 1-23, The MacMillan Company, New York, 1932.

Holloway, F.A. State-dependent effects of ethanol on active and passive avoidance learning. *Psychopharm*, 25(3): 238-261, 1972.

Hunt, P.S. and Richardson, R. Pharmacological dissociation of trace and long-delay fear conditioning in young rats. *Neurobiol. Learn Mem.*, 87(1): 86-92, 2007.

Izquierdo, I., Bevilaqua, L.R., Rossato, J.I., Bonini, J.S., Da Silva, W.C., Medina, J.H. and Cammarota, M. The connection between the hippocampal and the striatal memory systems of the brain: a review of recent findings. *Neurotox Res.*, 10(2): 113-121, 2006.

Jafari-Sabet, M. NMDA receptor blockers prevents the facilitatory effects of post-training intra-dorsal hippocampal NMDA and physostigmine on memory retention of passive avoidance learning in rats. *Behav. Brain Res.* 169(1): 120-127, 2006.

Kang, M., Spigelman, I., Sapp, D.W. and Olsen, R.W. Persistent reduction of GABA(A) receptor-mediated inhibition in rat hippocampus after chronic intermittent ethanol treatment. *Brain Res.* 709(2): 221-228, 1996.

Knight, D.C., Cheng, D.T., Smith, C.N. and Stein, E.A., Helmstetter, F.J. Neural substrates mediating human delay and trace fear conditioning. *J. Neurosci.*, 24(1): 218-28, 2004.

Knight, D.C., Nguyen, H.T. and Bandettini, P.A. The role of awareness in delay and trace fear conditioning in humans. *Cogn. Affect Behav. Neurosci.* 6(2): 157-62, 2006.

Knudsen, E.I. Fundamental components of attention. *Annu Rev Neurosci* 30: 57-78, 2007.

Koob, G.F. A role for GABA mechanisms in the motivational effects of alcohol. *Biochem. Pharmacol.* 68(8):1515-25, 2004.

Korte, S.M. Corticosteroids in relation to fear, anxiety and psychopathology. *Neurosci. Biobehav. Rev.*, 25(2): 117-142, 2001.

Kuziemka-Leska, M., Car, H. and Wisniewski, K. Baclofen and AII 3-7 on learning and memory processes in rats chronically treated with ethanol. *Pharmacol Biochem Behav*, 62(1): 39-43, 1999.

Land, C. and Spear, N.E. Fear conditioning is impaired in adult rats by ethanol doses that do not affect periadolescents. *Int. J. Dev. Neurosci.*, 22(5-6): 355-362, 2004.

LeDoux, J. The emotional brain, fear, and the amygdala. *Cell Mol. Neurobiol.*, 23(4-5): 727-38, 2003.

Lima-Landman, M.T. and Albuquerque, E.X. Ethanol potentiates and blocks NMDA-activated single-channel currents in rat hippocampal pyramidal cells. *FEBS Lett* 247(1): 61-67, 1989.

Little, H.J. The contribution of electrophysiology to knowledge of the acute and chronic effects of ethanol. *Pharmacol Ther.*, 84(3): 333-353, 1999.

Littleton, J. and Little, H. Current concepts of ethanol dependence. *Addiction* 89(11): 1397-1412, 1994.

Logue, S.F., Paylor, R. and Wehner, J.M. Hippocampal lesions cause learning deficits in inbred mice in the Morris water maze and conditioned-fear task. *Behav. Neurosci.*, 111(1): 104-133, 1997.

Lyon, R.J., Tong, J.E., Leigh, G. and Clare, G. The influence of alcohol and tobacco on the components of choice reaction time. *J. Stud. Alc*, 36(5): 587-596, 1975.

Markel, E., Nyakas, C. and Tal, E., Endroczi, E. Changes in avoidance behaviour following ethanol treatment in rats of different ages. *Acta Physiol. Hung*, 68(2): 175-181, 1986.

Martinez, I., Quirarte, G.L., Diaz-Cintra, S., Quiroz, C. and Prado-Alcala, R.A. Effects of lesions of hippocampal fields CA1 and CA3 on acquisition of inhibitory avoidance. *Neuropsychobiol*, 46(2): 97-103, 2002.

Matsushima, T., Izawa, E., Aoki, N. and Yanagihara, S. The mind through chick eyes: memory, cognition and anticipation. *Zoolog Sci.*, 20(4): 395-408, 2003.

Matthews, D.B. and Morrow, A.L. Effects of acute and chronic ethanol exposure on spatial cognitive processing and hippocampal function in the rat. *Hippocampus* 10(1): 122-30, 2000.

McBride, W.J. Central nucleus of the amygdala and the effects of alcohol and alcohol-drinking behavior in rodents. *Pharmacol Biochem. Behav* 71(3): 509-15, 2002.

McEchron, M.D., Bouwmeester, H., Tseng, W., Weiss, C. and Disterhoft, J.F. Hippocampectomy disrupts auditory trace fear conditioning and contextual fear conditioning in the rat. *Hippocampus* 8(6): 638-46, 1998.

McEchron, M.D. and Disterhoft, J.F. Hippocampal encoding of non-spatial trace conditioning. *Hippocampus* 9(4): 385-96, 1999.

McNally, G.P. and Westbrook, R.F. Predicting danger: the nature, consequences, and neural mechanisms of predictive fear learning. *Learn Mem.*, 13(3): 245-253, 2006.

Melia, K.R., Ryabinin, A.E., Corodimas, K.P., Wilson, M.C. and LeDoux, J.E. Hippocampal-dependent learning and experience-dependent activation of the hippocampus are preferentially disrupted by ethanol. *Neurosci.*, 74 (2): 313-322, 1996.

Melis, F., Stancampiano, R., Imperato, A., Carta, G. and Fadda, F. Chronic ethanol consumption in rats: correlation between memory performance and hippocampal acetylcholine release in vivo. *Neuroscience*, 74(1): 155-159, 1996.

Mhatre, M.C. and Ticku, M.K. Chronic ethanol administration alters gamma-aminobutyric acidA receptor gene expression. *Mol. Pharmacol.*, 42(3): 415-422, 1992.

Moye, T.B. and Rudy, J.W. Ontogenesis of trace conditioning in young rats: dissociation of associative and memory processes. *Dev. Psychobiol.*, 20(4): 405-414, 1987.

Muller, J., Corodimas, K.P., Fridel, Z. and LeDoux, J.E. Functional inactivation of the lateral and basal nuclei of the amygdala by muscimol infusion prevents fear conditioning to an explicit conditioned stimulus and to contextual stimuli. *Behav. Neurosci.* 111(4): 683-691, 1997.

Myhrer, T. Neurotransmitter systems involved in learning and memory in the rat: a meta-analysis based on studies of four behavioral tasks. *Brain Res Brain Res Rev* 41(2-3): 268-287, 2003.

Nader, K., Majidishad, P., Amorapanth, P. and LeDoux, J.E. Damage to the lateral and central, but not other, amygdaloid nuclei prevents the acquisition of auditory fear conditioning. *Learn Mem.* 8(3): 156-163, 2001.

National Institute on Alcohol Abuse and Alcoholism (2004): http://pubs.niaaa.nih.gov /publications/GettheFacts_HTML/Facts.pdf.

Naylor, J.C., Simson, P.E., Gibson, B., Schneider, A.M., Wilkins, E. and Firestone, A., Choy, M. Ethanol inhibits spontaneous activity of central nucleus of the amygdala neurons but does not impair retention in the passive-avoidance task. *Alc. Clin. Exp. Res.*, 25(11): 1683-1688, 2001.

Nevo, I. and Hamon, M. Neurotransmitter and neuromodulatory mechanisms involved in alcohol abuse and alcoholism. *Neurochem. Int.* 26(4) 305-336, 1995.

Nixon, K. and Crews, F.T. Binge ethanol exposure decreases neurogenesis in adult rat hippocampus. *J. Neurochem.*, 83(5): 1087-93, 2002.

Peris, J., Anderson, K.J., Vickroy, T.W., King, M.A., Hunter, B.E. and Walker, D.W. Neurochemical basis of disruption of hippocampal long term potentiation by chronic alcohol exposure. *Front Biosci.,* 2: d309-16, 1997a.

Peris, J., Eppler, B., Hu, M., Walker, D.W., Hunter, B.E., Mason, K. and Anderson, K.J. Effects of chronic ethanol exposure on GABA receptors and GABAB receptor modulation of 3H-GABA release in the hippocampus. *Alc Clin. Exp. Res.,* 21(6): 1047-1052, 1997b.

Phillips, R.G. and LeDoux, J.E. Differential contribution of amygdala and hippocampus to cued and contextual fear conditioning. *Behav. Neurosci.,* 106 (2): 274-285, 1992.

Pihl, R.O. and Peterson, J.B. Alcoholism: The role of different motivational systems. *J Psych Neurosci.,* 20(5): 372-397, 1995.

Popke, E.J., Allen, S.R. and Paule, M.G. Effects of acute ethanol on indices of cognitive-behavioral performance in rats. *Alcohol,* 20: 187-192, 2000.

Popovic, M., Caballero-Bleda, M., Puelles, L. and Guerri, C. Multiple binge alcohol consumption during rat adolescence increases anxiety but does not impair retention in the passive avoidance task. *Neurosci. Lett,* 357(2): 79-82, 2004.

Reid, L.D., Hunter, G.A., Beaman, C.M. and Hubbell, C.L. Toward understanding ethanol's capacity to be reinforcing: a conditioned place preference following injections of ethanol. *Pharmacol. Biochem. Behav.,* 22(3): 483-7, 1985.

Rezayof, A., Motevasseli, T., Rassouli, Y. and Zarrindast, M.R. Dorsal hippocampal dopamine receptors are involved in mediating ethanol state-dependent memory. *Life Sci,* 80(4): 285-292, 2007.

Rezvani, A.H. and Levin, E.D. Nicotine-alcohol interactions and attentional performance on an operant visual signal detection task in female rats. *Pharm. Biochem. Behav.,* 76: 75-83, 2003.

Riekkinen, P. Jr, Riekkinen, M. and Sirviö, J. Cholinergic drugs regulate passive avoidance performance via the amygdala. *J. Pharmacol Exp. Ther.* 267(3): 1484-1492, 1993.

Ripley, T.L., O'Shea, M. and Stephens, D.N. Repeated withdrawal from ethanol impairs acquisition but not expression of conditioned fear. *Euro. J. Neuro.,* 18: 441-448, 2003.

Roberto, M., Bajo, M., Crawford, E., Madamba, S.G. and Siggins, G.R. Chronic ethanol exposure and protracted abstinence alter NMDA receptors in central amygdala. *Neuropsychopharm,* 31(5): 988-996, 2006.

Roberto, M., Nelson, T.E., Ur, C.L. and Gruol, D.L. Long-term potentiation in the rat hippocampus is reversibly depressed by chronic intermittent ethanol exposure. *J. Neurophysiol.,* 87(5): 2385-2397, 2002.

Rodrigues, S.M., Schafe, G.E. and LeDoux, J.E. Molecular mechanisms underlying emotional learning and memory in the lateral amygdala. *Neuron.,* 44(1): 75-91, 2004.

Rudolph U. and Möhler H. GABA-based therapeutic approaches: GABAA receptor subtype functions. *Curr. Opin. Pharmacol.,* 6(1): 18-23, 2006.

Rudy, J.W., Barrientos, R.M., O'Reilly, R.C. Hippocampal formation supports conditioning to memory of a context. *Behav. Neurosci.,* 116(4): 530-538, 2002

Ryback, R.S. The continuum and specificity of the effects of alcohol on memory. *Q. J. Stud Alc,* 32: 996-1016, 1971.

Samson, H.H. and Harris, R.A. Neurobiology of alcohol abuse. *Trends Pharmacol. Sci.* 13(5): 206-211, 1992.

Sanna, E., Serra, M., Cossu, A., Colombo, G., Follesa, P., Cucceddu, T., Concas, A. and Biggio, G. Chronic ethanol intoxication induces differential effects on GABAA and NMDA receptor function in the rat brain. *Alc Clin. Exp. Res.*, 17(1): 115-123, 1993.

Santucci, A.C., Mercado, M., Bettica, A., Cortes, C., York, D. and Moody, E. Residual behavioral and neuroanatomical effects of short-term chronic ethanol consumption in rats. *Brain Res. Cogn. Brain Res.*, 20(3): 449-461, 2004.

Sasaki, H., Matsuzaki, Y., Nakagawa, T., Arai, H., Yamama, M., Sekizawa, K., Ikarashi, Y. and Maruyama, Y. Cognitive function in rats with alcohol ingestion. *Pharmacol. Biochem. Behav*, 52(4): 845-848, 1995.

Schummers, J., Bentz, S. and Browning, M.D. Ethanol's inhibition of LTP may not be mediated solely via direct effects on the NMDA receptor. *Alc Clin. Exp. Res.*, 21(3): 404-408, 1997.

Schummers J. and Browning M.D. Evidence for a role for GABA(A) and NMDA receptors in ethanol inhibition of long-term potentiation. *Brain Res. Mol. Brain Res.* 94(1-2): 9-14, 2001.

Shapiro N.R. and Riley E.P. Avoidance behavior in rats selectively bred for differential alcohol sensitivity. *Psychopharm*, 72(1): 79-83, 1980.

Sheela Rani, C.S. and Ticku, M.K. Comparison of chronic ethanol and chronic intermittent ethanol treatments on the expression of GABA(A) and NMDA receptor subunits. *Alcohol.* 38(2): 89-97, 2006.

Silveri, M.M. and Spear, L.P. Decreased sensitivity to the hypnotic effects of ethanol early in ontogeny. *Alc Clin. Exp. Res.*, 22(3): 670-676, 1998.

Snell, L.D., Tabakoff, B. and Hoffman, P.L. Radioligand binding to the NMDA receptor/ionophore complex: alterations by ethanol in vitro and by chronic in vivo ethanol ingestion. *Brain Res.*, 602: 91-98, 1993.

Snell, D. and Harris, R.A. Impairment of avoidance behavior following short-term ingestion of alcohol. *Psychopharm*, 63(3): 251-257, 1979.

Stephens, D.N., Brown, G., Duka, T. and Ripley, T.L. Impaired fear conditioning but enhanced seizure sensitivity in rats given repeated experience of withdrawal from alcohol. *Euro J. Neuro.*, 14: 2032-2031, 2001.

Stephens, D.N., Ripley, T.L., Borlikova, G., Schubert, M., Albrecht, D., Hogarth, L. and Duka, T. Repeated ethanol exposure and withdrawal impairs human fear conditioning and depresses long-term potentiation in rat amygdala and hippocampus. *Biol. Psych.*, 58: 392-400, 2005.

Suzdak, P.D. and Paul, S.M. Ethanol stimulates GABA receptor-mediated Cl- ion flux in vitro: possible relationship to the anxiolytic and intoxicating actions of alcohol. *Psychopharmacol. Bull*, 23(3): 445-451, 1987.

Tinsley, M.R., Quinn, J.J. and Fanselow M.S. The role of muscarinic and nicotinic cholinergic neurotransmission in aversive conditioning: comparing pavlovian fear conditioning and inhibitory avoidance. *Learn Mem.*, 11(1): 35-42, 2004.

Tohyama, K., Nabeshima, T., Ichihara, K. and Kameyama, T. Involvement of GABAergic systems in benzodiazepine-induced impairment of passive avoidance learning in mice. *Psychopharm* 105(1): 22-26, 1991.

Tokuda, K., Zorumski, C.F. and Izumi, Y. Modulation of hippocampal long-term potentiation by slow increases in ethanol concentration. *Neurosci.,* 146(1): 340-349, 2007.

Vago, D.R. and Kesner, R.P. Cholinergic modulation of Pavlovian fear conditioning in rats: differential effects of intrahippocampal infusion of mecamylamine and methyllycaconitine. *Neurobiol. Learn Mem.* 87(3): 441-449, 2007.

Vertes, R.P. Brain stem generation of the hippocampal EEG. *Prog Neurobiol,* 19: 159-186, 1982.

Vogel, R.A., Frye, G.D., Wilson J.H., Kuhn C.M., Koepke K.M., Mailman R.B., Mueller R.A. and Breese G.R. Attenuation of the effects of punishment by ethanol: comparisons with chlordiazepoxide. *Psychopharm,* 71(2): 123-129, 1980.

Wagner, A.F. and Hunt, P.S. Impaired trace fear conditioning following neonatal ethanol: reversal by choline. *Behav Neurosci,* 120(2): 482-487, 2006.

Wallace, G.B. The physiological action of alcohol. Emerson H. (Ed.), Alcohol and Man, 24-65, The MacMillan Company, New York, 1932.

Wanisch, K., Tang, J., Mederer A. and Wotjak C.T. Trace fear conditioning depends on NMDA receptor activation and protein synthesis within the dorsal hippocampus of mice. *Behav. Brain Res.,* 157(1): 63-69, 2005.

Wehner, J.M., Keller, J.J., Keller, A.B., Picciotto, M.R., Paylor, R., Booker, T.K., Beaudet, A., Heinemann, S.F. and Balogh, S.A. Role of neuronal nicotinic receptors in the effects of nicotine and ethanol on contextual fear conditioning. *Neuroscience* 129(1): 11-24, 2004.

Weiner, J.L. and Valenzuela, C.F. Ethanol modulation of GABAergic transmission: the view from the slice. *Pharmacol. Ther.* 111(3): 533-554, 2006.

Weitemier, A.E. and Ryabinin, A.E. Alcohol-induced memory impairment in trace fear conditioning: a hippocampus-specific effect. *Hippocampus,* 13: 305-315, 2003.

Wilensky, A.E., Schafe, G.E. and LeDoux J.E. The amygdala modulates memory consolidation of fear-motivated inhibitory avoidance learning but not classical fear conditioning. *J. Neurosci.,* 20(18): 7059-7066, 2000.

Wilkinson, D.A. and Poulos, C.X. The chronic effects of alcohol on memory: a contrast between a unitary and dual system approach. Galanter (Ed.), Rec Dev Alc. 5-26, Plenum Press, New York, 1987.

Wiltgen, B.J., Sanders, M.J., Ferguson C., Homanics G.E. and Fanselow M.S. Trace fear conditioning is enhanced in mice lacking the delta subunit of the GABAA receptor. *Learn Mem.,* 12(3): 327-333, 2005.

Wonnacott, S. Presynaptic nicotinic Ach receptors. *Trends Neurosci.,* 20(2): 92-98, 1997.

Woodward, J.J., Ron, D., Winder, D. and Roberto, M. From blue states to up states: a regional view of NMDA-ethanol interactions. *Alc Clin. Exp. Res.,* 30(2): 359-367, 2006.

Yamazaki, Y., Jia, Y., Hamaue, N. and Sumikawa, K. Nicotine-induced switch in the nicotinic cholinergic mechanisms of facilitation of long-term potentiation induction. *Eur J. Neurosci.,* 22(4): 845-860, 2005.

Yang, X., Criswell, H.E., Simson, P., Moy, S. and Breese, G.R. Evidence for a selective effect of ethanol on NMDA responses: ethanol affects a subtype of the ifenprodil-sensitive NMDA receptors. *J. Pharm. Exp. Ther.,* 278(1): 114-124, 1996.

In: Substance Withdrawal Syndrome
Editors: J. P. Rees and O. B. Woodhouse

ISBN 978-1-60692-951-3
© 2009 Nova Science Publishers, Inc.

Chapter VIII

Topographic Brain Mapping of Caffeine Use and Caffeine Withdrawal[*]

Roy R. Reeves[1] and Frederick A. Struve[2]
[1]Department of Mental Health at the G.V. (Sonny) Montgomery VA
Medical Center at the University of Mississippi School of Medicine, MS, USA
[2] Department of Psychiatry at Yale University School of Medicine and the New Haven
VA Connecticut Healthcare System, CT, USA

Abstract

Caffeine is a widely used psychoactive substance consumed daily by the majority of Americans. Saletu showed that 250 mg of caffeine can produce a transient reduction of EEG total absolute power in normal persons. Additional studies have confirmed this phenomenon. Overall, however, studies of EEG changes following caffeine exposure have reported variable results. Studies have been done in individuals who are not caffeine naïve and the effect of previous caffeine usage (often for years) on EEG is unknown. It is postulated that this confound may contribute to the variations in results between studies of caffeine exposure.

Several studies have shown that persons consuming even low or moderate amounts of caffeine (in some cases, as low as 100 mg per day) may develop a withdrawal syndrome with caffeine cessation with symptoms such as headaches, lethargy, muscle pain, impaired concentration, and physiological complaints such as nausea or yawning. Preliminary studies of individuals abstaining from caffeine have demonstrated significant changes relative to when they were consuming the drug in a number of EEG variables, including: 1.) increases in theta absolute power over all cortical areas, 2.) increases in delta absolute power over the frontal cortex, 3.) decreases in the mean frequency of both the alpha and beta rhythm, 4.) increase in theta relative power and decrease in beta relative power, and 5.) significant changes in interhemispheric coherence. Additionally, caffeine cessation appears to increase firing rates of diffuse paroxysmal dysrhythmias in

---

[*] A version of this chapter was also published as a chapter in *Caffeine and Health Research*, edited by Kenneth P. Chambers, published by Nova Science Publishers, Inc. It was submitted for appropriate modifications in an effort to encourage wider dissemination of research.

some individuals. Preliminary data also suggests that caffeine withdrawal has some effect on cognitive P300 auditory and visual evoked potentials.

Introduction

Caffeine, a naturally occurring member of the methylxanthine family with a chemical structure similar to theophylline, is generally believed to be the most widely consumed psychoactive agent in the world. It is ingested daily by millions of people in a variety of forms, and often in large quantities [1]. The amount consumed annually in the world probably exceeds several billion kilograms. Yet for most of the last century, caffeine seemed to interest neither clinicians nor investigators and was considered a relatively innocuous agent. Although history indicates that it has been consumed for a thousand years or more, it was not until the 1970s that attention began to be called to caffeine's pharmacological consequences.

Caffeine is easily available to most individuals, including children, and may be ingested in a variety of forms, including brewed coffee (100 mg per 6 oz); instant coffee (65 mg per 6 oz); tea (40 mg per 6 oz); carbonated soft drinks (50 mg per 6 oz); over the counter stimulants, analgesics, antihistamines, and weight loss aids (50 to 200 mg per tablet); and prescription analgesics and migraine medications (30 to 100 mg per tablet). Individuals taking over the counter medications are often unaware of their caffeine content. In North America 80 to 90% of adults use caffeine regularly, with almost half of them ingesting caffeine from multiple sources [2]. Average daily intake of caffeine consumers in the United States is approximately 280 mg per day with higher intakes estimated in some European countries [3]. Occasionally, however, patients are encountered who report intake as high as 2,000 to 5,000 mg per day [4]. After oral ingestion caffeine is rapidly and completely absorbed, with peak blood levels generally reached in 30 to 45 minutes [5] and is rapidly eliminated with a half life of 4 to 6 hours [6]. Once absorbed, caffeine is poorly bound (10 to 30%) to plasma albumin, promptly crosses the blood-brain barrier, and enters into relative equilibrium between the plasma and brain [7].

The primary mechanism of action of caffeine is antagonism of adenosine receptors. Adenosine receptors activate an inhibitory G protein, inhibiting the formation of the second messenger cyclic adenosine monophosphate (cAMP). Caffeine intake therefore results in an increase in intraneuronal cAMP concentrations in neurons that have adenosine receptors [8]. Caffeine, especially at high doses, may enhance dopamine activity and affect noradrenergic neurons [9]. It has been shown to elevate brain lactate among caffeine intolerant subjects [10]. Many studies [11-15] have found that caffeine causes global vasoconstriction, although this may not occur in the elderly. Tolerance does not develop to the vasoconstrictive effects, and cerebral blood flow shows a rebound effect after withdrawal from caffeine. In a placebo double blind study [16] in which subjects abstaining from caffeine were given either caffeine or placebo capsules, subjects receiving placebo had significantly increased mean velocity, systolic velocity, and diastolic velocity in all four cerebral arteries.

Caffeine produces a variety of physiological effects, including effects on the cerebral vascular system, blood pressure, respiratory functioning, gastric and colonic activity, urine volume, and exercise performance. Low to moderate doses of caffeine (20 to 200 mg) produce reports of increased well being, happiness, energy, alertness, and sociability, whereas higher doses are more likely to produce reports of anxiety, jitteriness, and upset stomach [17]. Physical dependence on caffeine has been documented in both pre-clinical and clinical research, and the physiological basis has been postulated to be increased functional sensitivity to endogenous adenosine [18]. Persons using caffeine regularly may develop a withdrawal syndrome 12-24 hours after abrupt caffeine cessation; this has been demonstrated using placebo double blind methods in which regular caffeine consumers were given either caffeine or placebo and monitored for signs and symptoms of withdrawal [19]. "Withdrawal" refers to time-limited effects due to cessation of a drug. Symptoms of caffeine withdrawal have been described in the literature for more than 170 years. A variety of symptoms occurring with caffeine withdrawal have been cited, including headache, tiredness/fatigue, decreased energy/activeness, decreased alertness, drowsiness/sleepiness, decreased contentedness/well being, decreased desire to socialize, flu-like symptoms, depressed mood, difficulty concentrating, irritability, lack of motivation for work, foggy/not clearheaded feelings, yawning, decreased self confidence, confusion/bewilderment, nausea/vomiting, muscle pain/stiffness, anxiety/nervousness, heavy feelings in arms and legs, increased night time sleep duration, need for analgesic use, craving for caffeine, blurred vision, lightheadedness/dizziness, anger/hostility, hot and cold spells, rhinorrhea, diaphoresis, and limb tremor [20]. Symptoms have occurred in some persons after cessation of doses as low as 100 mg of caffeine per day [21]. So significant has been the literature on the occurrence of withdrawal symptoms that it has been proposed that caffeine withdrawal be included in the Diagnostic and Statistical Manual of Mental Disorders (DSM) and the International Classification of Diseases (ICD) [22] (currently the DSM lists specific criteria for a diagnosis of caffeine intoxication). A recent excellent comprehensive review [20] identifies and summarizes a total of 57 experimental and 9 survey studies of caffeine withdrawal.

It is evident from the volume of both basic science and clinical research and literature that has accumlated that caffeine is likely to have a significant affect on neurophysiological functioning. This chapter will review electrophysiological studies of exposure to caffeine and of caffeine withdrawal.

The EEG during Caffeine Exposure

EEG variables are sensitive to the CNS effects of numerous pharmacological compounds, and interest in the effects of caffeine on the EEG began in the 1960s. In 1963, Goldstein and associates [23] showed that caffeine ingestion may decrease EEG voltage. Saletu [24] later demonstrated that a 250 mg caffeine dose can produce a transient reduction of EEG total power (in frequencies from 1.3 to 35 Hz) in normal healthy volunteers and Bruce et al [25] reported similar findings with 250 mg and 500 mg doses of caffeine. Kaplan et al [26] found that 250 mg of caffeine (a dose producing favorable subjective effects such as elation, peacefulness, and pleasantness) and 500 mg (a dose producing unpleasant effects such as tension, nervousness, anxiety, excitement, irritability, nausea, palpitations, and restlessness) both reduced electroencephalographic amplitude over the 4 Hz to 30 Hz spectrum, as well as in the alpha (8 to 11 Hz) and beta (12 to 30 Hz) ranges. However, these effects were not dose dependent. Seipman and Kirch [27] described total EEG power reduction over both hemispheres by 200 mg of caffeine with the effect more pronounced when the subjects had their eyes open than when they had their eyes closed. Gilbert et al [28] found that caffeine decreased EEG power across all conditions they studied and produced a wider range of EEG power decrease than did nicotine.

Patat et al [29] found that a 600 mg slow release caffeine formulation produced a significant decrease in delta and theta relative power and a significant increase in alpha and beta (12-40 Hz) relative power. Lundolt et al [30] found that administration of 200 mg of caffeine in the morning reduced sleep time and efficiency and EEG power the subsequent night. In another study conducted by Newman and associates [31], caffeine was associated with a significant increase in peak occipital alpha frequency and significant decreases in occipital alpha amplitude, central beta amplitude, and central theta amplitude both in subjects with panic disorder (who have been demonstrated to be more sensitive than normal individuals to the anxiogenic effects of caffeine) and in normal control subjects. Studies published in languages other than English by Krapivin and Veronina (drop in the absolute power of all frequency ranges) [32] and Kunkel (highly significant reduction of theta amplitude, decreased theta frequency, decreased alpha amplititude, and increased alpha frequency) [33, 34] also reported EEG power reduction secondary to caffeine exposure.

However, several other studies of EEG changes secondary to caffeine exposure have not yielded the same results. Pritchard and colleagues [35] using a dose of less than 200 mg found little in the way of caffeine effects on EEG. In an investigation of the physiological effects of smoking and caffeine, Hasenfratz and Battig [36] reported that caffeine increased blood pressure, finger vasoconstriction, motor activity, frontal EMG, and EEG theta power and decreased heart rate and EEG beta power. Dimfel [37] et al presented data that suggested that caffeine dependent decreases in theta power and delta power occurred under relaxation conditions after exposure to 400 mg of caffeine, but that these same EEG changes did not occur if subjects were engaged in the performance of tasks requiring mental concentration. Other studies of EEG change following caffeine exposure by Sule et al [38], Clubley et al [39], and Pollock et al [40] reported minimal or inconsistent effects.

Why should some studies of caffeine exposure show changes in EEG power while others did not? The reason is uncertain but a reasonable explanation might be related to the fact that the subjects exposed to caffeine were not caffeine naïve. In general, studies used subjects who had previously consumed caffeine and then underwent a period of abstinence during which they were exposed to caffeine for the EEG studies. The effect of previous caffeine usage (often in variable amounts and often for years) on EEG is unknown. It is postulated that this confound may contribute to the variations in results between studies of the effects of caffeine exposure on EEG. The ideal situation to assess the effects of caffeine exposure on EEG would be to find individuals who did not consume caffeine and study them during exposure to the drug. However, finding adults who have had no or minimal use of caffeine to consent to such studies is difficult (and possibly unethical according to some scientists and clinicians who believe caffeine to possess addictive potential).

The Quantitative EEG during Caffeine Withdrawal

An approach which avoid the confounds of previous caffeine use is to study subjects who regularly consume caffeine during abstinence or withdrawal from the drug. Two studies involving EEG have utilized this approach. Both studies have limitations and in a sense could be considered preliminary investigations, but both reveal pertinent neurophysiological findings. Jones and associates [16] investigated cerebral blood flow and quantitative EEG in caffeine withdrawal in a double blind study, but EEG applications were relatively limited. Reeves and colleagues [41, 42] performed a comprehensive analysis of EEG variables, but used an open (versus double blind) investigation.

Jones and associates [16] examined the effect of caffeine withdrawal on cerebral blood flow and quantitative EEG. Ten volunteers reporting moderate caffeine intake (mean 333 mg per day) participated in this double blind study. Subjects were studied while maintaining their normal diet (baseline period) and during two 1-day periods during which they consumed caffeine free diets and received capsules containing placebo (placebo test session) or caffeine (caffeine test session) in amounts equal to their baseline daily caffeine consumption. Blood flow velocity was determined for right and left middle cerebral arteries and right and left anterior cerebral arteries using pulsed transcranial Doppler sonography. Placebo (i.e., the caffeine withdrawal state) significantly increased the mean velocity, systolic velocity, and diastolic velocity in all four cerebral arteries.

Three minutes of EEG were recorded from eight electrode sites and assessment of theta power differences between the placebo condition and the caffeine condition were performed. A significant limitation of the EEG methodology used would be the relatively short recording time and the use of eight versus a larger number of electrodes. However, even in these short recordings the placebo condition (caffeine withdrawal) demonstrated significantly increased EEG theta power.

Reeves and colleagues [41, 42] investigated caffeine withdrawal focusing primarily on comprehensive assessment of EEG variables using an open study. EEGs utilized recording from 21 electrode sites for 30-45 minutes. Thirteen subjects who consumed 300 mg or more of caffeine daily underwent quantitative EEG studies during their usual caffeine consumption (baseline). They then underwent a 4-day period of abstinence from caffeine and were studied on days 1, 2, and 4 of abstinence. The severity of withdrawal was rated at each visit on a scale of 1+ to 4+. Serum caffeine levels were performed on the day of each study to verify abstinence. The project was conducted as an open study and was not a double blind protocol, although the individual who performed analyses of the EEGs was not aware of whether the EEGs were obtained from subjects consuming caffeine or at some point in the period of abstinence. Each subject served as his or her own control with EEG data obtained on caffeine abstinence days compared to the pre-withdrawal baseline measures. In addition to the EEGs obtained at baseline and on days 1, 2, and 4 of abstinence, 10 of the subjects underwent a second EEG on day 4 after being given caffeine. To accomplish this, the final EEG of the abstinence period was obtained, and with the EEG electrodes still in place, the subject was given 2 cups of brewed coffee (200 mg of caffeine) over 15 minutes. Afterward EEG was recorded for an additional 30 minutes.

For each EEG, 25 artifact free 2.5 second epochs were selected for analysis. An analog to digital conversion digitized each epoch into 512 individual points and multiple epochs were averaged together. Spectra subdivision into four basic EEG bandwidths was accomplished with a Fast Fourier Transform. A comprehensive analysis of multiple quantitative variables, including estimates of absolute power, relative power, and mean frequency for the four major EEG frequency bands (alpha: 7.5 to 12.5 Hz; beta: greater than 12.5 Hz; theta: 3.5 to 7.5 Hz; and delta: less than 3.5 Hz) was performed for each EEG study during the abstinence period and compared to the variables obtained at baseline for each subject. Interhemispheric coherence and power asymmetry were also obtained for the four standard EEG frequency bands using homologous central, posterior, temporal, parietal, and occipital electrode pairs, and the baseline and withdrawal conditions compared.

Even before quantitative analysis was performed, changes in the analog (visual) could be seen, demonstrating an effect from caffeine abstinence and resumption. Generalized increase of alpha and theta voltage, particularly over the frontal cortex was observable during withdrawal from caffeine. Figure 1 demonstrates samples of raw analog EEG tracings from a subject showing representative voltage increases from baseline to a point during caffeine withdrawal, and then again approximately 30 minutes after resumption of caffeine consumption. As seen here, in most cases it was possible to visually recognize voltage increases during caffeine withdrawal and a return of voltage to previous levels with caffeine resumption.

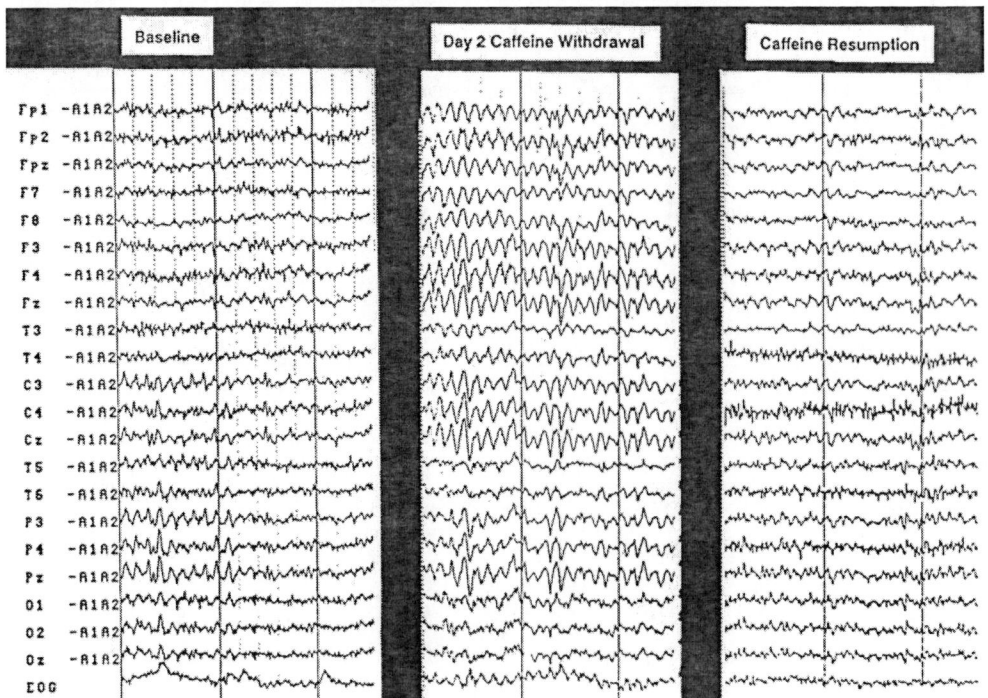

Figure 1. Analog EEG samples during baseline, caffeine withdrawal, and caffeine resumption.

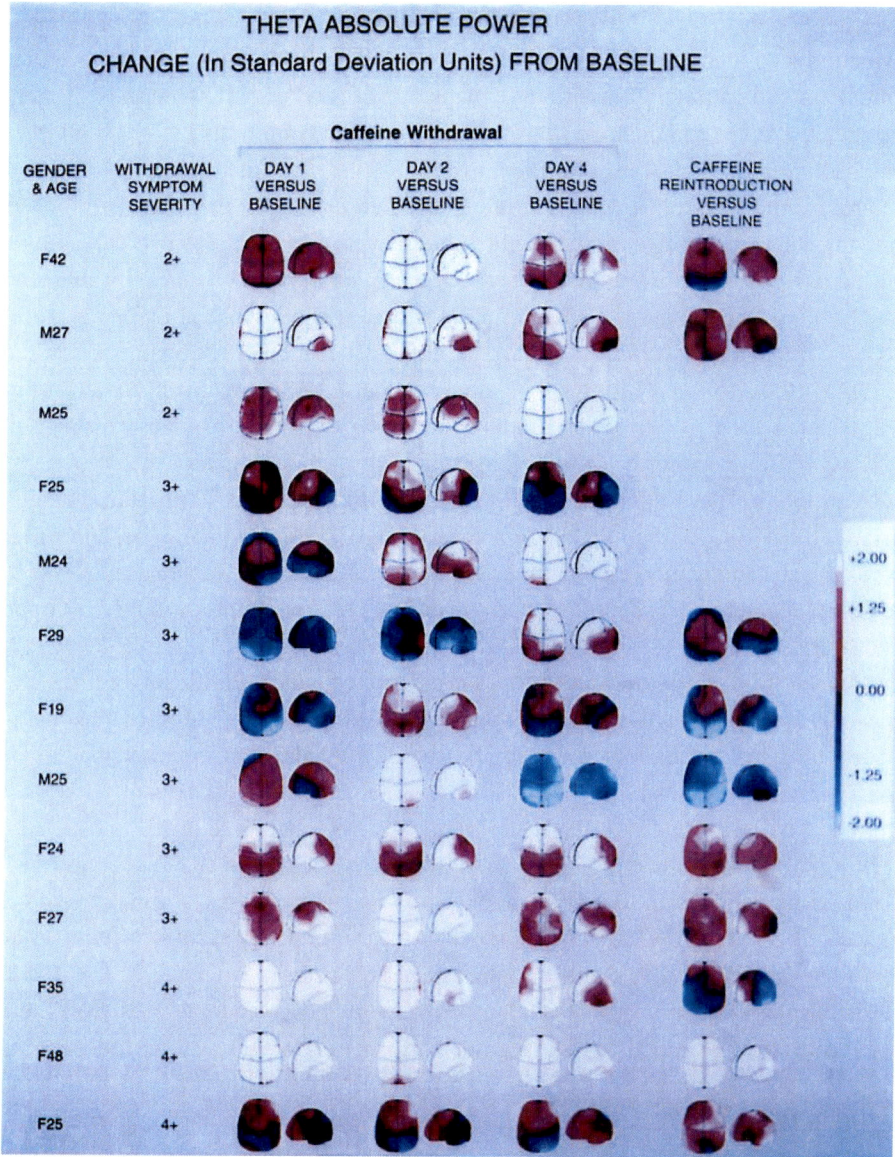

Figure 2. Changes in theta absolute power (in Standard Deviation Units) relative to baseline during caffeine withdrawal and with caffeine reintroduction.

For the results of the quantitative EEG comparisons, the most striking changes occurred with the absolute power of theta. 38.5% of subjects showed statistically significant increases of theta power on withdrawal day 1 and this nearly doubled to 76.9% on withdrawal day 2. Fully 92.3% of subjects showed statistically significant increases of theta absolute power over the frontal cortex at some point during caffeine withdrawal. Significant voltage increase of theta activity following caffeine withdrawal appears to be a highly robust effect.

This finding was confirmed by the study by Jones et al [16] mentioned above showing increased theta power during 1-day periods of caffeine abstinence. Caffeine's effect is dramatically illustrated by topographic maps of change in theta absolute power (in Standard

Deviation units) on days 1, 2, and 4 relative to baseline conditions (Figure 2). Caffeine abstinence-induced increase in theta voltage is particularly noticeable over the frontal cortex and is most marked on day 2. Topographic maps of EEGs recorded within only 30 minutes of caffeine reintroduction demonstrate return to near baseline conditions in almost all instances.

For absolute power of delta, significant changes were confined primarily to increases at the bilateral frontal electrodes, with a single additional electrode, the left posterior temporal, also showing a significant decrease in delta voltage over time. Group statistical analyses from baseline across the withdrawal period indicated no significant changes in alpha absolute power or beta absolute power as a function of caffeine withdrawal. For alpha absolute power considerable intersubject variation occurred, with some subjects showing a marked EEG change while others showed little or no change. Because the intersubject variability in alpha power attenuated the EEG effect for collapsed group data, mean changes in alpha absolute power during caffeine withdrawal were not significant for the group as a whole.

Neither alpha relative power nor delta relative power showed significant change during the period of caffeine withdrawal when compared with pre-abstinent baseline measures. There was a substantial increase of theta relative power for the subjects as a whole. Beta relative power tended to substantially decrease during caffeine withdrawal days as opposed to baseline values.

Withdrawal from caffeine appears to be associated with significant reductions in the frequency of the alpha rhythm (alpha slowing). At all 21 electrode sites the mean alpha frequency decreased throughout the caffeine withdrawal days as contrasted with baseline measures. As with theta absolute power, for most subjects who underwent QEEG after the reinstitution of caffeine on day 4, the mean frequency of the alpha returned to baseline values within 30 minutes. With the exception of only a few electrode sites (FP_1, F_8, and O_2), there was a small but significant decrease in mean beta frequency as a function of caffeine withdrawal. There were no significant changes in mean frequency across caffeine withdrawal days for either theta frequency bands or delta frequency bands.

Interhemispheric coherence measures, expressed as Z-score departures from normative database means were obtained across baseline and caffeine withdrawal periods. Eight (25%) of the 32 coherence measures showed significant change with caffeine withdrawal. Of interest is the observation that coherence values increased during caffeine withdrawal over the frontal cortex but decreased over the posterior cortex. Both alpha coherence and theta coherence increased sharply over the frontal cortex (FP_1/FP_2 and F_3/F_4) throughout the first two days of caffeine abstinence and moved back toward baseline levels by day 4 of caffeine withdrawal. When coherence data following caffeine reinstitution was compared with baseline values, no significant differences were obtained. This suggests that coherence values that did undergo significant change had returned to baseline levels. Both theta coherence (T_5/T_6, P_3/P_4), and delta coherence (C_3/C_4 and O_1/O_2) decreased significantly over posterior cortex during the caffeine withdrawal period. As before, when caffeine was reintroduced following the withdrawal period, coherence measures were no longer significantly different from baseline values.

Interhemispheric asymmetry as a function of caffeine withdrawal was examined for the four traditional EEG frequency bands at all 21 electrode sites. These analyses did not reveal any significant differences between baseline and withdrawal or reinstitution parameters. This suggests that caffeine withdrawal does not produce significant changes in interhemispheric symmetry for any of the frequency bands at any of the cortical regions.

Other EEG Occurrences during Caffeine Withdrawal

In addition to the findings described above, it was observed that patients who have diffuse paroxysmal slowing (DPS) on EEG may have increased bursts of DPS during caffeine withdrawal [43]. DPS is a minor EEG dysrhythmia that is sometimes seen in normal individuals and may be more common in persons with migraine. In six individuals with DPS at baseline (normal consumption), bursts of slowing increased by 88.3% on day 1 of caffeine abstinence, and peaked on day 2 at a 106.4% increase. After the subjects were given caffeine on day 4, the DPS firing rate for all subjects returned to, or below baseline levels.

Cognitive Evoked Potential and Caffeine Withdrawal

The only study currently in the literature on the effects of caffeine withdrawal on cognitive evoked potentials is an extention of the 4 day EEG study of caffeine withdrawal described above. On the same days these subjects underwent quantitative EEG studies, cognitive auditory and visual P300 evoked potentials were also performed. Results [44] indicated that there were no significant differences in auditory P300 latencies from baseline through caffeine withdrawal days 1, 2, and 4. However, there were significant decreases in auditory P300 amplitudes across the caffeine withdrawal days. In contrast to the results from the auditory P300 measures, caffeine withdrawal produced a different effect on visual P300 measurements. Findings indicated a statistically significant decrease in the visual P300 latency and no differences in P300 amplitude as a function of caffeine withdrawal. Why there would be differences in the types of responses of auditory and visual evoked potentials to the caffeine withdrawal state remains to be explained.

Significance of Electrophysiological Effects of Caffeine Exposure and Withdrawal

A number (but not all) of EEG studies of caffeine exposure demonstrate decreased power (voltage). The lack of this finding by some studies is postulated to be related to the confound of the effect of previous usage of caffeine among subjects. In spite of these inconsistencies, there appear to be adequate studies [23-34] supporting decreased EEG power with caffeine exposure to conclude that this is a valid phenomenon. Supporting this finding are a number of SPECT and PET studies [11-15] demonstrating cerebral blood flow decreases following caffeine exposure. It is easily plausible that decreased EEG voltage could occur as a result of decreased cerebral blood flow caused by vasoconstriction induced by caffeine exposure.

Quantitative EEG parameters that show significant changes as a result of caffeine withdrawal can be summarized as follows: 1.) increases in theta absolute power over all cortical areas; 2.) increases in delta absolute power over the frontal cortex; 3.) decreases in the mean frequency of both the alpha and beta rhythm; 4.) increase in theta relative power and decrease in beta relative power; and 5.) significant changes in interhemispheric coherence. Since caffeine exposure can result in alpha frequency increase [30], decreases in mean alpha frequency during withdrawal would not be unexpected. Increased EEG voltage during caffeine withdrawal is consistent with the postulate that caffeine exposure causes cerebral vasoconstriction followed by rebound cerebral vasodilitation during caffeine withdrawal. In fact, decreased cerebral blood flow during caffeine withdrawal has been shown to be reversed within 2 hours after caffeine intake [16]. These findings would be consistent with the report of occurrence of headache in 77% of studies of caffeine withdrawal [20]. It would appear that, at least in some cases, these headaches may be vascular in nature. The increase in DPS dysththymia [43] in some individuals may then be related to vascular headache as DPS occurs more often in migraine sufferers than in the general population.

Caffeine withdrawal related vasodilitation would appear, at least for some individuals, to be reversed with caffeine consumption. In addition to the cerebral blood low study mentioned above, Reeves et al [42] showed that, in most cases theta absolute power quickly returns to essentially baseline conditions within 30 minutes of caffeine resumption (see Figure 2). However, this vascular phenomenon may be limited to younger persons as it did not occur in the single patient in their study who was over 30 years old (age 48).

EEG changes including relative power as well as mean frequency measures are less clearly understood in terms of a vasodilitation hypothesis. The implications of caffeine withdrawal induced changes in interhemispheric coherence, particularly the directional differentiation of change between the anterior and posterior cortex remain obscure. Similarly, the findings of decreases in auditory P300 evoked potentials amplitudes and no significant differences in auditory latencies, but decreases in visual P300 latencies and no significant differences in visual amplitudes during caffeine withdrawal are difficult to explain. The anatomic and/or neurophysiological substrate involved in the regulation of coherence during caffeine withdrawal are not well understood.

The fact that in nearly every case reinstitution of caffeine following withdrawal tended to return altered QEEG values to baseline levels supports the contention that caffeine withdrawal was truly the operative variable in the EEG changes seen in the studies of caffeine withdrawal discussed here. It is interesting that despite the fact that post-caffeine reintroduction QEEGs were completed before peak levels of caffeine were likely to have been obtained (i.e., 30 to 45 minutes post ingestion), the majority of EEG variables did return to baseline following caffeine reintroduction [42]. More importantly, for most subjects, at all electrode sites the caffeine withdrawal changes in alpha rhythm returned completely to baseline levels within 30 minutes following caffeine reintroduction. This was also true for all electrodes for which beta mean frequency was altered by caffeine withdrawal. Thus it appears that caffeine withdrawal is a detectable and to some degree measureable phenomenon which can be reversed at some levels by reinstitution of caffeine. However, in spite of EEG or cerebral blood flow normalization with caffeine reinstitution, many of the clinical symptoms of caffeine withdrawal may not immediately resolve.

Conclusions

There would seem to be little question that caffeine exposure and caffeine withdrawal have neurophysiological effects which are detectable and quantifiable by EEG methods. A number of physiological responses to caffeine exposure and caffeine withdrawal may be theoretically explained by the phenomenon of cerebral vasoconstriction during caffeine exposure and rebound cerebral vasodilitation with abrupt cessation of caffeine. However, some of the effects of caffeine and its withdrawal are poorly understood, and for some effects (e.g., differences in directional changes in interhemispheric coherence in different areas of the brain and differences in effects on amplitudes and latencies of auditory and visual cognitive evoked potentials during caffeine withdrawal), no explanation is available as to why they occur.

Although there is a signicant collection of research on the electrophysiological effects of caffeine exposure, studies of caffeine withdrawal done to date could at best be described as preliminary. These studies present fascinating data but are limited in design and numbers of subjects. A number of needs and possibilities for further research are readily obvious. Particularly important would be placebo double blind studies to confirm data from previous open studies. Future work should attempt to extend the caffeine abstinence over additional days as this would permit assessment of the duration of neurophysiological caffeine withdrawal effects over longer periods of time. In addition, assessment of caffeine reinstitution should be done in a double blind paradigm with placebo or measurable doses of caffeine given in tablet form, and the time period of response should be carefully recorded and be sufficiently long (i.e., over 30 to 45 minutes) to allow peak caffeine blood levels to be obtained. It might be particularly interesting in view of previous findings to combine a cerebral blood flow study with a comprehensive quantitative EEG and evoked potentials study using a double blind placebo protocol for caffeine withdrawal and reinstitution. Assessing EEG parameters in combination with other research tool such as magnetic resonance spectroscopy could also be of value. For example, a proton spectroscopic study [10] has demonstrated globally and regionally specific brain lactate increases in caffeine intolerant subjects when they were exposed to caffeine; quantitative EEG changes in combination with spectroscopic data in such individuals could provide further insight into caffeine's effects. Finally, the relevance of the EEG findings to date, if confirmed, might largely depend on whether or not subjective symptoms of caffeine withdrawal can be shown to significantly co-vary over time with alterations of electrophysiological measures.

References

[1]   Gilbert RM. Caffeine consumption. In: Spiller GA, editor. *The Methylxanthine Beverages and Foods: Chemistry, Consumption, and Health Effects*. New York: Alan R. Liss; 1984, pp 185-213.

[2]   Hughes JR, Oliveto AH. A systematic survey of caffeine intake in Vermont. *Exp. Clin. Psychopharmacol.* 1997; 5:393-398.

[3]   Barone JJ, Roberts HR. Caffeine consumption. *Food Chem. Toxicol.* 1996; 34:119-129.

[4]   Molde DA. Diagnosing caffeineism. *Am. J. Psychiatry* 1975; 132:202-205.

[5]   Mumford GK, Benowita NL, Evans SM. Kaminski BJ, Preston KL, Sannerud CA, Silverman K, Griffiths RR. Absorption rates of methylxanthines following capsules, cola, and chocolate. *Euro. J. Clin. Pharmacol.* 1996; 51 :319-325.

[6]   Liguori A, Hughes JR, Grass JA. Absorption and subjective effects of caffeine from coffee, cola, and capsules. *Pharmacol. Biochem. Behav.* 1997; 58:721-726.

[7]   Kaplan GB, Greenblatt DJ, LeDuc BW, Thompson ML, Shader RI. Relationships of plasma and brain concentrations of caffeine and metabolites to benzodiazepine receptor binding and locomotor activity. *J. Pharmacol. Exp. Ther* 1989; 248:1078-1083.

[8]   Snyder SS, Katims JJ, Annau Z. Adenosine receptors and behavioral actions of methylxanthines. *Proc. Natl. Acad. Sci. USA* 1981; 78:3260-3264.

[9]   Goldstein A, Kaiser S, Whitby O. Psychotropic effects of caffeine in man. IV. Quantitative and qualitative differences associated with habituation to caffeine. *Clin. Pharmacol. Ther.* 1969; 10:489.

[10] Dager SR, Layton ME, Strauss W, Richards TL, Heide A, Friedman SD, Artru AA, Hayes CE, Posse S. Human brain metabolic response to caffeine and the effects of tolerance. *Am. J. Psychiatry* 1999; 156:229-237.

[11] Cameron OG, Model JG, Hariharan M. Caffeine and human cerebral blood flow: A positron emission topographic study. *Life Sci.* 1990; 47:1141-1146.

[12] Mathew RJ, Wilson WH. Caffeine-induced changes in cerebral circulation. *Stroke* 1985; 16:814-817.

[13] Mathew RJ, Wilson WH. Caffeine consumption, withdrawal and cerebral blood flow. *Headache* 1985; 25:305-309.

[14] Mathew RJ, Barr DL, Weinman ML. Caffeine and cerebral blood flow. *Brit. J. Psychiatry* 1983; 143:604-608.

[15] Couterier ECM, Laman DM, van Dujin MAJ, van Dujin H. Influence of caffeine and caffeine withdrawal on headache and cerebral flow velocities. *Cephalgia* 1997; 17:188-190.

[16] Jones HE, Herning RI, Cadet JL, Griffiths RR. Caffeine withdrawal increases cerebral blood flow and alters quantitative electroencephalography (EEG) activity. *Psychopharmacol.* 2000; 147:371-377.

[17] Griffiths RR, Juliano LM, Chausmer AL. Caffeine pharmacology and clinical effects. In: Graham AW, Schultz TK, Mayo-Smith M, Ries K, Wilford BB, editors. Principles of Addiction Medicine, 3rd edition. Chevy Chase: American Society of Addiction Medicine; pp 193-224.

[18] Griffiths RR, Mumford GK. Caffeine reinforcement, discrimination, tolerance, and physical dependence in laboratory animals and humans. In: Schuster CR, Kuhar MJ, editors. Pharmacological Aspects of Drug Dependence: Toward an Integrated Neurobehavioral Approach (Handbook of Experimental Pharmacology). Berlin Heidelberg New York: Springer; pp 315-341.

[19] Silverman K, Evans SM, Strain EC, Griffiths RR. Withdrawal syndrome after the double-blind cessation of caffeine consumption. *New Eng. J. Med.* 1992; 327:1109-1114.

[20] Juliano LM, Griffiths RR. A critical review of caffeine withdrawal: empirical validation of symptoms and signs, incidence, severity, and associated features. *Psychopharmacology* (Berl) 2004; 76:1-29.

[21] Griffiths RR, Evans SM, Heightman SJ. Low-dose caffeine dependence in humans. *J. Pharmacol. Exp.* 1990; 225:1123-1132.

[22] Hughes JR, Oliveto AH, Helzer JE, Higgins ST, Bickel WK. Should caffeine abuse, dependence, or withdrawal be added to DSM-IV and ICD-10? *Am. J. Psychiatry* 1992; 149:33-40.

[23] Goldstein L, Murphree HB, Pfeiffer CC. Quantitative electroencephalography in man as a measure of CNS stimulation. *Ann. NY Acad. Sci.* 1963; 107:1045-1056.

[24] Saletu B. EEG imaging of brain activity in clinical psychopharmacology. In: Mauer K, editor. *Topographic Brain Mapping of EEG and Evoked Potentials.* New York: Springer Verlag; 1989, pp 482-506.

[25] BruceM, Scott N, Ladner M, Marks V. The psychopharmacological and electrophysiological effects of single doses of caffeine in human subjects. *Br. J. Pharmacol.* 1986; 22:81-87.

[26] Kaplan GB, Greenblatt DJ, Ehrenberg BL, Goddard JE, Cotreau MM, Harmatz JS, Shader RI. Dose-dependent pharmacokinetics and psychomotor effects of caffeine in humans. *J. Clin. Pharmacol.* 1997; 37:693-703.

[27] Seipman M, Kirch W. Effects of caffeine on topographic quantitative EEG. *Neuropsychobiology* 2002; 45:161-166.

[28] Gilbert DG, Dibb WD, Plath LC, Hiyane SG. Effects of nicotine and caffeine, separately and in combination, on EEG topography, mood, heart rate, cortisol, and vigilance. *Psychophysiology* 2000; 37:583-595.

[29] Patat A, Rosenzweig P, Enslen M, Trocherie S, Miget N, Bozon MC, Allain H, Gandon JM. Effects of a new slow release formulation of caffeine on EEG, psychomotor and cognitive functions in sleep-deprived subjects. *Hum. Psychopharmacol.* 2000; 15:153-170.

[30] Landolt HP, Werth E, Borbely AA, Dijik DJ. Caffeine intake (200 mg) in the morning affects human sleep and EEG power spectra at night. *Brain Res.* 1995; 675:67-74.

[31] Newman F, Stein MB, Trettau JR, Coppola R, Uhde TW. Quantitative electroencephalographic effects of caffeine in panic disorder. *Psychiatric Res* 1992; 45:105-113.

[32] Krapivin SV, Voronina TA. Comparative quantitative pharmacological-EEG anakysis of the effects of psychostimulants [article in Russian]. *Vestn. Ross Akad. Med. Nauk* 1995; 6:7-16.

[33] Kunkel H. EEG spectral analysis of caffeine effects [article in German]. *Arzneimittelforschung* 1976; 26:462-465.

[34] Kunkel H. Multichannel EEG spectral analysis of the caffeine effect [article in German]. *Z. Ernahrungswiss* 1976; 15:71-79.

[35] Pritchard WS, Robinson JH, DeBethizy JD, Davis RA, Stiles MF. Caffeine and smoking: subjective performance and psychophysiological effects. *Psychophysiology* 1995; 32:19-27.

[36] Hasenfratz M, Battig K. Action profiles of smoking and caffeine: Stroop effect, EEG, and peripheral physiology. *Pharmacol. Biochem. Behavior* 1992; 42:155-161.

[37] Dimfel W, Schober F, Spuler M. The influence of caffeine on human EEG under resting conditions and during mental loads. *Clin. Investig* 1993; 71:197-207.

[38] Sule J, Brozek G, Cmiral J. Neurophysiological effects of small doses of caffeine in man. *Activitas Nervosa Superior* (Praha) 1974; 16:217-218.

[39] Clubley M, Bye CE, Henson TA, Peck AW, Riddington CJ. Effects of caffeine and cyclizine alone and in combination on human performance, subjective effects, and EEG activity. *Brit. J. Pharmacol.* 1979; 7:157-163.

[40] Pollock VE, Teasdale T, Stern J. Effects of caffeine on resting EEG and response to sine wave modulated light. *Electroencephalogr Clin. Neurophysiol.* 1981; 51:470-476.

[41] Reeves RR, Stuve FA, Patrick G, Bullen JA. Topographic quantitative EEG measures of alpha and theta power changes during caffeine withdrawal: Preliminary findings from normal subjects. *Clin. Electroencephalogr* 1995; 26:154-162.

[42] Reeves RR, Struve FA, Patrick G. Topographic quantitative EEG response to acute caffeine withdrawal: A comprehensive analysis of multiple quantitative variables. *Clin. Electroencephalogr* 2002; 178-188.

[43] Patrick G, Reeves RR, Struve FA. Does caffeine cessation increase firing rates of diffuse of diffuse paroxysmal slowing dysrhythmia? A serendipitous observation. *Clin. Electroencephalogr.* 1996; 27:78-83.

[44] Reeves RR, Struve FA, Patrick G. The effects of caffeine withdrawal on cognitive P300 auditory and visual evoked potentials. *Clin. Electroencephalogr.* 1999; 30:24-27.

In: Substance Withdrawal Syndrome
Editors: J. P. Rees and O. B. Woodhouse

ISBN 978-1-60692-951-3
© 2009 Nova Science Publishers, Inc.

Short Communication

Craving, Leptin and Metabolic Assessment in Subjects with Cocaine Abuse Dependence: Results from an Original Study

S. Andreoli, G. Martinotti, M. Mazza, M. Di Nicola, F. Tonioni and L. Janiri

Department of Psychiatry, University of Sacred Heart, Rome, Italy

Abstract

Introduction: Leptin is a 16-kDa protein secreted from white adipocytes; it acts by binding to specific hypothalamic receptors to alter the expression of several neuropeptides regulating neuroendocrine function, food intake and the body's entire energy balance. Leptin receptors have been found in several brain areas, including the cerebellum, cortex, hippocampus, thalamus and in peripheral tissues including the liver, pancreas, adrenals, ovaries, and hematopoietic stem cells. Leptin regulates and is regulated by several neuropeptides and hormones, such as Neuropeptide Y, melanocyte-stimulating-hormone, Agouti-related-hormone, pro-opiomelanocortin, orexin, cocaine-and amphetamine-regulated transcript, melanin-concentrating-hormone, insulin, IGF-system, sympathetic/parasympathetic tone, immune function and hemopoiesis (cytokines), the hypothalamic-pituitary-gonadal axis and the thyroid and adrenal axes (CRH, TSH). Actually, leptin is considered a modulator of withdrawal-induced craving in alcoholic subjects. During detoxification, craving can shift towards other kinds of craving (e.g., food or smoking), but if plasma leptin increases during withdrawal this shift can be attenuated, and consequentially appetite decreases and alcohol craving can be enhanced, determining possible relapses in alcohol consumption. Leptin is involved in the brain reward circuitry together with the CART-system, regulated by leptin itself; CART may be an important connection between food- and drug-related rewards. We studied the hypothesis that leptin might modulate cocaine craving in cocaine-detoxified addicts, evaluating any possible correlation with metabolic, hormonal and psychometric parameters.

Methods: A sample of 12 cocaine-dependent subjects, according to DSM-IV-TR, was evaluated as follows: height, weight (BMI), blood pressure, heart rate, substance and drug consumption, triglicerides, cholesterol, plasma leptin value, cortisol, insulin, ACTH, FT3, FT4, and TSH; and SHAPS, VASc/f/s (Visual-Analogue-Scale for cocaine/food/sex), CCQ (Cocaine-Craving-Questionnaire), Barratt Impulsiveness Scale, HAM-D, and HAM-A at baseline and after 15 days of abstinence.

Results: Leptin results positively correlated with VASc, CCQ and HAM-A; VASc was positively correlated with CCQ and HAM-D. VASf was negatively correlated with cholesterol (as attended) and positively with VASs and TSH. CCQ was positively related with HAM-D and the plasma leptin mean levels in the male subsample were higher with respect to controls. Data is expressed as mean, standard deviation and Pearson correlation coefficiency.

Conclusions: In our sample, leptin correlates with cocaine craving measured by VASc and CCQ independently from BMI or the hypothalamic-pituitary-adrenal axis. At baseline, VASc (mean) was less than VAS f and s mean score, confirming the shifting craving phenomenon. Cocaine craving is correlated with depressive symptoms and leptin correlates with anxious symptoms. Although our data confirm the correlation between leptin and cocaine craving, further studies are requested.

Introduction

Leptin, a 16-kDa protein secreted from white adipocytes, is involved in the complex neuroendocrinological network; it has been implicated in the regulation of food intake, energy expenditure and whole-body energy balance. Leptin plays an important role in the brain reward circuitry [Fulton et al., 2000]; in fact, it has been involved in the complex craving phenomenon for substances of abuse, especially for alcohol abuse (independently from weight and Body Mass Index, BMI) [Kiefer 2001, 2004], food [Berridge, 1996; Halaas et al., 1995; Pelleymounter et al., 1995] and, hypothetically, for sexual behaviour. Leptin regulates and is regulated by several neuropeptides and hormones, such as Neuropeptide Y, melanocytes-stimulating-hormone, Agouti-related-hormone, pro-opiomelanocortin, orexin, cocaine- and amphetamine-regulated transcript (CART), melanin-concentrating-hormone, insulin, IGF-system, sympathetic/parasympathetic tone, immune function and hemopoiesis (cytokines), the hypothalamic-pituitary-gonadal axis and the thyroid and adrenal axes (CRH, TSH). In addition, leptin can modulate gene expression: for example, CRH and POMC genes in the hypotalamic area, strengthening its correlation with the brain reward system (Inui, 1999). Many authors have contributed to clarify possible correlations between leptin and stress hormones [Casanueva and Dieguez, 1999; Leal-Cerro, 1996; Slieker et al., 1996; Gong et al., 1996]. It has been demonstrated that cortisol can increase plasma leptin levels [Newcomer et al., 1998]. Some peripheral factors, including leptin, are able to regulate the hypothalamic gene expression of CART (whose peptide is particularly concentrated in the hypothalamus): CART peptides can stimulate energy expenditure and decrease food appetite [Murphy, 2005]. Not only are dopamine, norepinephrine and serotonin involved in the regulation of feeding, but even several peptides such as NPY, orexin, ghrelin and, with an anorectic effect, CART peptide, thyrotropin-releasing hormone (TRH), corticotropin-releasing hormone (CRH), amylin and leptin. Such a neuroendocrinological network is translated into satiety or appetite signals in the hypothalamus [Brunetti et al., 2005]. Regarding substance-related behaviours, Da Silveira et al. reported the importance of cocaine craving as a predictive factor of possible relapses, together with the substance use modalities [Da Silveira et al., 2006]. Sinha et al. reported that stress-induced cocaine craving is related to a shorter abstinence period; moreover, CRH and cortisol hormonal responses are able to predict an increase in consumed cocaine each time [Sinha et al., 2006]. From a metabolic point of view, many authors have described the central role of leptin; it can mediate the metabolic effects of many well-known hormones, such as insulin, probably because leptin originates from fat tissue and is involved in liver functionality [Valtuena et al., 2005]. Leptin, moreover, may be able, at least experimentally, to modulate the hypothalamic (not only) concentrations of some neuronal factors such as serotonin, dopamine, and norepinephrine through unknown mechanisms. The role of leptin has also been individuated experimentally in oxidative stress through depletion of antioxidant agents such as vitamins C and E, and increase of lipoperoxidation, especially in the liver; thus, leptin can contribute to alcohol-induced liver damage [Balasubramaniyan, 2006]. Finally, the role of leptin is well known as an anorectic agent in the balancing of feeding. The correlation between craving and leptin suggests a possible direct or indirect effect of leptin itself on the motivational brain systems; several clinical studies on alcoholics reveals how craving during withdrawal tends to shift towards food (especially carbohydrates) or tobacco in order to substitute the substance of abuse [Junghanns et al., 2000] with a compensative reward mechanism. This could be the explanation for why, in alcoholic subjects with elevated plasma leptin levels, the 'substitutive' craving results are attenuated [Fulton, 2000] with an appetite reduction and an increase of alcohol craving, strengthening the hypothesis of an interrelationship between craving subtypes and metabolism. We studied the hypothesis that leptin could modulate cocaine craving in cocaine-detoxified addicts; our research tried to investigate a possible correlation among cocaine craving, leptin plasma levels, hormonal parameters, food and sex craving.

Methods

We studied a sample of 12 patients with the following features:

10 males, 2 females; mean age ± SD: 37.7 ± 6.1 years;
weight 80 ± 16.1 Kg; height: 1.77 ± 0.08 m; BMI: 25.6 ± 3.8 Kg/m2;

They were cocaine abusers or dependents according to DSM-IV-TR criteria. The subjects were recruited in the Day Hospital of Psychiatry, General Hospital 'A. Gemelli' in Rome. Among the exclusion criteria, selected subjects were not to use any other drug (actually or lifetime) except nicotine; treatments with neuroleptics, antidepressants, benzodiazepines, antihypertensive or hypoglicemic drugs during the previous three months before the recruitment were also not allowed. Recruited patients were screened for the following parameters at baseline (the beginning of the detoxification): routine laboratory parameters including blood cell count, triglycerides, cholesterol, plasma leptin, plasma cortisol, CRH,

FT3, FT4, TSH, blood insulin, Body Mass Index (BMI). Patients were also evaluated with the following psychometric tests: SHAPS (Snaith Hamilton Pleasure Scale); VAS (Visual Analogue Scale) for cocaine (VASc), food (VASf) and sex (VASs); Cocaine Craving Questionnaire or CCQ, Barratt Impulsiveness Scale, Hamilton Rating Scale for Depression, and Hamilton Rating Scale for Anxiety. Our aim was to describe any statistically significant correlation among substance-related behaviours, anhedonic-depressive symptoms and the hormonal and metabolic parameters. Such correlations have been already found in alcoholics, but they have not yet been explored in cocaine addicts.

Primary aim: evaluating any possible correlation among leptin, metabolic and hormonal pattern (even in stress condition such as withdrawal syndrome) and craving for cocaine, food and sex.

Secondary aim: evaluating among those measured psychopathologic parameters (such as anxiety, impulsiveness, depressive and anhedonic symptoms) which can be considered predictors of future relapse.

Procedure

Patients are evaluated at the beginning of the detoxification (T0):

- Anamnesis, physical examination: diagnosis of cocaine abuse/dependence according to DSM IV criteria;
- Vital signs: weight, height, blood pressure (BP), heart rate (HR), Body Mass Index (BMI);
- Toxicological anamnesis: substance of abuse, methods and quantities of consumption;
- Pharmacological anamnesis;
- Standard laboratory parameters: blood cell count, triglycerides, cholesterol, liver and renal function, plasma leptin, blood cortisol, CRH, FT3, FT4, TSH, blood insulin;
- Electrocardiogram (ECG);

Psychometric tests: SHAPS (Snaith Hamilton Pleasure Scale); VAS (Visual Analogue Scale) for cocaine (VASc), food (VASf) and sex(VASs); Cocaine Craving Questionnaire or CCQ, Barratt Impulsiveness Scale, Hamilton Rating Scale for Depression, Hamilton Rating Scale for Anxiety.

Leptin Dosage Procedure

The DRG® Leptin Enzyme Immunoassay Kit provides materials for the quantitative determination of Leptin in serum and plasma. The DRG® Leptin ELISA Kit is a solid phase enzyme-linked immunosorbent assay (ELISA) based on the sandwich principle.

Population ng/ml Males 3.84 ± 1.79 Females 7.36 ± 3.73

Data Analysis

All data are expressed as mean ± standard deviation. Correlations are analyzed using Pearson's correlation coefficients. Statistical significance is accepted if a p-value less than 0.05 is obtained.

Preliminary descriptive sample data

(Expressed as mean and standard deviation) at baseline

Patients 12 (10 males, 2 females)
Age 37.7 ± 6.1 years;
Weight 80.5 ± 16.1 Kg;
Height 1.77 ± 0.08 m;
BMI 25.6 ± 3.8 Kg/m2
First substance use age 23.75 ± 11.03 years
Daily consumed cocaine quantity 2.02 ±1.88 gr
ACTH 20.40 ± 16.47 pg\ml (n.r. 10–55)
Cortisol 167.33 ± 72.41 ng\ml (n.r. 80–220)
FT3 3.73 ± 0.65 pg\ml (n.r. 2.3–4.2)
FT4 12.46 ± 1.75 pg\ml (n.r. 8.5–15.5)
TSH 1.72 ± 1.16 microUI\ml (n.r. 0.35–2.80)
Blood insulin 16.00 ± 10.82 microUI\ml (n.r. 5.0–20.0)
Triglycerides 191.63 ± 87.27 mg\dl (n.r. 20–170)
Cholesterol 207.25 ± 65.45 mg\dl (n.r. 130–200)
Plasma leptin 10.92 ± 11.98 ng/ml (n.r. ♂ 3.84 ± 1.79)
Male subsample plasma leptin 8.56 ± 9,94 ng/ml (n.r. ♀ 7.36 ± 3.73)

Method of consumption:
7 via sniffing; 1 via smoking, 2 e.v. + sniffing; 1 smoked+sniffing; 1 e.v.

Results

At baseline (i.e., at the beginning of detoxification) the following correlations have been found in the recruited subjects with cocaine abuse/dependence (parameters taken into account and analyzed are: leptin, ACTH, cortisol, TSH, FT3, FT4, insulin, cholesterol, triglycerides, BMI, SHAPS, VAS, VASc, VASf, VASs, CCQ, Barratt Impulsiveness Scale, HAM-D, HAM-A):

- Leptin positively correlates with VAS for cocaine (VASc) (r=0.98), CCQ (r=0.93) and HAM A (r=0.89)
- TSH positively correlates with ACTH (r=0.91) and VAS for food (VASf) (r=0.90)

- Cholesterol negatively correlates with VAS for food VASf (r=-0.96) and VAS for sex (VASs) (r=-0.91)
- BMI positively correlates with the Barratt Impulsiveness Scale (r=0.90)
- SHAPS and VAS don't correlate with any parameter
- VASc correlates with leptin, as already noted (r=0.98), and positively correlates with CCQ (r=0.96) and HAM-D (r=0.90)
- VASf positively correlates with TSH (r=0.90), negatively with cholesterol (r=-0.96), and positively with VASs (r=0.93)
- CCQ positively correlates with VASc, as already said (r=0.96), and with HAM-D (r=0.98)

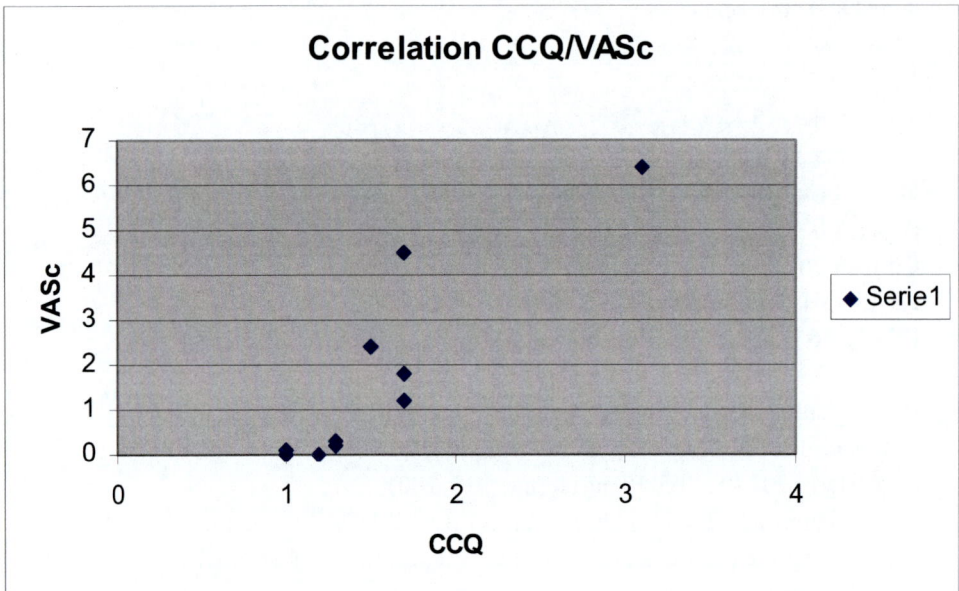

Correlation CCQ/VASc

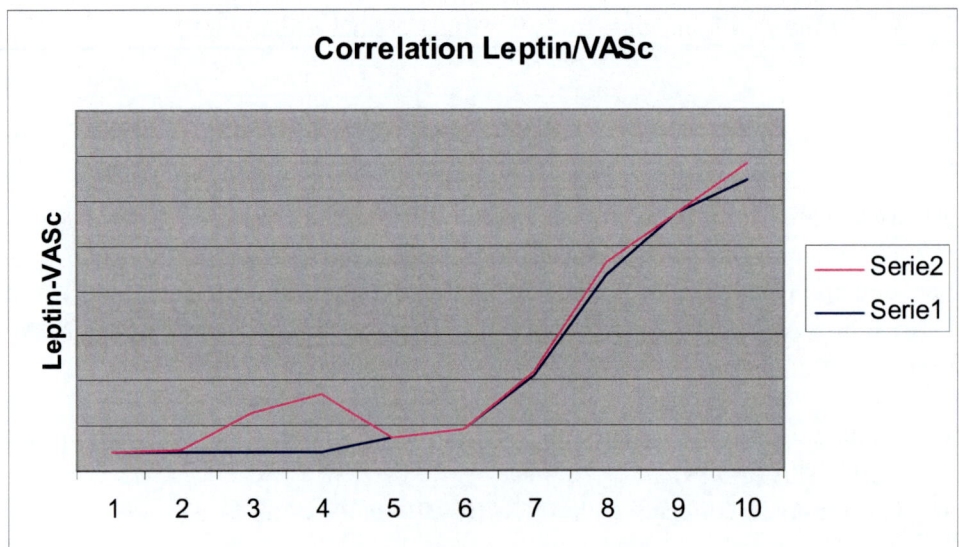

Correlation Leptin/VASc

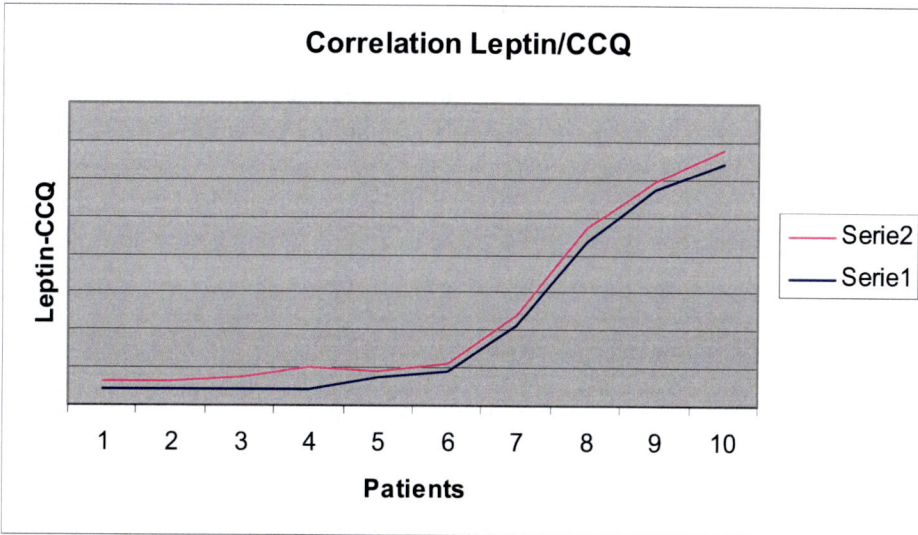

Correlation Leptin/CCQ

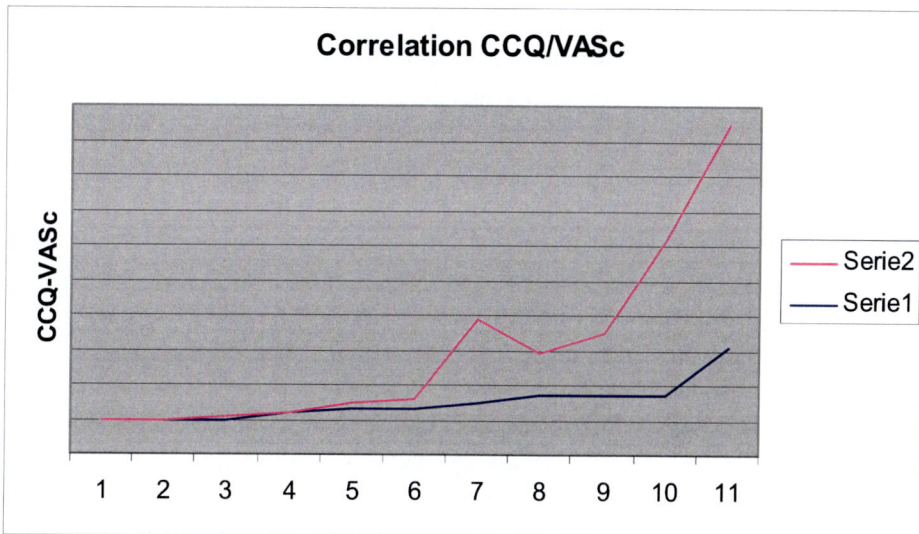

Correlation CCQ/VASc

- Among the psychometric tests, SHAPS and VAS do not correlate with other parameters
- chortisol, FT3, insulin and triglycerides do not correlate among themselves, nor with other parameters
- in the male subsample mean leptin values result high with respect to standard leptin values (male subsample mean leptin value: 8.56 ± 9.94 ng/ml; attended male mean leptin value in the general population: 3.84 ± 1.79 ng/ml)
- in the general population mean leptin values (± SD) are 10.92 ± 11.98 ng/ml

Conclusion

Our working hypothesis was to correlate the cocaine craving phenomenon with plasma leptin levels and some laboratory parameters, including the hormonal ones. A statistically significant correlation between leptin (whose mean values are high in our little sample with respect to general population) and VASc and CCQ (tests that specifically measure cocaine craving) has been found.

Our hypothesis was based on previous studies executed on alcoholic subjects [Kiefer et al., 2001]: it has been demonstrated that at the beginning of the detoxification very high leptin levels were found; such values were correlated with alcohol craving, independently from BMI and the activation of the hypothalamic-pituitary-surrenal axis. We have observed the same phenomenon in our sample, although it is limited in size: cortisol and ACTH do not correlate with leptin, craving or psychopathological symptoms (for example, withdrawal symptoms). Moreover, leptin does not correlate with BMI, even if we attended such correlation, nor with other parameters except the Barratt Impulsiveness Scale. Thus, even in our small-size sample, leptin correlates with cocaine craving independently from BMI and acute activation of the hypothalamic-pituitary-surrenal axis, which we can observe in the withdrawal syndrome. Although it is well known that cortisol induces leptin, in our sample there is no correlation between the two parameters. A possible explanation is that short-term physiological variations of cortisol do not modify circulating leptin levels, whereas a chronic activation of the 'stress' axis is able to activate directly the transcription of leptin promoter [Gong et al., 1996; Slieker et al., 1996]. TSH positively correlates with ACTH; the mean of both these values are normal. The other laboratory parameters (cortisol, FT3, FT4, insulin) are normal; two parameters result over the mean: cholesterol (207.25 ± 65.45 mg/dl; normal range 130–200) and triglycerides (191.63 ± 87.27 mg/dl; normal range 20–170). TSH correlates with VAS for food, probably for its stimulating action on the thyroid, which can influence feeding. Cholesterol (whose mean value is high in our sample) negatively correlates with both VAS for food and VAS for sex: elevated fat stores and circulating lipids inhibit feeding and caloric intake through food craving reduction; leptin, in fact, can reduce food intake through its anorectic effect, and leptin mean value results elevated in our sample (male subsample plasma leptin: 8.56 ± 9.94 ng/ml, n.r.: ♂ 3.84 ± 1.79; ♀ 7.36 ± 3.73). Moreover, addicts at the beginning of the abstinence often show a shift of craving towards substitutive behaviours, such as food or sex: in our sample, VASc mean value (2.08±2.77) is less at baseline than VASf mean value (5.03±3.63) and VASs mean value (5.67±3,30). In our sample, in fact, cocaine addicts at the beginning of abstinence seem to prefer food consumption or sex- related behaviours; this can confirm not only the shifting craving phenomenon towards subtypes of craving with compensative and supplying aims, but even the overlap of rewarding corticomesolimbic circuitries. Although craving can shift, the elevated leptin mean values we observed in our small sample can attenuate the substitutive craving (towards food, for example), strengthening substance-related craving (i.e., cocaine in our sample). It would be interesting to evaluate even in cocaine addicts future relapses with respect to baseline and possible correlations with plasma leptin; this could confirm the hypothesis of a correlation among substance of abuse, leptin and craving; craving, in fact, is one of the major risk factors for relapse, so eventual prevention strategies could focus on it.

As already reported, VASc and CCQ correlate with leptin, but they correlate with each other and with HAM-D as well: this confirms the validity of CCQ (short items version) with respect to the original version, as supported by recent studies [Sussner et al., 2005]. In addition, these data correlate cocaine craving with depressive symptoms, which usually can be observed at the beginning of detoxification, by the way depressive symptoms score: the HAM-D score is 12.67±8.15. Moreover, leptin correlates with HAM-A; this suggests a possible role of leptin related to craving and anxious symptoms that emerge during withdrawal syndrome. Although our data confirm the initial hypothesis of a correlation between cocaine craving and leptin, the recruited sample size is small, so further studies are requested to confirm these preliminary data.

Acknowledgments

We wish to thank Sigma Tau and Dr Menotti Calvani for providing The DRG® Leptin Enzyme Immunoassay Kit, which allowed us to realize this study. Many thanks are given to Dr. Anna Caprodossi for her punctual work.

References

Balasubramaniyan V, Nalini N. Effect of hyperleptinaemia on chronic ethanol-induced hepatotoxicity in mice. *Fundam. Clin. Pharmacol.* 2006 Apr;20(2):129-36.

Berridge KC. Food reward: brain substrates of wanting and liking. *Neurosci Behave Rev* 1996;20:1-25.

Brunetti L, Di Nisio C, Orlando G, Ferrante C, Vacca M. The regulation of feeding: a cross talk between peripheral and central signalling. *Int. J. Immunopathol. Pharmacol.* 2005 Apr-Jun;18(2):201-12

Casanueva FF, Dieguez C. Neuroendocrine regulation and actions of leptin. *Front Neuroendocrinol.* 1999 Oct;20(4):317-63. Review.

Da Silveira DX, Doering-Silveira E, Niel M, Jorge MR. Predicting craving among cocaine users. *Addict. Behav.* 2006 Mar 28.

Fulton S, Woodside B, Shizgal P. Modulation of brain reward circuitry by leptin. *Science* 2000;287:125–128.

Gong DW, Bi S, Pratley RE, Weintraub BD. Genomic structure and promoter analysis of the human obese gene. *J. Bioch.* 1996;271:3971-4.

Halaas JL, KS Gajiwala, M Maffei, SL Cohen, BT Chait, D Rabinowitz, R L Lalone, SK Burley, and JM Friedman. Weight reducing effects of the plasma protein encoded by the obese gene. *Science* (Wash DC) 1995;269:543-546.

Inui A. Feeding and body-weight regulation by hypothalamic neuropeptides- mediation of the actions of leptin. *TiNS* 1999;22:62-67.

Junghanns K, Veltrup C, Wetterling T. Craving shift in chronic alcoholics. *Eur. Addict. Res.* 2000 Jun;6(2):64-70.

Kiefer F, Jahn II, Jaschinski M, Holzbach R, Wolf K, Naber D, Wiedemann K. Leptin: a modulator of alcohol craving? *Biol. Psychiatry.* 2001;49:782-787.

Leal-Cerro A, Considine RV, Peino R, Venegas E, Astorga R, Casanueva FF, Dieguez C. Serum immunoreactive-leptin levels are increased in patients with Cushing's syndrome. *Horm. Metab. Res.* 1996 Dec;28(12):711-3.

Murphy KG. Dissecting the role of cocaine- and amphetamine-regulated transcript (CART) in the control of appetite. *Brief Funct. Genomic Proteomic.* 2005 Jul;4(2):95-111.

Newcomer JW, Selke G, Melson AK, Gross J, Vogler GP, Dagogo-Jack S. Dose-dependent cortisol-induced increases in plasma leptin concentration in healthy humans. *Arch. Gen. Psychiatry.* 1998 Nov;55(11):995-1000.

Pelleymounter MA, MJ Cullen, MB Baker, R Hecht, D Winters, T Boone, and F Collins. Effects of the obese gene product on body weight regulation in ob/ob mice. *Science* (Wash DC) 1995; 69:540-543.

Sinha R, Garcia M, Paliwal P, Kreek MJ, Rounsaville BJ. Stress-induced cocaine craving and hypothalamic-pituitary-adrenal responses are predictive of cocaine relapse outcomes. *Arch. Gen. Psychiatry.* 2006 Mar;63(3):324-31.

Slieker LJ, Sloop KW, Surface PL, Kriauciunas A, LaQuier F, Manetta J. Regulation of expression of ob mRNA and protein by glucocorticoids and cAMP. *J. Biol. Chem.* 1996;271:5301-5304.

Sussner BD, Smelson DA, Rodrigues S, Kline A, Losonczy M, Ziedonis D. The validity and reliability of a brief measure of cocaine craving. *Drug Alcohol Depend.* 2005 Dec 26.

Vicentic A and Jones DC. The CART system in appetite and drug addiction. *J. Pharmacol Exp Ther.* 2006.

Valtuena S, Numeroso F, Ardigo D, Pedrazzoni M, Franzini L, Piatti PM, Monti L, Zavaroni I. Relationship between leptin, insulin, body composition and liver steatosis in non-diabetic moderate drinkers with normal transaminase levels. *Eur. J. Endocrinol.* 2005 Aug;153(2):283-90.

Index

5

5-hydroxytryptophan, 55

A

abdominal cramps, 86
abnormalities, 127, 132, 146
absorption, 128, 129
abstinence, xi, xii, xiii, 7, 15, 16, 18, 86, 113, 114,
    115, 116, 117, 119, 120, 121, 124, 125, 126, 128,
    129, 130, 131, 132, 133, 134, 135, 137, 139, 140,
    141, 142, 143, 144, 145, 146, 147, 148, 149, 150,
    152, 153, 154, 155, 157, 161, 162, 164, 166, 168,
    179, 193, 200, 201, 202, 203, 204, 205, 207, 212,
    213, 218
academic, vii, 1, 10, 21, 23
academics, 6, 10, 23, 24, 25, 27
accidents, 133, 136
acetaldehyde, 118, 122, 127, 130, 149, 162
acetate, 118
acetylation, 136, 149
acetylcholine, 184, 185, 186, 188, 189, 192
Ach, 195
acid, 94, 118, 120, 121, 122, 123, 127, 128, 129,
    142, 143, 154, 156, 158, 184
acidity, xi, 114, 122, 123
ACTH, xiii, 212, 215, 218
activated receptors, 149
activation, xi, 35, 45, 52, 114, 118, 125, 134, 135,
    137, 138, 139, 161, 167, 186, 189, 190, 192, 195,
    218
activators, 134, 135, 137
activity level, 146

acute, vii, viii, x, xi, xii, 2, 3, 6, 7, 15, 16, 17, 18, 19,
    20, 31, 33, 37, 44, 45, 50, 53, 67, 94, 95, 98, 99,
    100, 101, 103, 105, 108, 109, 111, 112, 113, 114,
    115, 118, 119, 122, 125, 132, 136, 137, 138, 140,
    141, 142, 144, 152, 154, 160, 161, 167, 168, 169,
    170, 171, 173, 174, 176, 177, 179, 180, 181, 182,
    183, 184, 185, 186, 190, 191, 192, 193, 210, 218
acute coronary syndrome, x, xi, 94, 95, 99, 103, 105,
    108, 109, 111, 112, 114, 125, 132, 137, 161, 168
ad hoc, 97
adaptation, 115, 123
addiction, viii, ix, 2, 9, 11, 15, 18, 23, 24, 32, 33, 65,
    81, 82, 120, 138, 171, 174, 188
adducts, 130
adenine, 118
adenosine, 198, 199
ADH, 118, 130, 149, 168
adhesion, 132, 135, 139, 141, 142, 157, 164
adipocytes, xiii, 211, 212
adiponectin, 148, 164, 167
adjudication, 102
administration, vii, viii, xii, 2, 6, 8, 9, 10, 14, 21, 22,
    30, 31, 44, 49, 56, 120, 140, 163, 169, 170, 171,
    172, 174, 176, 177, 178, 179, 180, 181, 182, 183,
    184, 186, 190, 192, 200
adolescence, 178, 190, 193
adolescents, 163
ADP, 133
adult, 41, 59, 67, 170, 178, 191, 192
adults, 56, 154, 157, 158, 165, 168, 178, 198, 200
adverse event, x, 39, 40, 41, 55, 56, 94, 99, 100, 103,
    104
aerobic, 121
affect, 128, 150
affective disorder, 47, 49, 56, 58, 60
Africa, vii, viii, 1, 2, 6, 15, 16, 31

Afrikaans, 31
after abrupt cessation, 86
Ag, xi, 114, 135, 137, 138, 139, 140, 144
age, ix, xii, 16, 18, 61, 65, 69, 72, 73, 84, 94, 96,
    130, 138, 140, 142, 148, 161, 169, 178, 187, 206,
    213, 215
agent, 9, 18, 20, 21, 22, 28, 31, 33, 51, 65, 85, 94,
    96, 132, 139, 198, 213
agents, 9, 11, 19, 21, 38, 54, 67, 94, 105, 108, 109,
    111, 112, 160, 213
aggregation, 132, 133, 139, 142, 160, 162
agonist, viii, 2, 31, 44, 56
agoraphobia, 42, 54, 55, 57, 58
agranulocytosis, 15
aid, 6, 83, 154, 172, 178
air, 8
airways, 147
Alabama, 85, 86, 89, 90
alanine, 124
alanine aminotransferase, 124
albumin, 131, 198
alcohol abuse, xi, xii, 30, 114, 117, 119, 120, 121,
    124, 125, 126, 128, 131, 132, 133, 134, 136, 137,
    138, 141, 142, 145, 148, 149, 150, 153, 170, 171,
    172, 179, 187, 192, 194, 212
alcohol consumption, xiii, 114, 115, 117, 119, 122,
    126, 129, 130, 131, 133, 135, 136, 142, 147, 148,
    151, 153, 154, 157, 159, 160, 161, 162, 164, 166,
    167, 170, 186, 188, 193, 211
alcohol dependence, 12, 114, 121, 124, 125, 127,
    129, 130, 131, 138, 140, 141, 142, 143, 149, 156,
    157, 159, 166
alcohol research, 28, 186
alcohol use, 33, 115, 116, 119, 122, 125, 133, 145,
    163, 166
alcohol withdrawal, vii, xi, xii, 1, 5, 8, 14, 20, 24,
    26, 28, 29, 30, 31, 32, 33, 34, 35, 113, 114, 116,
    117, 125, 126, 127, 128, 129, 130, 131, 133, 134,
    135, 136, 138, 139, 140, 141, 142, 143, 144, 145,
    148, 151, 154, 159, 160, 164, 165
alcoholic cirrhosis, 152
alcoholic liver disease, 115, 125, 147, 152
alcoholics, 4, 115, 116, 117, 118, 120, 122, 123, 124,
    125, 126, 127, 128, 129, 131, 132, 133, 134, 135,
    136, 137, 138, 139, 140, 142, 143, 144, 145, 146,
    147, 148, 149, 150, 151, 152, 154, 155, 160, 161,
    163, 165, 170, 181, 213, 214, 219
alcoholism, 24, 31, 116, 131, 133, 140, 151, 152,
    154, 155, 160, 170, 178, 187, 189, 192
alcohols, 120

ALDH2, 143, 145, 165
alertness, 199
alexithymia, 78, 122, 123, 152, 155
algorithm, 108
alkaline, 122
allele, 145
allergy, 95
alpha, xi, xii, 112, 114, 117, 124, 125, 130, 131, 135,
    140, 141, 142, 146, 148, 156, 162, 164, 165, 167,
    197, 199, 200, 202, 204, 206, 210
ALT, 124, 125, 132, 142
alteplase, 137
alternative, ix, 39, 62
alternatives, 53
alters, 172, 173, 180, 185, 186, 189, 192, 208
amelioration, 18, 19, 147
American Heart Association, 94, 112
American Psychiatric Association, 30, 76, 151
amino, 59, 147
amino acid, 59, 147
amino acids, 59, 147
amnesia, 116
amphetamine, xiii, 17, 52, 211, 212, 220
amplitude, 117, 122, 123, 155, 199, 200, 205
Amsterdam, 55, 57, 79
amygdala, 172, 173, 187, 191, 192, 193, 194, 195
amylase, 122
anaesthesia, 3, 4, 5, 6, 7, 20, 22, 29
analgesia, 29, 32
analgesic, 3, 14, 15, 23, 30, 31, 32, 33, 34, 199
analgesics, 198
analog, 202
analysis of variance, 72
androgens, 149
anemia, 146
anesthesiologists, 22
anger, 199
angina, 69, 111, 147, 166, 167
angioplasty, 142
animal models, 152
animal studies, 17, 86
animals, 83, 87, 172, 174, 176, 177, 178, 179, 182,
    183, 209
anorexia, 88
antagonism, 23, 198
antagonist, 31, 44, 45, 165, 185
antagonistic, 6
antagonists, 184
anterior, 201, 206
antianxiety drugs, 49, 58

anti-atherogenic, 128, 149

anticoagulant, 107, 135

anticoagulants, 94, 137

anticonvulsants, viii, 61, 62

antidepressant, viii, 37, 38, 39, 40, 41, 42, 43, 44, 45, 46, 47, 48, 49, 50, 51, 52, 53, 54, 55, 56, 57, 58, 59

antidepressant medication, 39, 47, 59

antidepressants, viii, 37, 40, 42, 46, 47, 48, 51, 52, 54, 56, 57, 58, 64, 67, 76, 78, 213

antigen, xi, 114, 135, 161

antihistamines, 198

anti-inflammatory drugs, 105

antinociception, 30

antioxidant, 139, 213

anti-platelet, 132, 137

antipsychotic, 85

Antithrombin, 161

antrum, 119

anxiety, ix, x, 17, 30, 38, 39, 40, 41, 42, 47, 49, 53, 55, 56, 59, 61, 62, 63, 69, 70, 73, 74,75, 77, 78, 81, 86, 87, 88, 116, 139, 152, 155, 170, 191, 193, 199, 214

anxiety disorder, 38, 41, 42, 47, 49, 53, 55, 59, 62, 69

anxiolytic, 62, 63, 64, 65, 66, 67, 74, 171, 194

apolipoprotein A-I, 125

appetite, xiii, 39, 62, 64, 128, 211, 212, 220

application, viii, 2, 28, 59, 77, 78, 126

appraisals, 74

arginine, 141, 163

argument, 35

Arizona, 89, 90

arrhythmia, 116, 125, 146, 148

arrhythmias, 39

ART, 212

arterial hypertension, 115

arteries, 122, 136, 142, 147, 155, 167, 198, 201

artery, x, 93, 94, 95, 96, 97, 99, 100, 103, 104, 105, 106, 107, 109, 110, 111, 112, 126, 128, 129, 130, 133, 136, 141, 145, 148, 157, 159, 167

Asian, 143

aspartate, 45, 138, 190

aspiration, 147

aspirin, x, 26, 93, 94, 95, 96, 97, 98, 99, 100, 101, 102, 103, 104, 105, 106, 107, 108, 109, 110, 111, 112, 132

assessment, 13, 39, 40, 42, 56, 72, 73, 78, 98, 133, 149, 153, 165, 167, 201, 207

association, 99, 103, 115, 136, 138, 142, 143, 161

asthenia, 40

asymmetry, 202, 204

asymptomatic, 118, 135

ataxia, 88, 116

atherogenesis, 139

atherosclerosis, xi, 114, 121, 126, 130, 132, 135, 137, 138, 141, 142, 143, 144, 146, 147, 157, 161, 166

atherothrombotic, x, 94, 107

ATP, 147

atrial fibrillation, 125

attacks, 25, 26, 28, 39, 57, 110

attention, 141, 198

attenuated, 204

attitudes, 3

atypical, 122, 123, 166

auditory hallucinations, 63, 116

authority, 88

autonomic nervous system, xi, 113, 114, 123, 144, 145, 146, 152, 155

availability, 42, 141

avoidance, xii, 169, 171, 172, 173, 174, 177, 178, 179, 180, 182, 183, 184, 185, 186, 187, 188, 189, 190, 191, 192, 193, 194, 195

avoidance behavior, 177, 188, 194

awareness, viii, 37, 45, 51, 52, 89, 176, 191

B

back pain, 82, 86

bacteria, 118, 121, 122

bacterial, 118, 121, 122, 124, 125, 139, 140, 142, 154

bacterial contamination, 125

Badia, 142, 164

barbiturates, 9, 83

barrier, 122, 140, 142, 198

basal forebrain, 187

basal nuclei, 192

Beck Depression Inventory (BDI), 123, 143

beer, 120, 121, 134, 145

behavior, xii, 57, 87, 167, 169, 174, 177, 179, 180, 188, 189, 192, 194

behavior therapy, 57

behavioral change, 170, 181, 186

behavioral effects, 60, 170, 180, 183, 184, 185

behaviours, 213, 214, 218

beneficial effect, 17, 105, 170

benefits, x, xii, 10, 49, 76, 93, 99, 114, 116, 130, 149

benign, 42, 118

benzodiazepine, ix, 9, 11, 12, 13, 19, 34, 53, 61, 62, 63, 64, 65, 67, 68, 69, 70, 71, 72, 73, 74, 76, 77, 85, 89, 195, 208

benzodiazepines, viii, ix, 2, 7, 9, 11, 13, 14, 19, 21, 22, 33, 42, 61, 62, 63, 64, 65, 66, 67, 69, 76, 77, 81, 82, 84, 85, 213

Best Practice, 152, 153

beta, xii, 197, 199, 200, 202, 204, 206

beverages, 120, 121, 130, 132, 134, 140, 142, 153, 154, 155, 163

bias, 39, 97, 102, 103, 104

bilateral, 204

bile, 67, 128, 129

bile acids, 128

bile duct, 67

bilirubin, 131

binding, xiii, 56, 118, 128, 139, 147, 152, 194, 208, 211

binge drinking, 131, 138, 172, 181

biopsies, 121, 124

biopsy, 105

biosynthesis, 162

bipolar, viii, 37, 38, 43, 44, 48, 49, 58, 59, 85

bipolar disorder, viii, 37, 38, 43, 48, 49, 58, 59, 85

bipolar illness, 48

bismuth, 154

blackouts, 170

bladder, 67

bleeding, x, 93, 94, 95, 97, 98, 100, 104, 105, 106, 107, 108, 109, 110, 111, 117, 119, 133, 137

blocks, 191

blood, xi, xiii, 13, 63, 95, 100, 114, 116, 125, 126, 131, 134, 135, 136, 137, 138, 139, 143, 144, 146, 147, 152, 157, 158, 159, 162, 165, 166, 178, 183, 198, 200, 201, 206, 207, 208, 212, 213, 214

blood flow, 135, 146, 147, 198, 201, 205, 206, 207, 208

blood monocytes, 152

blood pressure, 95, 116, 126, 131, 138, 139, 143, 144, 146, 157, 158, 159, 165, 166, 198, 200, 214

blood pressure, 166, 167

blood transfusion, 100

blood-brain barrier (BBB), 198

body, 116, 122, 127, 131, 134, 137, 138, 139, 143, 144, 146, 148, 159, 167

body aches, 86

body composition, 220

body mass index (BMI), xiii, 143, 146, 148, 167, 212, 213, 214, 215, 216, 218

body temperature, 116

body weight, 144, 159, 220

bone marrow, 132

border crossing, 85

borderline, 123, 145

bowel, 122, 155

brain, xiii, 34, 56, 65, 83, 115, 118, 123, 124, 141, 148, 152, 163, 164, 171, 172, 173, 174, 176, 178, 180, 181, 184, 185, 186, 187, 188, 191, 194, 198, 207, 208, 209, 211, 212, 219

brain activity, 209

brain natriuretic peptide, 148

Brazil, 120, 154

Brazilian, 153

breathing, 16, 19, 116

breathing rate, 116

broad spectrum, 104

bronchus, 67

bupropion, 51

burn, 154

bypass, x, 94, 99, 105, 106, 109, 110

bypass graft, x, 94, 99, 105, 106, 109

C

Ca^{2+}, 144

CAD, 126, 127, 129, 131, 136, 143, 144

caffeine, xii, 197, 198, 199, 200, 201, 202, 203, 204, 205, 206, 207, 208, 209, 210

calcitonin, 147, 167

calcium, 64, 147, 165

calcium channel blocker, 64

calcium channels, 165

caloric intake, 218

cAMP, 198, 220

cancer, 115, 151

cannabinoids, 19

cannabis, vii, 2, 6, 7, 18, 19, 20, 31, 32

capacity, xi, 113, 114, 118, 146, 147, 166, 193

Cape Town, 35

carbohydrate, 132

carbohydrates, 213

carbon, 8

carbon dioxide, 8

carcinogenesis, 119, 121

cardiac arrhythmia, 39, 125

cardiac autonomic function, 152, 166

cardiac surgery, 65, 103

cardiology, 160

cardiomyocytes, 147

cardiomyopathy, 115, 147
cardiovascular disease, xi, 94, 109, 111, 114, 115, 126, 151, 157, 158, 159, 160, 161, 165
cardiovascular risk, 97, 105, 109, 126, 127, 130, 131, 138, 139, 159, 160, 161, 162
cardiovascular system, xi, xii, 113, 114, 125, 126, 131, 148
carrier, 149, 163
catalase, 118
cataract, 105, 108
cataract surgery, 105, 108
catatonia, 39
catecholamine, 122
Catholic, 93
Caucasian, 167
CDT, 158
cell, 116, 118, 134, 139, 142, 162, 213, 214
central nervous system (CNS), 123, 170, 199, 209
cerebellum, xiii, 211
cerebral arteries, 198, 201
cerebral blood flow, 198, 201, 205, 206, 207, 208
cerebral cortex, 123
cerebral hemorrhage, 95
cerebrovascular, 112
cerebrovascular disease, 112
channels, 144, 165, 187
chemical, 198
childhood, 120
children, 56, 198
chloride, 187
chocolate, 208
cholecystokinin, 31, 123, 124
cholesterol, xi, xiii, 114, 116, 125, 126, 127, 129, 130, 131, 132, 139, 146, 156, 157, 158, 163, 212, 213, 214, 215, 216, 218
cholinergic, 38, 44, 123, 176, 184, 185, 187, 194, 195
chronic diseases, 115
chronic renal failure, 67
cigarette smoking, 18, 30, 33, 148
cigarettes, 17
circulation, 24, 121, 123, 136, 154, 208
cirrhosis, 118, 152, 168
citalopram, 43, 44, 50, 56, 58
classes, 16, 42
classical, 4, 5, 19, 170, 171, 195
classification, 89, 119
clients, 19
clinical, 199, 207, 208, 209
clinical diagnosis, 136

clinical symptoms, 74, 119, 207
clinical trial, 7, 14, 26, 41, 54, 59, 79, 86, 95, 106, 109, 129, 138
clinical trials, 14, 41, 59, 86, 106, 109, 129, 138
clinically significant, 63, 116
clinician, 40, 159
clinicians, 198, 200
clinics, ix, 19, 62, 64, 73, 76, 77
clonidine, 32, 33
clopidogrel, 94, 106, 108, 109, 110, 111, 132
CNS, 32, 54, 58, 59, 79, 83, 156, 199, 209
Co, 133, 160
coagulation, xi, 114, 134, 135, 136, 137, 138, 161, 162
coagulation factor, 134, 135, 136, 161
coagulation factors, 134, 135, 136, 161
cocaine, vii, ix, xiii, 2, 6, 7, 14, 16, 17, 19, 20, 30, 33, 34, 52, 81, 83, 84, 85, 139, 190, 211, 212, 213, 214, 215, 218, 219, 220
cocaine abuse, 17, 213, 214, 215
cocaine use, ix, 81, 219
Cochrane Database of Systematic Reviews, 76, 163
coefficient of variation, 152
coffee, 198, 201, 208
cognition, 170, 174, 176, 180, 183, 185, 186, 192
cognitive, xii, xiii, 39, 47, 50, 57, 59, 73, 115, 116, 169, 170, 171, 172, 180, 183, 184, 186, 192, 193, 198, 205, 207, 209, 210
cognitive behavior therapy, 57
cognitive behavioral therapy, 47
cognitive deficit, 170
cognitive deficits, 170
cognitive function, 170, 209
cognitive impairment, 39, 116, 170
cognitive process, xii, 169, 170, 171, 184, 186, 192
cognitive processing, 170, 192
cognitive therapy, 50
coherence, xiii, 197, 202, 204, 206, 207
coherence measures, 204
cohort, 4, 5, 11, 12, 13, 18, 22, 102, 151, 158, 161
collaboration, 27, 94, 95, 97, 108, 121
collagen, 132, 133, 142
colon, 115
colonization, 117, 120, 123, 125, 142
colonoscopy, 109
common symptoms, 39
communication, 5, 22, 26, 78, 172
community, 10, 89, 114
competence, 126, 146, 147, 148
compliance, 37, 46, 95

complications, 41, 105, 110, 115, 124, 126, 129, 131, 132, 133, 134, 135, 136, 137, 138, 141, 144, 146, 148

components, 115, 127, 132, 144, 145, 148, 191

composition, 155

compounds, 199

computing, 97

concentration, vii, xi, xii, 1, 3, 4, 5, 6, 7, 13, 15, 21, 22, 27, 48, 59, 114, 116, 117, 118, 121, 124, 125, 126, 127, 128, 129, 130, 131, 134, 135, 137, 139, 140, 142, 146, 147, 149, 150, 158, 162, 164, 195, 197, 200, 220

conception, 28

conditioned stimulus, 171, 192

conditioning, xii, 169, 170, 171, 172, 173, 174, 176, 177, 178, 179, 180, 181, 182, 183, 184, 185, 186, 187, 188, 189, 190, 191, 192, 193, 194, 195

conduct, 97, 106

confidence, x, 73, 94, 97, 103, 104, 199

confidence interval, x, 73, 94, 97, 103, 104

confidence intervals, 73, 97

conflict, 28

conflict of interest, 28

confusion, 23, 39, 49, 116, 199

congestive heart failure, 109, 125

Congress, 24

conjugated dienes, 133

Connecticut, 197

consciousness, 3

consensus, 160

consent, 11, 12, 69, 200

consolidation, 172, 173, 174, 177, 179, 187, 190, 195

consulting, 25

consumers, 136, 198, 199

consumption, xiii, 33, 87, 115, 120, 122, 126, 129, 130, 131, 133, 134, 136, 141, 142, 144, 147, 148, 151, 153, 154, 157, 158, 159, 160, 161, 162, 164, 165, 166, 167, 168, 170, 178, 180, 183, 185, 186, 187, 188, 189, 192, 193, 194, 201, 202, 205, 206, 208, 209, 211, 212, 214, 215, 218

contamination, 125

contractions, 117, 122, 123, 155

control, 15, 42, 43, 64, 69, 70, 72, 88, 95, 98, 99, 119, 121, 122, 123, 124, 128, 131, 132, 134, 137, 139, 140, 141, 142, 145, 146, 148, 150, 156, 200, 201, 220

control group, 69, 70, 72, 98, 121, 122, 124, 128, 132, 134, 140, 142, 145, 146, 150

controlled studies, 90

controlled substance, x, 82, 90, 91

controlled substances, ix, 81, 84, 85, 89

controlled trials, vii, 2, 108

conversion, 137, 202

coronary arteries, 122, 147, 155, 167

coronary artery bypass graft, x, 94, 99, 105, 106, 109

coronary artery disease, x, 93, 94, 95, 96, 97, 99, 103, 104, 105, 106, 107, 109, 111, 112, 126, 128, 129, 130, 133, 135, 141, 145, 148, 157, 159, 167

coronary bypass surgery, 110

coronary heart disease, 94, 109, 111, 115, 151, 156, 157, 161, 163, 166

correlation, xiii, 46, 129, 139, 140, 178, 192, 211, 212, 214, 215, 218

correlation coefficient, 215

correlations, 63, 130, 150, 212, 214, 215, 218

cortex, xii, xiii, 123, 172, 173, 176, 197, 202, 203, 204, 206, 211

cortical, xii, 197, 205, 206

corticotropin, 52, 124, 212

cortisol, xiii, 60, 209, 212, 213, 214, 215, 218, 220

cost-effective, vii, 1, 94, 116

costs, ix, 61, 76, 114

cotinine, 18

crack, 16

craving, viii, xiii, 2, 3, 16, 18, 19, 20, 31, 33, 86, 190, 199, 211, 212, 214, 218, 219, 220

C-reactive protein, 141, 142, 164

credibility, 21, 22, 23, 24, 27, 28

credit, 48

CRH, xiii, 211, 212, 213, 214

critical period, 188

criticism, 13, 25

cross-sectional, 154

cross-sectional study, 154

CRP, 141, 142

cues, 171, 174, 190

culture, 137

currency, 48

Cushing's syndrome, 220

CVD, 115

cyanide, 26

cycling, 48

cyclothymic disorder, 43

cytochrome, 118

cytokine, xi, 114, 117, 124, 125, 130, 132, 134, 141, 142, 165

cytokines, xiii, 122, 124, 130, 139, 141, 159, 167, 211, 212

cytosol, 118

cytosolic, 118
cytotoxic, xi, 114, 122, 140, 142
cytotoxic action, xi, 114
Czech Republic, 120, 153

D

damage, 116, 117, 135
danger, viii, 2, 9, 192
data analysis, 77
database, 39, 84, 96, 204
de novo, 105
death, xi, 7, 94, 97, 98, 99, 100, 102, 108, 113, 115, 116, 118, 126, 133, 144, 145, 146, 151
deaths, 85, 90, 94, 100, 101, 126
debt, 29
decisions, 106
defense, 122
deficiency, 116, 132, 149, 162
deficit, 56, 186
deficits, xii, 169, 170, 172, 173, 174, 178, 180, 181, 182, 183, 185, 186, 190, 191
definition, 54, 72, 107, 130
degradation, 137
degree, 206
dehydrogenase, 118, 149
dehydrogenases, 118, 122
delayed gastric emptying, 122
delirium, 7, 12, 88, 116, 131, 142
delirium tremens, 12, 88, 116, 131, 142
delta, xii, 197, 200, 202, 204, 206
delusions, 63
demoralization, 53
dendritic spines, 188
denial, 48
density, 45, 118, 147, 152, 157, 163, 180, 185, 186
dentate gyrus, 173, 187
dentist, 6, 25
dentists, 3, 22, 35
Department of Health and Human Services, 90
depersonalization, 62, 87
deposits, 137
depressed, 42, 46, 47, 50, 53, 59, 64, 76, 77, 178, 193, 199
depression, viii, 16, 37, 38, 40, 42, 45, 46, 47, 48, 49, 51, 52, 53, 55, 56, 57, 58, 59, 62, 64, 67, 68, 69, 70, 73, 74, 77, 78, 117, 122, 123, 127, 143, 146, 148, 152, 155, 170, 185, 189
depressive disorder, 41, 42, 43, 44, 55, 57, 59

depressive symptoms, xiii, 44, 46, 47, 48, 50, 55, 116, 212, 214, 219
dermatologic, 110
dermatology, 65
desensitization, 44, 185
desipramine, 49, 59
desire, 199
detection, 97, 193
detoxification, xiii, 9, 10, 12, 87, 88, 211, 213, 214, 215, 218
developed countries, 94, 126
developmental change, 178
deviation, 97, 145
diabetes, 67, 69, 109, 126, 138, 148
diabetes mellitus, 67, 69, 148
diagnosis, 199
Diagnostic and Statistical Manual of Mental Disorders, 62, 199
diagnostic criteria, 78, 116
diaphoresis, 87, 199
diarrhea, 40, 87, 117, 121
diastolic blood pressure, 143
dienes, 133
diet, 124, 126, 129, 131, 137, 182, 201
diets, 201
differentiation, 130, 206
digestive tract, 119, 122, 123, 139, 155
disability, 77, 115, 144, 151
discomfort, 117, 121
discriminant analysis, 159
discrimination, 209
diseases, xi, 114, 118, 122, 136
disorder, 42, 43, 47, 48, 56, 116, 154, 155, 200, 209
disseminated intravascular coagulation, 136
dissociation, 191, 192
distillation, 121
distress, 41, 63, 116, 155
dizziness, 39, 40, 41, 82, 199
DNA, 118
dogs, 86, 155
domain, 143, 145
dopamine, 6, 16, 18, 19, 34, 35, 190, 193, 198, 212
dopaminergic, 189
dopaminergic neurons, 189
Doppler, 201
dosage, 13, 26, 47, 48, 49, 58, 74, 82, 86, 87, 88
dosing, 22
double blind study, 198, 201
double-blind trial, 9, 10, 13, 32
down-regulation, 44, 142, 185, 186

draft, 26
drainage, 99
drinking, vii, xi, xii, 114, 115, 117, 122, 123, 124,
    126, 127, 128, 130, 131, 132, 133, 134, 136, 137,
    138, 140, 141, 142, 143, 144, 145, 146, 147, 148,
    149, 150, 151, 159, 166, 170, 172, 181, 192
drinking pattern, 127, 131, 144, 148
dropouts, 50
drowsiness, 199
drug abuse, 30, 88
drug addiction, 159, 220
drug dependence, 45, 91
drug interaction, 77
drug reactions, 39
drug therapy, 49, 53, 56, 110
drug treatment, viii, 37, 38, 45, 46, 48, 50, 58, 91
drug use, 91, 174
drug withdrawal, 34, 104
drug-induced, 48
drug-related, xiii, 49, 90, 211
drugs, viii, ix, 37, 38, 42, 43, 45, 46, 47, 48, 49, 50,
    51, 52, 53, 54, 56, 60, 81, 83, 84, 85, 88, 91, 101,
    105, 129, 132, 137, 139, 152, 170, 193, 213
DSM, xiii, 12, 42, 43, 62, 63, 64, 69, 73, 77, 78, 152,
    199, 209, 212, 213, 214
DSM-III, 78
DSM-IV, xiii, 12, 42, 43, 62, 63, 64, 69, 73, 77, 78,
    152, 209, 212, 213
duodenal ulcer, 122
duration, ix, 4, 41, 43, 46, 48, 61, 72, 73, 74, 103,
    106, 107, 120, 123, 124, 125, 129, 145, 146, 148,
    179, 184, 187, 190, 199, 207
dyspepsia, 122
dysphoria, 15, 39, 62, 86
dysregulation, 164
dysthymia, 49, 59

E

ECM, 208
education, 10
educational programs, 76
EEG, xii, 190, 195, 197, 199, 200, 201, 202, 203,
    204, 205, 206, 207, 208, 209, 210
EEG activity, 210
EKG, 166
elderly, 39, 115, 151, 167, 198
electrodes, 201, 204, 206
electroencephalography, 208, 209
electrolytes, 146
electromyography, 5
electrophysiological, 199, 207, 209
electrophysiology, 191
ELISA, 214
embolism, 143
EMG, 200
emission, 208
emotional, xii, 3, 43, 69, 123, 155, 169, 170, 191,
    193
emotional disorder, 123, 155
encapsulated, 23
encoding, 192
endocrine, xi, 113, 121, 149
endocrine glands, 121
endogenous, 199
endogenous depression, 47
endoscopy, 119
endothelial cell, 118, 134, 137, 140, 142, 157, 162,
    164
endothelial cells, 118, 137, 140, 142, 157, 162, 164
endothelial dysfunction, 135, 139, 142, 144, 161,
    162
endothelium, 135, 141
endotoxemia, 121, 122, 124
endotoxins, 118, 140, 142
energy, xiii, 116, 146, 147, 199, 211, 212
energy supply, 147
England, 109
English, 200
enthusiasm, 24
environment, 87, 177, 188
environmental factors, 123, 177
environmental stimuli, 171
enzymatic, 133
enzyme-linked immunosorbent assay, 214
enzymes, 31, 127, 129, 159
epidemiology, 59, 112, 151
epidermal growth factor, 122, 155
epilepsy, 140
epinephrine, 133
epistaxis, 95
epithelium, 140
equilibrium, 198
escitalopram, 41, 42, 55
esophageal varices, 154
esophagitis, 119, 153, 156
esophagus, 115, 121, 122, 123
ester, 127
esterase, 137
esters, 127

estradiol, 149, 150
ethanol, xii, 9, 31, 33, 115, 118, 121, 122, 127, 132, 138, 139, 140, 142, 144, 147, 149, 153, 154, 155, 158, 162, 163, 164, 166, 167, 168, 169, 170, 171, 172, 173, 174, 175, 176, 177, 178, 179, 180, 181, 182, 183, 184, 185, 186, 187, 188, 189, 190, 191, 192, 193, 194, 195, 196, 219
ethanol metabolism, 118, 122, 141, 149
ethics, 35, 65, 69
ethyl alcohol, 170
Euro, 188, 193, 194, 208
European, 198
evening, 24, 87
evening news, 24
evidence, 96, 103, 104, 107, 109, 110, 111, 116, 126, 127, 152, 154
evoked potential, xiii, 198, 205, 206, 207, 210
examinations, xi, 78, 114, 121, 123
excision, 105
excitation, 3, 4, 5, 14
excitement, 199
excitotoxic, 187
exclusion, 27, 42, 98, 100, 124, 150, 213
excuse, 21
exercise, xi, 113, 126, 137, 143, 144, 146, 147, 148, 158, 166, 167, 198
exercise performance, 148, 198
expert, 23, 24, 27, 111
exposure, xii, 8, 9, 11, 15, 20, 24, 31, 42, 43, 55, 57, 120, 122, 164, 165, 166, 168, 174, 176, 181, 192, 193, 194, 197, 199, 200, 205, 206, 207
expression, 123, 133, 157, 164, 168
extracellular matrix (protein) (ECM), 208
eyes, 64, 192, 200

F

face validity, 10
factor VII, 136
factorial, 129, 130, 150
failure, 5, 32, 38, 46, 50, 100, 102, 118, 124, 135, 141, 143, 146, 148, 167, 168
false belief, 27
familial, 157
family, 41, 43, 88, 140, 198
family history, 43, 140
fasting, 126, 128, 129, 131, 146, 149
fasting glucose, 146, 149
fat, 118, 148, 167, 213, 218
fatalities, 26

fatigue, 39, 43, 199
fatty acids, 118, 147, 163
FDA, 82, 89
fear, xii, 23, 169, 171, 172, 173, 174, 176, 177, 178, 179, 180, 181, 182, 183, 184, 185, 186, 187, 188, 189, 190, 191, 192, 193, 194, 195
fee, 6
feedback, 42, 172
feeding, 212, 218, 219
feelings, 87, 199
females, 16, 115, 149, 150, 161, 213, 215
fermentation, 121
fibrin, 135, 137
fibrinogen, xi, 114, 134, 136, 137, 138, 139, 142, 161
fibrinolysis, xi, 114, 125, 134, 136, 137, 138, 139, 160, 162, 163
fibrosis, 118
finance, 126
Finland, vii, viii, 1, 2, 10, 14, 20, 21, 23, 24, 25, 34
Finns, 28
first degree relative, 130, 131
fitness, 165
flatulence, 117
flavonoids, 132
flora, 142
flow, 106, 122, 135, 146, 147, 155, 167, 198, 201, 206, 207, 208
flow rate, 122, 155
flu, 199
fluoxetine, 38, 39, 40, 43, 46, 47, 48, 50, 54, 57, 58, 79
fluvoxamine, 39, 43, 44, 47, 64, 78
focusing, 99, 103, 104, 105, 201
folate, 31
follicle-stimulating hormone, 149
follicular, 150
food, xiii, 211, 212, 214, 215, 216, 218
Food and Drug Administration (FDA), 82
food intake, xiii, 211, 212, 218
forebrain, 187
Fourier, 202
France, 99
free radical, 141
free radicals, 141
freezing, 177
frontal cortex, xii, 197, 202, 203, 204, 206
FSH, 149, 150
functional changes, xi, 114, 117, 122
functional magnetic resonance imaging, 188

funding, 28

G

G protein, 198
GABA, 52, 56, 179, 182, 184, 185, 186, 190, 191,
    193, 194
GABA$_B$, 193
GABAergic, 173, 176, 184, 186, 187, 188, 195
GABRA2, 130
Gamma, 158, 165
gamma-aminobutyric acid, 184, 192
gamma-glutamyltransferase, 124, 158, 167
gas, viii, 2, 3, 6, 7, 8, 9, 11, 12, 13, 15, 21, 26, 28,
    29, 30, 32, 35
gases, vii, viii, 1, 2, 7, 8, 9, 10, 11, 23
gastric, xi, 95, 114, 117, 118, 119, 121, 122, 123,
    125, 142, 147, 153, 154, 155, 198
gastric mucosa, 117, 118, 120, 122, 123, 125, 142,
    153
gastrin, 121, 124
gastritis, 119, 136, 153
gastroesophageal reflux, 119, 122, 155
gastroesophageal reflux disease, 119, 155
gastrointestinal, xi, 39, 95, 113, 114, 115, 117, 118,
    119, 121, 122, 123, 124, 152, 153, 154, 155
gastrointestinal bleeding, 95, 117
gastrointestinal tract, xi, 113, 114, 117, 118, 119,
    121, 122, 123, 124, 153, 154
gel, 120
gender, 96, 133, 150, 160, 165, 166
gene, 67, 128, 130, 137, 142, 143, 147, 162, 164,
    167, 192, 212, 219, 220
gene expression, 137, 162, 164, 192, 212
general anesthesia, 4
general practitioner, 115
general practitioners, 115
general surgery, 65
generalizations, 67
generation, 76, 122, 125, 134, 136, 195
genes, 128, 158, 188, 212
genetics, xii, 169, 174, 178, 179, 187
genotypes, 145, 165
Georgia, 89
geriatric, 57
Germany, 99
gestalt, 189
GGT, 124, 128, 129, 130, 131, 140, 143, 144, 146,
    148, 150, 158
glass, 134

glatiramer acetate (GA), 208
glucocorticoids, 220
glucose, 131, 143, 146, 147, 148, 167
glucose regulation, 167
glucose tolerance test, 149
glutamate, 45, 52, 182, 184, 185, 186, 189
glutamatergic, 45, 174, 176, 184
glycine, 52, 59
glycoprotein, 95, 109, 133, 135
goals, 3
gold, 5, 14, 22
gonads, 149
google, 96
government, 23
grafting, x, 94, 99, 105, 106, 109
gram-negative bacteria, 118
granules, 133
graph, 27
gravity, 156
groups, 8, 11, 13, 14, 40, 42, 46, 64, 67, 69, 70, 72,
    103, 123, 129, 150, 178
growth, 122, 142, 154, 155
growth factor, 122, 155
guidance, 5, 95
guidelines, 35, 77, 96, 105
guilt, 16
gut, 118, 123, 124, 152, 153, 154

H

H. pylori, 120, 122, 123, 154
habituation, vii, 52, 90, 208
haemostasis, 112, 132, 133
half-life, 13, 29, 38, 39, 41, 63, 104, 106
hallucinations, x, 63, 81, 87, 88, 116
hands, vii, 1, 4, 5, 6, 10, 24, 25, 28, 29
happiness, 199
harmful effects, xii, 114, 116
Harvard, 14, 56
Hawaii, 89
hazards, x, 93, 95, 96, 99, 100, 104
HDL, xi, 114, 116, 118, 125, 126, 127, 128, 129,
    131, 139, 157
headache, 40, 44, 74, 86, 199, 206, 208
healing, 100, 102
health, xi, xii, 3, 4, 14, 21, 23, 25, 69, 78, 91, 113,
    114, 141, 146, 147, 153, 159, 167
Health and Human Services, 84, 90
health care, 14, 114
health care costs, 114

health problems, 115, 146

heart, xi, xiii, 67, 93, 94, 108, 109, 110, 111, 112, 114, 115, 123, 125, 126, 135, 141, 143, 144, 145, 146, 147, 148, 151, 152, 155, 156, 157, 158, 159, 160, 161, 162, 163, 165, 166, 167, 200, 209, 211, 212, 214

heart attack, 110

heart disease, 94, 109, 111, 115, 151, 156, 157, 158, 161, 163, 166

heart failure, 67, 109, 135, 141, 143, 146, 148, 167

heart rate (HR), xi, xiii, 113, 114, 123, 143, 145, 146, 155, 165, 166, 167, 200, 209, 212, 214

Heart rate variability (HRV), 144, 166

heartburn, 117

heavy drinkers, 118, 120, 126, 128, 129, 131, 138, 141, 142, 154, 164

heavy drinking, 115, 130, 131, 142

heavy smoking, 124

height, xiii, 212, 213, 214

Helicobacter pylori, xi, 114, 117, 120, 125, 142, 153, 154, 156, 166

hematocrit, 146, 148

hematopoietic, xiii, 211

hematopoietic stem cell, xiii, 211

hematopoietic stem cells, xiii, 211

hematuria, 95

hemisphere, 21

hemodynamics, 145

hemorrhage, 95, 99, 119

hemorrhagic stroke, 133

hemostasis, 105, 133, 136, 160, 161

hemostatic, 125, 134, 160, 161

hepatitis, 35, 118, 168

hepatitis a, 118

hepatocellular, 118

hepatocytes, 118

hepatomegaly, 118

hepatotoxicity, 159, 219

heroin, 19, 35, 190

heterogeneity, 97, 103, 104

heterogeneous, 96

heterozygotes, 143, 145

high density lipoprotein, 152

high risk, x, 93, 94, 95, 102, 104, 107, 108

high-density lipoprotein, 163

high-risk, 127, 156

hip, 126, 143

hippocampal, 173, 176, 188, 189, 191, 192, 193, 195

hippocampus, xiii, 56, 170, 172, 173, 176, 180, 184, 185, 189, 191, 192, 193, 194, 195, 211

hips, 139

histidine, 59

homeostasis, 17, 149, 165

homework, 42

homocysteine, 129

homogeneity, 106

homogenous, 96

homologous, 202

hormone, xiii, 149, 168, 211, 212

hormones, xi, xiii, 60, 114, 149, 150, 211, 212

hospital, ix, 62, 64, 65, 66, 67, 69, 76, 77, 99, 101, 102, 140, 151

hospitalization, 38, 67

hospitalizations, 151

hospitalized, 87, 140, 143

hospitals, ix, 62, 67, 76, 115

host, 119

hostility, 199

HPA, 52

HPA axis, 52

HRV, 124, 143, 144, 146, 147

human, 34, 86, 97, 133, 137, 138, 139, 142, 155, 157, 159, 164, 171, 181, 188, 190, 191, 194, 208, 209, 210, 219

human brain, 34

human subjects, 209

humans, 86, 91, 153, 154, 155, 191, 209, 220

hydro, 115

hydrochloric acid, 120, 121

hydrophilic, 115

hyperactivity, 43, 56, 63, 116

hypercholesterolemia, 158

hyperlipidemia, 69, 118, 126, 129, 138, 146, 148, 156

hypersensitive, 122

hypersensitivity, 62

hypersplenism, 132

hypertension, 69, 115, 121, 126, 138, 143, 144, 146, 147, 148, 165, 166, 167

hypertensive, 123

hypertrophy, 143

hypnotic, 62, 63, 65, 194

hypothalamic, xiii, 52, 150, 168, 211, 212, 218, 219, 220

hypothalamic receptors, xiii, 211

hypothalamic-pituitary-adrenal axis, xiii, 212

hypothalamus, 212

hypothesis, xiii, 6, 7, 32, 38, 40, 44, 45, 69, 96, 103, 104, 107, 127, 130, 140, 144, 145, 159, 206, 211, 213, 218 hypothyroidism, 130

I

ICD, 67, 69, 199, 209
id, 8, 16, 23, 45, 69, 91, 104, 206
identification, 131, 171
IGF, xiii, 211, 212
IL-6, 130, 141
illusion, 3
illusions, 116
imaging, 188, 209
imbalances, 52
immobilization, 133, 136
immune function, xiii, 211, 212
immune response, 130
immunological, 139
immunomodulation, 152
immunomodulator, 142
impairments, xii, 169, 170, 174, 179, 180, 181, 182
implementation, 30
impulsiveness, 74, 214
in vitro, 105, 137, 164, 194
in vivo, xi, 59, 105, 114, 134, 136, 137, 187, 188, 192, 194
inactivation, 172, 192
inactive, 148
incidence, x, 39, 41, 48, 73, 82, 89, 94, 101, 105, 108, 111, 115, 120, 209
independent variable, 150
India, 83, 86, 91
Indian, 159
indication, 14, 28, 96
indicators, 120, 125
indices, 143, 145, 159, 165, 193
indirect effect, 213
individual differences, 149
induction, 147, 195
inductor, 139
industry, 39
infants, 41
infarction, 97, 98, 99, 100, 101, 102, 108, 109, 156, 157, 160, 167
infection, xi, 15, 114, 117, 120, 125, 153, 154, 156
infertility, 150
inflammation, 117, 118, 119, 123, 164, 167
inflammatory, 105, 120, 121, 124, 130, 132, 139, 140, 141, 162, 164
inflammatory disease, 141

influence, xi, 114, 116, 117, 120, 122, 123, 124, 126, 127, 128, 129, 130, 131, 134, 136, 139, 140, 142, 143, 144, 145, 146, 147, 149, 153, 160, 167
informed consent, 11, 12
ingestion, 82, 86, 118, 167, 194, 198, 199, 206
inhalation, vii, 1
inhibition, 35, 44, 48, 58, 138, 142, 163, 173, 186, 187, 191, 194
inhibitor, ix, xi, 31, 48, 54, 55, 61, 71, 78, 79, 114, 134, 135, 137, 139, 162, 163
inhibitors, viii, ix, 37, 38, 41, 42, 44, 51, 54, 55, 57, 59, 62, 76, 77, 78, 79, 95, 109, 134, 135, 137, 139, 161
inhibitory, 44, 45, 51, 52, 123, 133, 171, 184, 191, 194, 195, 198
inhibitory effect, 45, 51, 52, 133
initiation, 50, 59, 118
injection, 187
injections, 193
injuries, 114
injury, 115, 117, 118, 120, 121, 124, 125, 128, 132, 133, 136, 140, 142, 147, 149, 150, 154
iNOS, 139
insects, 88
insight, 207
insomnia, 39, 40, 41, 53, 63, 86, 87, 88, 116
institutions, 21, 28, 67, 74
insulin, xiii, 67, 146, 148, 162, 164, 168, 211, 212, 214, 215, 217, 218, 220
insulin resistance, 146, 148
insulin sensitivity, 148, 164, 168
insurance, vii, 2, 6
integrity, 119, 120, 140, 154
intensity, 4, 62, 63, 106, 119, 120, 123, 125, 126, 142, 177
intensive care unit, 115, 151
interaction, 118, 152
interaction process, 118
interactions, 77, 96, 138, 185, 189, 193, 195
intercellular adhesion molecule, 157
interleukin-1, 156
interleukin-6, 141, 152
interleukin-8, 156, 164
internal validity, 102
International Classification of Diseases, 199
internet, 87
internists, ix, 62, 64, 67, 73, 77
interpretation, 122, 135, 138, 145, 152
interrelations, 124
interrelationships, 149

interval, x, 94, 103, 104, 106, 121, 145, 146, 148, 152

intervention, 14, 20, 51, 68, 69, 95, 99, 101, 103, 105, 107, 109, 131, 160

interview, 55, 69, 77, 87, 89

interviews, 69, 73

intestine, 128, 155, 164

intoxication, 82, 163, 170, 187, 190, 194, 199

intracranial, 95, 105

intraoperative, 105

intravascular, 125, 135, 136

intravenous (IV), 9, 95, 208, 209

intrinsic, 137, 138

invasive, x, 93, 95, 104, 106, 124

irritability, 39, 41, 43, 62, 74, 86, 199

irritable bowel disease, 122

irritable bowel syndrome, 155

ischaemia, 136, 147, 166

ischaemic heart disease, 158

ischemia, 100, 101, 108

ischemic, 133, 147

ischemic stroke, 133

isoforms, 132, 140

Italy, 37, 93, 99, 107, 211

J

JAMA, 57, 77, 78, 91, 108, 109, 110, 112, 151, 156, 162

Japan, ix, 61, 64, 65, 67, 76, 77

Japanese, ix, 62, 64, 65, 66, 67, 73, 74, 76, 77, 78, 145, 163, 165

Jefferson, 85, 90

journalists, 24

Jun, 219

K

kappa, 17, 34

Kentucky, 89, 90

knowledge, xi, 113

Korean, 168

L

labour, 3

Lactobacillus, 159

Langerhans cells (LC), 209

language, x, 94, 96

laryngospasm, 4

larynx, 115

latency, 171, 205

later life, 46

laughing, 32, 33

LDL, xi, 114, 116, 118, 125, 126, 127, 128, 129, 131, 139, 141, 146, 156

lead, 100, 105, 115, 116, 118, 134, 135

learning, xii, 169, 170, 171, 172, 173, 174, 176, 177, 178, 179, 181, 182, 183, 184, 185, 186, 189, 190, 191, 192, 193, 195

learning process, 173

learning task, 171, 185, 186

lecithin, 127

left ventricular, 143, 166

leptin, xiii, 211, 212, 213, 214, 215, 216, 217, 218, 219, 220

lesions, 119, 122, 151, 187, 188, 191

lethargy, xii, 39, 197

leukocytes, 139

licensing, 85

life expectancy, 159

life style, 132

life-threatening, xi, 113

lifetime, 148, 213

likelihood, 39, 40, 46, 48, 50, 53, 104

limitation, 43, 124, 143, 201

limitations, 74, 105, 141, 201

linear, 115, 129, 150

links, 115, 156

lipase, 127

lipemia, 127, 148, 157, 158, 167

lipid, 126, 127, 129, 130, 131, 133, 152, 156, 157, 160

lipid peroxidation, 133

lipid profile, 130

lipids, 118, 125, 126, 127, 128, 129, 130, 131, 133, 138, 139, 142, 143, 148, 149, 156, 157, 159, 162, 218

lipophilic, 115

lipopolysaccharide, 118, 152

lipopolysaccharides, 152

lipoprotein, 118, 127, 134, 137, 139, 156, 157, 158, 159, 163

lipoproteins, 118, 119, 127, 128, 129, 149, 152, 157, 160, 163

liquids, 134

literature, 199, 205

lithium, 48, 49, 58, 129

lithotripsy, 112

liver, xi, xiii, 67, 83, 113, 114, 115, 117, 118, 119, 121, 124, 125, 128, 129, 131, 132, 134, 136, 141, 142, 147, 148, 149, 150, 152, 154, 159, 160, 164, 168, 211, 213, 214, 220
liver cells, 118
liver cirrhosis, 118
liver damage, 213
liver disease, 115, 118, 125, 136, 141, 147, 152, 154, 159, 160
liver enzymes, 129, 159
liver failure, 124, 168
liver function tests, xi, 114, 118, 124, 131, 132, 134, 149
locomotion, 170, 178
locomotor activity, 178, 208
locus, 44, 56, 123
London, 76
long period, 125, 145, 179
long-term memory, 171, 189, 190
long-term potentiation, 34, 187, 193, 194, 195
Los Angeles, 85, 119
loss of control, 85
losses, 115
Louisiana, 85
lovastatin, 158
low risk, 95, 102, 106
low-density, 118, 157
low-density lipoprotein, 157
low-dose aspirin, 105, 110, 111
lower esophageal sphincter, 122, 124
LPS, 118, 119, 142
LTP, 194
lumen, 117, 121, 122
lung, 67
luteinizing hormone, 149
lymphocytosis, 15

M

machinery, 115
macrophage, 142
macrophages, 118, 152
magnetic resonance imaging, 188
magnetic resonance spectroscopy (MRS), 207
maintenance, 4, 38, 40, 48, 49, 53, 56, 57, 58, 134
major depression, viii, ix, 37, 42, 46, 48, 49, 50, 52, 53, 56, 59, 61, 64, 68, 69, 70, 73, 78
major depressive disorder, 41, 42, 43, 44, 55, 57, 59
males, 16, 95, 115, 126, 145, 149, 150, 161, 213, 215
malignant, 45, 67

malondialdehyde (MDA), 164
malpractice, 24
management, x, 30, 31, 34, 46, 56, 93, 94, 104, 106, 107, 115, 121
mania, 38, 47, 54, 55, 58
manic, 44, 48, 58
manic episode, 48
manual workers, 166
MAO, 38, 133
marijuana, 85
market, 74
marketing, 39, 55, 86
marrow, 132
mask, 136
mass, 127, 131, 134, 137, 138, 144
Massachusetts, 39, 89
MAST, 142
mast cell, 139
mast cells, 139
maternal, 41, 55
MDA, 45
meals, 128, 148, 155, 167
mean, xii, 197, 198, 201, 202, 204, 206
measurement, 42
measures, 159, 185, 201, 204, 205, 206, 207, 210
media, 23, 24, 25, 27, 28
median, 97, 101
mediation, 123, 219
mediators, 123
medical care, 78, 126
medication, 5, 12, 22, 38, 39, 40, 46, 50, 74, 82, 84, 87
medications, viii, ix, 2, 9, 22, 38, 40, 43, 47, 59, 61, 62, 63, 74, 81, 85, 112, 198
medicine, ix, 14, 22, 53, 62, 64, 65, 66, 67, 69, 72, 73, 74, 77, 78, 107, 108
MEDLINE, 112
melanin, xiii, 211, 212
membership, 64
memory, ix, xii, 29, 61, 62, 64, 116, 169, 170, 171, 172, 173, 174, 176, 178, 184, 185, 186, 187, 188, 189, 190, 191, 192, 193, 195
memory deficits, 172, 185, 186, 187
memory performance, 192
memory processes, 184, 191, 192
men, 65, 69, 94, 108, 111, 133, 143, 144, 145, 148, 151, 157, 158, 161, 162, 163, 165, 166, 168
menstrual cycle, 149, 150
menstruation, 150
mental disorder, 63, 76, 77, 116, 151

mental health, 53, 69, 76

mental illness, 87

mental load, 210

meta-analysis, x, 93, 94, 96, 101, 103, 104, 107, 108, 109, 115, 129, 151, 167, 192

metabolic, xi, xiii, 113, 114, 116, 118, 126, 129, 138, 143, 144, 147, 148, 163, 165, 167, 168, 208, 211, 213, 214

metabolic disturbances, 118

metabolic pathways, 129

metabolic syndrome, 143, 144, 148, 168

metabolism, 38, 116, 118, 122, 127, 129, 132, 133, 134, 141, 146, 147, 148, 149, 158, 164, 213

metabolite, ix, 48, 81, 82, 83, 84, 88, 122, 124

metabolites, xi, xii, 39, 52, 56, 83, 88, 114, 123, 135, 140, 141, 143, 163, 164, 208

metallic taste, 62

methodology, 167

metropolitan area, 64

metyrapone test, 58

Mexican, 85

Mexico, 82, 85, 89

mg, xii, 197, 198, 199, 200, 201, 209

mice, 16, 30, 158, 163, 171, 177, 178, 187, 188, 189, 190, 191, 195, 219, 220

Michigan Alcoholism Screening Test, 140, 142

microcirculation, 120

microorganism, 120

microorganisms, 121

middle-aged, 161, 162, 165, 166, 167

migraine, 198, 205, 206

migration, 139

milnacipran, 64

misconception, 3

misconceptions, 3

misidentified, 53

misleading, 53

Mississippi, 81, 85, 91, 197

mitochondria, 147

mitochondrial, 118

MK-80, 185, 187, 190

modalities, 53, 213

modality, 46

models, xii, 152, 169, 171

modulation, 7, 162, 163, 164, 172, 189, 193, 195

molecular changes, 179, 182

molecular mechanisms, 139

molecules, 141, 142, 159

monitoring, 121, 123, 125, 143

monkeys, 166

monoamine oxidase, 48, 54, 58, 133, 160

monocyte, 142

monocytes, 118, 142, 152, 164

mood, 3, 38, 39, 42, 43, 47, 48, 49, 54, 156, 199, 209

mood disorder, 42, 47, 49

morbidity, 94, 115, 126, 144, 151

morning, 200, 209

morphine, 16, 30, 158

morphological, xi, 113, 114, 119, 125, 126, 139, 155

morphology, 117, 120, 146

mortality, 94, 99, 101, 102, 105, 108, 109, 110, 115, 116, 125, 126, 127, 130, 136, 138, 144, 151, 157, 158, 159, 160, 161

mortality rate, 116

MOS, 78

motion, 86

motivation, 146, 199

motor activity, 121, 200

motor control, 189

motor function, 122

motor vehicle crashes, 133

mouse, 178, 188

mouth, 64

movement, 136

mRNA, 182, 220

mucosa, 117, 118, 120, 122, 123, 125, 142, 153

mucosal barrier, 120

multiple factors, xii, 169

multiple regression analysis, 125, 140, 143

multivariate, 142, 153

muscarinic receptor, 44

muscle, viii, ix, x, xii, 5, 61, 62, 64, 81, 82, 83, 87, 88, 90, 139, 146, 197, 199

muscle cells, 139

muscle relaxant, viii, 61, 62

muscle relaxation, 83

muscle spasms, 82

muscles, 116, 147

musculoskeletal, 82

music, 87

mutant, 189

mutation, 143, 145

myalgia, 87

myocardial infarction, 67, 97, 98, 99, 100, 101, 102, 108, 146, 147, 156, 157, 160, 167

myoclonus, 41

myocyte, 139

N

NADH, 118
naloxone, 19, 32
narcotic, 35
narcotics, 87
National Academy of Sciences, 163
natural, 46, 48
nausea, xii, 39, 40, 62, 63, 72, 74, 86, 87, 116, 117, 121, 197, 199
necrosis, 124, 130, 141, 152, 156, 164, 167
needles, 64
needs, 125, 136, 141
negative attitudes, 3
negative relation, 126, 135, 139
neonatal, 176, 195
neonates, 41
neoplasm, 67
neoplastic, 127
nerve, xi, 114, 116, 126, 145, 146, 147
nervous system, xi, 67, 113, 114, 116, 123, 144, 145, 146, 147, 155
nervousness, 40, 199
Netherlands, 93
network, 212
neural function, xii, 169, 186
neural mechanisms, 192
neural network, 186
neural networks, 186
neuroadaptation, 189
neurodegeneration, 189
neuroendocrine, xiii, 211
neurogenesis, 192
neurohormonal, 167
neurokinin, 123
neuroleptic, 54
neuroleptics, 213
neurons, 44, 52, 56, 83, 189, 192, 198
Neuropeptide Y, xiii, 211, 212
neuropeptides, xiii, 211, 212, 219
neuroprotective, 29
neuropsychiatry, 32
neurotic, 55, 64
neurotoxic, 187
neurotransmission, 52, 123, 194
neurotransmitter, 52, 123, 139, 141, 172, 173, 184, 185, 186
neurotransmitters, 52, 118, 184
neutralization, 118
neutrophils, 152

New England, 109
New Jersey, 82
New Mexico, 89
New York, 29, 30, 31, 32, 33, 34, 35, 190, 195, 208, 209
NGO, 15
nicotinamide, 118
nicotine, vii, 2, 6, 7, 17, 18, 19, 20, 30, 34, 138, 139, 189, 190, 193, 195, 200, 209, 213
nitrate, 59, 164
nitrates, 155
nitric oxide (NO), xi, xii, 114, 123, 125, 135, 139, 140, 141, 143, 155, 156, 163, 164
nitric oxide synthase, 139, 163, 164
nitrogen, 52
nitrous oxide, vii, 1, 2, 3, 4, 5, 6, 7, 8, 9, 12, 13, 14, 15, 16, 17, 20, 21, 22, 23, 25, 26, 27, 28, 29, 30, 31, 32, 33, 34, 35
NMDA, 45, 56, 138, 163, 179, 188, 190, 191, 193, 194, 195, 196
NMDA receptors, 163, 188, 193, 194, 196
N-methyl-D-aspartate, 45, 138, 190
nociception, 123
noise, 64, 74
non-human, 97
non-pharmacological, 131, 143
non-steroidal anti-inflammatory drugs, 105
noradrenaline, ix, 62, 148
norepinephrine, 41, 44, 56, 212
normal, xii, 44, 83, 121, 122, 123, 127, 132, 134, 148, 149, 150, 155, 197, 199, 200, 201, 205, 210, 218, 220
normalization, 131, 207
North America, 152, 198
Norway, 86
NOS, 139, 140
NR2B, 163
nuclei, 192
nucleus, 6, 19, 172, 173, 187, 192
nucleus accumbens, 6, 19
nurse, vii, 1, 7, 9, 11
nurses, viii, 2, 6, 9, 10
nursing, 9
nutrition, xi, 114
nutritional deficiencies, 115

O

obese, 219, 220
obesity, 146, 148, 162, 164

observations, 9, 14, 19, 45, 47, 48, 111, 124, 128, 131, 133, 134, 138, 139, 140, 143, 144, 150
obsessive-compulsive disorder, 42, 50, 58, 59
occipital, 200, 202
occlusion, 142
occupational, 40, 63, 116, 167
odds ratio, 73, 97, 148
Oklahoma, 89
olanzapine, 56, 85, 87
old age, 90
omeprazole, 154
operator, 7
opiates, 83, 87, 159
opioid, viii, 2, 6, 7, 15, 16, 18, 19, 29, 30, 31, 32, 33, 34, 35, 123, 190
opioids, vii, 2, 6, 7, 17, 20, 29, 89, 129, 139
opposition, vii, 1, 6, 23, 24, 25, 27, 28, 34, 136
oral, 13, 65, 82, 105, 109, 110, 115, 182, 183, 198
oral cavity, 115
organ, xi, 113, 115, 125, 132, 148, 149
organic, 12, 118
organic disease, 118
orthostatic hypotension, 82
outpatient, 14, 16, 20, 34
outpatients, viii, 2, 9, 10, 14, 20, 42, 59, 64, 65, 67, 69, 74, 76, 77
output, 120, 121, 122, 154
ovaries, xiii, 211
overproduction, 141
ovulation, 150
oxidation, 118, 139
oxidative stress, 118, 162, 213
oxide, vii, xii, 1, 2, 3, 4, 5, 6, 7, 8, 9, 12, 13, 14, 15, 16, 17, 20, 21, 22, 23, 25, 26, 27, 28, 29, 30, 31, 32, 33, 34, 35, 52, 114, 123, 125, 135, 139, 140, 141, 143, 148, 155, 156, 163, 164
oxygen, vii, viii, 1, 2, 3, 4, 5, 7, 8, 11, 12, 15, 16, 18, 19, 20, 21, 27, 30, 31, 32, 33, 34, 146, 147

P

P300, xiii, 152, 198, 205, 206, 210
paclitaxel, 107
PAI-1, xi, 114, 134, 135, 137, 138, 139, 140, 144, 162
pain, xii, 15, 33, 69, 82, 86, 117, 121, 122, 123, 136, 166, 180, 189, 197, 199
palpitations, 87, 199
PAN, vii, viii, 1, 2, 3, 4, 5, 6, 7, 8, 9, 10, 11, 12, 13, 14, 15, 16, 17, 18, 19, 20, 21, 22, 23, 24, 25, 26, 27, 28, 29, 30, 33, 34
pancreas, xi, xiii, 113, 117, 128, 211
pancreatitis, xi, 114, 115, 136, 141, 162
panic attack, 39, 57
panic disorder, 42, 43, 44, 47, 54, 55, 57, 62, 76, 78, 79, 200, 209
panic symptoms, 44
paradox, 21, 130
paradoxical, viii, 37, 47, 53
paralysis, 116
parameter, 124, 127, 148, 216
paraoxonase, 127
parasympathetic, xiii, 143, 144, 145, 211, 212
parenteral, 107
parents, 157
paresthesias, 39, 62
parkinsonism, 39
paroxetine, 38, 39, 40, 41, 42, 43, 44, 45, 54, 55, 64, 68, 69, 72, 73, 74, 77, 78, 79
paroxysmal, xiii, 197, 205, 210
particles, 127
passive, xii, 169, 171, 172, 173, 174, 177, 178, 179, 180, 182, 183, 184, 185, 186, 187, 188, 189, 190, 191, 192, 193, 195
pathogenesis, xi, 6, 16, 18, 19, 48, 114, 118, 121, 122, 124, 127, 131, 132, 137, 138, 141, 151
pathology, 12, 120
pathophysiological, 38, 51, 122, 132, 133
pathways, 51, 118, 129, 137, 138, 157
patient management, 34
patterning, 188
Pavlovian, 171, 190, 195
Pavlovian conditioning, 190
peak concentration, 13
peers, 28
peptic ulcer, 95, 136
peptide, 147, 155, 156, 167, 212
peptides, 212
perception, 53, 123, 189
perceptions, 2, 3, 69
performance, 97, 102, 148, 170, 177, 187, 190, 192, 193, 198, 200, 210
perfusion, 146
perinatal, 41
peripheral arterial disease, 112
peripheral blood, 146, 152
peripheral nervous system, 123
peristalsis, 122, 142

permeability, 120, 124, 142

permit, 207

peroxidation, 118, 133

peroxisomes, 118

personal, 3, 5, 22, 26, 28, 85, 130, 131, 136

personal communication, 5, 22, 26

personal history, 130, 131, 136

perspective, 159

perturbation, 185

PET, 205

pH, xi, 114, 117, 119, 121, 122, 123, 125, 142, 153, 154

pH values, 121

pharmaceutical, 20, 21, 28, 39, 53, 74, 85, 152

pharmaceutical industry, 39

pharmacies, 85

pharmacists, 85

pharmacokinetic, 13, 38, 48, 77

pharmacokinetics, 22, 33, 209

pharmacological, viii, 2, 3, 10, 21, 22, 30, 31, 34, 37, 41, 48, 50, 51, 56, 131, 137, 198, 199, 209

pharmacological treatment, 51

pharmacology, 35, 82, 208

pharmacotherapy, xi, 74, 109, 114, 128, 129, 141, 143

pharynx, 115

phenotype, 127, 156, 157

phenotypes, 157, 188

Philadelphia, 33, 169

physical activity, 126, 131, 146, 148

physical exercise, 126

physical fitness, 165

physicians, viii, ix, 2, 10, 21, 22, 62, 64, 67, 72, 76, 83, 84, 85, 87

physiological, vii, xii, 29, 123, 152, 167, 190, 195, 197, 198, 200, 207, 218

physiology, 210

pilot study, 77, 152

pituitary, xi, xiii, 52, 114, 128, 130, 149, 150, 168, 211, 212, 218, 220

placebo, 8, 10, 11, 12, 13, 14, 16, 20, 26, 29, 34, 39, 40, 41, 42, 46, 47, 48, 49, 55, 56, 59, 70, 74, 77, 78, 79, 95, 129, 158, 198, 199, 201, 207

planning, 74

plaque, 142

plasma, xi, xii, xiii, 59, 114, 116, 117, 118, 119, 123, 124, 125, 126, 127, 128, 129, 130, 131, 133, 134, 135, 136, 137, 138, 139, 140, 142, 143, 146, 148, 149, 155, 157, 158, 160, 161, 162, 163, 164, 198, 208, 211, 212, 213, 214, 215, 218, 219, 220

plasma levels, 213

plasma proteins, 127, 161

plasminogen, xi, 114, 134, 135, 137, 139, 161, 162, 163

plastic, 65

plastic surgery, 65

plasticity, 52, 188

platelet, 105, 106, 109, 116, 132, 133, 134, 135, 160, 162

platelet aggregation, 162

platelets, xi, xii, 104, 114, 125, 132, 133, 134, 135, 136, 137, 138, 139, 142, 146, 148

play, 122, 132, 135, 141, 178

pneumonia, 15

Poland, 113

polarity, 48

politics, 23

polymorphism, 128, 130, 142, 159

polymorphisms, 128, 164

polypeptide, 123

polyphenols, 133, 160

poor, 15, 141

poor health, 141

population, 38, 67, 78, 101, 111, 115, 117, 120, 122, 136, 144, 153, 154, 155, 158, 167, 170, 206, 217, 218

portal hypertension, 147, 167

ports, 12

positive correlation, 130, 140

positive relation, 68

positive relationship, 68

positron, 208

post traumatic stress disorder, 122

posterior cortex, 204, 206

postoperative, 105, 108

postsynaptic, 44, 52

poverty, 120

power, xii, 23, 96, 104, 120, 197, 199, 200, 201, 202, 203, 204, 205, 206, 209, 210

preclinical, 52

pre-clinical, 199

predictors, xii, 96, 108, 110, 111, 114, 119, 122, 131, 135, 138, 214

preference, 16, 17, 30, 174, 189, 193

prefrontal cortex, 172, 173, 176

pregnancy, 41

prejudice, 3

pressure, xiii, 95, 116, 122, 126, 131, 138, 139, 143, 144, 146, 157, 158, 159, 165, 166, 167, 198, 200, 212, 214

prevention, x, 15, 20, 53, 56, 94, 95, 97, 99, 103, 104, 108, 109, 110, 111, 127, 137, 141, 156, 163, 218
primary care, ix, 41, 53, 55, 62, 67, 68, 77, 82
primary medical care, 78
primates, 6
prisoners, 86, 92
private, 19, 26
private practice, 19
pro-atherogenic, xi, 114
probation, 85
probe, 33, 35
probiotics, 159
producers, 150
production, 88, 124, 125, 142, 156, 164, 165
progenitor cells, 180
progesterone, 149, 150
prognosis, 45
prognostic value, 145
program, ix, 12, 61, 63, 68, 69, 70, 71, 72, 73, 74, 76, 77, 87, 88
pro-inflammatory, 124, 167
prolactin, 149, 150
proliferation, 139, 142
promote, 114
promoter, 218, 219
propaganda, 53
propagation, 23
prophylactic, 48, 58, 126, 127
prophylaxis, 56, 58, 143
prostate, 105
prostatectomy, 105, 111
protection, 133, 163
protective mechanisms, 156
protective role, x, 93
protein, xiii, 118, 122, 127, 134, 135, 138, 152, 162, 179, 195, 198, 211, 212, 219, 220
protein synthesis, 179, 195
proteins, 52, 118, 128, 133, 149, 161
prothrombin, 134, 161
protocol, 13, 25, 42, 69, 72, 180, 187, 201, 207
protocols, 67, 179
psychiatric disorder, 31, 43, 59, 127
psychiatric disorders, 31, 59, 127
psychiatrist, 42, 43, 53
psychiatrists, 42
psychoactive, xii, 197, 198
psychoactive drug, 52, 60
psychological problems, 67
psychologist, 42

psychopathology, 191
psychopharmacological, 209
psychopharmacology, 209
psychophysiological, 210
psychosis, 39
psychosocial factors, 53
psychosomatic, xi, 61, 65, 73, 78, 113, 122, 123
psychostimulants, 139, 209
psychotherapy, 49, 141
psychotic symptoms, 88
psychotropic drug, 43, 56, 139
psychotropic drugs, 43, 139
psychotropic medications, 38
public, ix, 62, 67
public health, ix, 62, 67
pulmonary hypertension, 121, 147
pulse, 63, 116, 149
punishment, 195
pyramidal cells, 191

Q

qualitative differences, 208
quality of life, 69, 115, 155
quercetin, 133
questionnaire, 64, 69, 142
questionnaires, 72

R

R and D, 78
race, 161, 176
random, x, 11, 94, 97, 101, 103, 104
range, 4, 16, 19, 39, 44, 83, 97, 99, 101, 121, 123, 126, 134, 150, 170, 177, 178, 181, 200, 218
rat, 56, 168, 187, 188, 191, 192, 193, 194
rating scale, 55, 78
ratings, 13, 75
rats, 16, 17, 31, 33, 133, 143, 163, 165, 171, 176, 177, 178, 183, 188, 189, 191, 192, 193, 194, 195
reactant, 118
reaction time, 191
reactivity, 144, 165
reading, 53
reasoning, 9, 64
recall, 170, 173, 174, 177
receptor, 208
receptor agonist, 184

receptors, xiii, 44, 45, 51, 59, 83, 123, 129, 134, 147, 148, 149, 163, 174, 185, 186, 188, 189, 190, 193, 194, 195, 196, 198, 208, 211
recovery, viii, 2, 10, 16, 46, 48, 50, 57, 59, 60, 116, 183
recreational, xii, 115, 169
rectum, 115
recurrence, 38, 46, 58, 62, 88
red wine, 130, 133, 138, 142, 145, 159, 160, 162, 163
reduction, ix, xii, 15, 16, 61, 63, 69, 70, 71, 72, 116, 120, 126, 129, 143, 149, 158, 191, 197, 199, 200, 213, 218
reflexes, 4
reflux esophagitis, 156
refractoriness, 49, 54, 58
refractory, 48, 49, 50, 51, 59, 143
regional, 195
registered nurses, 6
regression, 72, 73, 96, 125, 140, 143
regression analysis, 72, 73, 125, 140, 143
regression method, 140
regular, 63, 119, 122, 126, 131, 133, 170, 199
regulation, 44, 52, 119, 139, 141, 142, 144, 146, 147, 149, 162, 167, 185, 186, 206, 212, 219, 220
rehabilitation, viii, 2, 10, 30, 65
rehabilitation program, 30
reinforcement, 209
rejection, 2
relapse, viii, xi, xii, 20, 37, 38, 43, 45, 46, 47, 48, 50, 51, 52, 53, 56, 57, 59, 113, 114, 116, 123, 126, 129, 131, 137, 140, 141, 143, 144, 164, 214, 218, 220
relapses, xiii, 20, 211, 213, 218
relationship, 38, 47, 64, 68, 74, 115, 120, 125, 126, 150, 154, 159, 160, 194
relationships, xi, 114, 115, 119, 124, 126, 127, 130, 133, 134, 136, 138, 139, 140, 144, 145, 147, 154, 159, 165
relatives, 130, 131
relaxation, 4, 6, 8, 83, 85, 139, 144, 200
relevance, 207
reliability, 63, 220
remission, 42, 46, 48, 50, 51, 57
renal, 65, 67, 100, 102, 214
renal disease, 65
renal failure, 100, 102
renal function, 214
reperfusion, 160

research, vii, 1, 3, 22, 26, 27, 28, 29, 50, 51, 53, 56, 72, 74, 78, 88, 93, 105, 113, 124, 169, 171, 172, 177, 179, 183, 184, 185, 186, 197, 199, 207, 213
research funding, 28
researchers, 3
resilience, 52
resins, 129
resistance, viii, 10, 27, 37, 38, 45, 49, 50, 52, 59, 132, 146, 148
resolution, 88, 120
resources, 19, 110
respiratory, 41, 139, 146, 198
response, 207, 208, 210
responsiveness, 49
restenosis, 135, 142
retention, 191, 192, 193
reticulum, 118, 147
returns, 206
revascularization, x, 94
rewards, xiii, 211
rhinorrhea, 199
rhythm, xii, 126, 144, 145, 146, 147, 197, 204, 206
risk, ix, x, xi, 38, 41, 46, 47, 81, 82, 89, 93, 94, 95, 96, 97, 98, 99, 100, 101, 102, 103, 104, 105, 106, 107, 108, 109, 110, 111, 114, 115, 116, 118, 125, 126, 127, 128, 129, 131, 132, 133, 134, 135, 136, 137, 138, 139, 141, 143, 144, 145, 146, 148, 151, 155, 156, 157, 158, 159, 160, 161, 162, 163, 165, 166, 167, 168, 178, 218
risk factors, xi, 114, 118, 126, 130, 131, 138, 143, 144, 148, 151, 156, 159, 161, 162, 163, 165, 167, 178, 218
risks, 62, 97, 99, 105, 106, 109
road map, 51
rodents, 6, 20, 192
Rome, 93, 211, 213
Russian, 209
rye, 127

S

SAD, 42
safety, 20, 21, 41, 55, 76, 95, 105, 110, 132
SAI, 40
sales, 64
saliva, 122, 124, 155
sample, xiii, 12, 18, 50, 65, 68, 69, 72, 73, 77, 97, 120, 153, 212, 213, 215, 218
SAS, 65, 72, 77
savings, viii, 2

SBU, 30
scavenger, 128
schemas, 35
schizophrenia, 35, 42, 55, 58
Schmid, 110
science, 199
scientific knowledge, 3
scientists, 3, 26, 200
scores, ix, 16, 17, 18, 40, 42, 46, 61, 72, 73, 123
search, 14, 96, 112
searches, 96, 98
secretin, 124
secretion, 120, 121, 124, 125, 128, 135, 139, 140,
    142, 147, 149, 150, 154, 168
sedation, vii, 1, 3, 4, 5, 8, 13, 30, 32, 35, 83, 115
sedative, viii, ix, 2, 7, 9, 15, 19, 21, 61, 62, 63, 81
sedative medication, viii, 2, 9, 15
sedatives, 9, 19, 84
seizure, 63, 194
seizures, 41, 88, 115, 138, 163, 190
selecting, 104
selective serotonin reuptake inhibitor, viii, ix, 37, 42,
    54, 55, 59, 61, 62, 77, 78, 79
self-report, 69
sensations, 78
sensitivity, 48, 52, 55, 56, 60, 109, 123, 149, 164,
    168, 178, 180, 185, 188, 189, 194, 199
sensitization, 17, 52, 53, 59, 60, 189
sensors, 121
sequelae, 7, 11, 21
series, 83, 84, 97, 100, 166
serine, 52, 59
serotonergic, 47, 123, 155
serotonin, viii, ix, 37, 41, 42, 44, 51, 54, 55, 56, 57,
    59, 60, 62, 76, 77, 78, 79, 212
sertraline, 39, 40, 43, 47, 51
serum, xi, 83, 114, 129, 148, 156, 158, 159, 164,
    167, 188, 214
serum cholinesterase, 188
severity, 41, 42, 48, 69, 105, 116, 118, 124, 125,
    129, 130, 131, 140, 143, 154, 201, 209
sex, ix, xiii, 61, 72, 73, 108, 149, 150, 161, 168, 212,
    213, 214, 216, 218
sex hormones, 149, 150
sexual behaviour, 212
shape, 168
shear, 135
shock, 171, 172, 176, 177, 180
short-term, 166, 170, 171, 176, 181, 194, 218
short-term memory, 170, 176

sialic acid, 127, 132
side effects, 50, 72, 82, 85
sign, 15, 45
signal transduction, 51
signaling, 51, 159, 162, 171, 172, 173, 184, 219
signals, 213
signs, 5, 8, 15, 53, 116, 117, 139, 147, 163, 182, 199,
    209, 214
sine wave, 210
sinus, 145, 146, 155, 166
sinus rhythm, 145
sites, 10, 87, 115, 201, 204, 206
skeletal muscle, ix, 81, 82, 83, 90, 147
skin, 105, 106
sleep, 39, 59, 62, 83, 116, 199, 200, 209
sleep disturbance, 39, 116
small intestine, 155, 164
smokers, 17, 20, 159, 166
smoking, vii, xiii, 17, 18, 30, 33, 123, 131, 133, 134,
    137, 138, 141, 145, 147, 148, 160, 162, 163, 166,
    200, 210, 211, 215
smoking cessation, 137, 139, 145, 163, 166
smooth muscle, 139
smooth muscle cells, 139
sociability, 199
social anxiety, 42
social phobia, 42
social problems, xi, 113
socioeconomic, 120
soft drinks, 198
solid phase, 214
somatic symptoms, 39, 53, 77, 78, 183
somatosensory, 78
somnolence, 39
South Africa, vii, viii, 1, 2, 6, 10, 12, 15, 16, 23, 30,
    31, 32, 33, 34, 35
spatial, 189, 192
spatial learning, 188
spatial memory, 188
species, 118, 171
specificity, xii, 169, 186, 193
SPECT, 205
spectra, 209
spectral analysis, 152, 210
spectroscopy, 207
spectrum, 44, 51, 104, 105, 118, 145, 199
speed, 20, 46
sphincter, 122, 124, 156
spinal anesthesia, 35
spinal cord, 83, 123

spines, 188
spirometry, 146
sponsor, 28
sports, 115
sprouting, 59
SRIs, 62, 74
stabilization, 51
stabilizers, 38
stable angina, 166, 167
stages, 31, 72, 118, 119
standard deviation, xiii, 65, 97, 145, 212, 215
standards, 33, 96, 152
statin, 159
statins, 127, 129, 132, 156
statistical analysis, 8
stenosis, 119
stent, x, 94, 99, 100, 101, 102, 103, 106, 107, 108, 109, 111
stents, x, 94, 99, 100, 105, 106, 107, 110, 111
stiffness, 199
stimulant, 84
stimulants, 198
stimulus, 52, 171, 192
stomach, 87, 115, 117, 118, 119, 121, 122, 199
strain, 178
strains, 178, 188
strategies, 50, 51, 57, 94, 96, 109, 112, 218
stratification, 138
streptokinase, 137
stress, 3, 52, 56, 118, 122, 129, 143, 144, 146, 160, 162, 164, 212, 214
stretching, 53
striatum, 172, 173, 190
stroke, 97, 100, 102, 108, 109, 111, 115, 125, 133, 135, 143
subgroups, 53, 101, 104
subjective, 199, 207, 208, 210
substance abuse, 3, 6, 7, 15, 16, 17, 19, 21, 23, 27, 29, 33, 35, 84, 85, 91, 178
substance use, 213, 215
substances, vii, 2, 19, 20, 85, 89, 91, 118, 120, 121, 124, 139, 140, 212
substitution, 40, 43, 98, 101
substrates, xii, 141, 169, 171, 172, 173, 176, 179, 180, 181, 183, 184, 186, 191, 219
success rate, ix, 61, 69, 73, 76
suffering, 5, 7, 12, 16, 121, 122
suicidal, 47, 74, 127
suicidal ideation, 74
suicide, 84, 116, 156

superiority, 9
supervision, vii, 1, 6, 72, 95, 96
supply, 11, 147
suppression, 142
surgery, 14, 65, 66, 67, 98, 99, 100, 101, 103, 105, 106, 107, 110, 133, 136
surgical, 3, 29, 101, 105, 110
surprise, 5
survival, 170, 180
susceptibility, 149, 150, 178
Sweden, vii, 1, 23, 120
switching, viii, 37, 50, 51, 58, 78
symmetry, 205
sympathetic, xiii, 5, 146, 147, 166, 211, 212
sympathetic nervous system, 147
symptom, 8, 13, 16, 41, 46, 55, 64, 146
symptoms, vii, viii, ix, xii, xiii, 15, 16, 17, 32, 34, 37, 38, 39, 41, 42, 43, 44, 45, 46, 47, 48, 50, 53, 54, 55, 56, 59, 62, 63, 73, 74, 77, 78, 79, 81, 82, 86, 87, 88, 89, 115, 116, 117, 119, 120, 121, 123, 136, 141, 146, 152, 155, 165, 170, 179, 181, 183, 186, 197, 199, 207, 209, 212, 214, 218
synapses, 189
synaptic plasticity, 52
synaptic transmission, 173
syndrome, ix, x, xii, 15, 29, 35, 37, 38, 41, 43, 44, 45, 54, 55, 56, 61, 62, 63, 74, 75, 76, 78, 79, 81, 82, 86, 87, 88, 89, 91, 99, 114, 115, 120, 125, 139, 141, 143, 144, 146, 148, 155, 167, 168, 197, 199, 209, 214, 218
synergistic, 154, 162
synthesis, 97, 105, 118, 124, 128, 129, 135, 139, 140, 141, 142, 147, 149, 179, 195
systematic, 208
systems, 6, 7, 16, 18, 52, 116, 117, 134, 138, 139, 172, 176, 184, 185, 191, 192, 193, 195, 213
systolic blood pressure, 144, 146

T

tachycardia, 141, 146, 148
tactics, 23
tannins, 133
targets, 156, 173
tariff, vii, 2, 6
task force, 160
taste, 64
tea, 198
Technology Assessment, 30
teenagers, 85

telephone, 24, 89

temperament, 58

temperature, 116

temporal, 133, 202, 204

tension, 199

terminals, 147

testosterone, 149, 150

Texas, 76

textbooks, 25

thalamus, xiii, 211

theft, 85

theory, 28, 170

therapeutic approaches, 193

therapeutics, 31

therapy, vii, viii, x, xi, 1, 2, 3, 6, 10, 15, 21, 23, 24, 25, 26, 28, 34, 37, 38, 40, 47, 52, 54, 57, 58, 59, 77, 93, 94, 96, 99, 101, 106, 107, 108, 110, 112, 113, 125, 126, 127, 129, 132, 137, 143, 144

theta, xii, 189, 197, 200, 201, 202, 203, 204, 206, 210

thinking, 189

Third World, vii, 1, 30

threshold, 72, 123, 185

thresholds, 64

thrombin, xi, 114, 125, 133, 134, 135

thrombocytopenia, 132

thrombomodulin, xi, 114, 134, 135, 138, 139, 161

thrombosis, 99, 100, 101, 102, 109, 110, 111, 134, 135, 136, 162

thrombotic, 100, 103, 104, 105, 106, 116, 133, 134, 135, 136, 137, 138

thromboxane, 105, 112

thrombus, 134, 135

thyroid, xi, xiii, 114, 128, 130, 149, 211, 212, 218

thyrotropin, 212

timing, 39, 51

tissue, xi, 114, 120, 135, 137, 158, 161, 162, 163, 213

tissue plasminogen activator, 161, 163

title, 97, 98

titration, vii, 1, 4, 7, 8, 17, 22

TNF, xi, 114, 117, 124, 125, 130, 131, 140, 141, 142, 146, 148, 156, 162, 164

TNF-alpha, xi, 114, 117, 124, 125, 130, 131, 140, 141, 142, 146, 148, 162, 164

tobacco, 18, 20, 31, 126, 191, 213

Tokyo, 61, 64, 69

tolerance, viii, 37, 38, 45, 48, 49, 50, 51, 52, 53, 60, 83, 115, 139, 140, 146, 147, 148, 149, 167, 170, 185, 187, 208, 209

total cholesterol, 127, 132

toxic, 122

toxicity, 41, 55

toxins, 142

training, vii, 1, 4, 5, 10, 14, 24, 25, 26, 28, 29, 53, 107, 143, 146, 148, 165, 171, 172, 174, 177, 179, 180, 187, 188, 191

transaminases, 131

transcranial Doppler sonography, 201

transcript, xiii, 211, 212, 220

transcription, 137, 218

transcriptional, 139, 162

transfer, 127

transferrin, 132

transformation, 83

transfusion, 95, 105

transition, 182

transitions, xii, 169

translation, 171

transmission, 35, 44, 83, 123, 173, 195

transport, 128

transurethral prostatectomy, 105, 111

trauma, 151

travel, 22, 28

treatment programs, 170

tremor, 62, 63, 116, 199

trend, 44, 46, 131, 160

trial, 7, 8, 9, 11, 12, 16, 17, 18, 20, 26, 29, 33, 35, 40, 43, 47, 49, 50, 51, 54, 55, 74, 77, 79, 95, 104, 111, 156, 168, 171

tricyclic antidepressant, 62

tricyclic antidepressants, 47, 54, 57, 67

triglyceride, 128, 157, 158

triglycerides, 118, 127, 130, 139, 213, 214, 215, 217, 218

TSH, xiii, 129, 130, 131, 211, 212, 214, 215, 216, 218

tumor, 124, 130, 141, 156, 164, 167

tumor necrosis factor, 124, 130, 141, 156, 164

type 2 diabetes, 109

U

ulcer, 95, 122, 136

ulceration, 119

ultrasonography, xi, 114

UN, 156

uncertainty, 96

unconditioned, 171, 172

United Kingdom (UK), 35, 39, 76, 82

United States, 64, 82, 94, 115, 151, 170, 198
univariate, 101
universities, 28
urease, 120
uric acid, 129, 143
uric acid levels, 129
urinary, 112, 139
urine, 83, 84, 198
urokinase, 137
urology, 65

V

vagal nerve, xi, 114, 126, 145, 146, 147
validation, 209
validity, 10, 14, 97, 102, 219, 220
values, xi, 97, 114, 117, 120, 121, 122, 124, 125,
    126, 128, 129, 130, 131, 132, 134, 135, 143, 144,
    145, 146, 149, 204, 206, 217, 218
variability, xi, 74, 113, 114, 116, 123, 143, 144, 145,
    146, 152, 155, 165, 166, 167, 183, 204
variable, xii, 4, 45, 106, 177, 183, 186, 187, 197,
    200, 206
variables, xii, 43, 97, 150, 162, 163, 197, 199, 201,
    202, 206, 210
variance, 72, 73, 97, 101
variation, 151, 152, 204
vascular, 198, 206
vascular headache, 206
vascular system, 134, 198
vasoactive intestinal peptide, 155
vasoactive intestinal polypeptide (VIP), 123, 124
vasoconstriction, 142, 198, 200, 206, 207
vasomotor, 141
vein, 44
velocity, 198, 201
venlafaxine, 41, 42, 51, 53, 55
verapamil, 165
Vermont, 208
vessels, 126, 128, 136, 148, 162
victims, 34
viscosity, 136, 146
visible, 174
vision, 199
visual, xiii, 198, 202, 205, 206, 207, 210
Visual Analogue Scale, 214
vitamin B1, 31

vitamin B12, 31
vitamins, 213
VLA, 142
VLDL, 118, 130
vomiting, 39, 63, 88, 116, 117, 120, 136, 199
vulnerability, viii, 37, 38, 45, 46, 47, 188

W

walking, 148, 167
warfarin, 94, 108, 110
water, 183, 191
water maze, 191
weakness, 44
wealth, 104
wear, 22
web, 54
weight loss, 198
Western Cape Province, 15
white-collar workers, 78
WHO, 77
WHR, 143
wild cards, 107
wildfire, 21
wine, 120, 121, 133, 134, 145, 154, 159
women, 69, 95, 108, 111, 142, 143, 145, 150, 152,
    160, 162, 163, 166, 167
work, 96, 104, 106, 107, 127, 129, 133, 138, 142,
    144, 145, 147, 148
work absenteeism, 38
workers, 3, 4, 5, 14, 15, 23, 25, 26, 28, 29, 73, 85,
    166
working memory, 171, 176, 189
wound healing, 100, 102
writing, 25

X

xenon, 29

Y

yawning, xii, 197, 199
yield, 38, 42, 43, 46, 51, 52, 53
young adults, 165
young men, 148